THIS TEXT
IS PROVIDED
AS A PROFESSIONAL
SERVICE BY

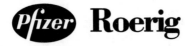

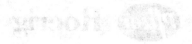

**Edited by Philip B. Mead, MD
and W. David Hager, MD**

INFECTION

PROTOCOLS

FOR

OBSTETRICS

AND

GYNECOLOGY

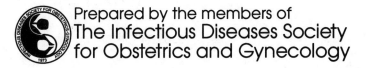

Prepared by the members of
The Infectious Diseases Society
for Obstetrics and Gynecology

**A publication of
CONTEMPORARY OB/GYN**

Supervising editor: James E. Swan
Manuscript editors: Mary Hale
                    Michael Lipton
Production editors: Ann Marie Kachler
                    Rosemary Kline
Art director: A. Michael Velthaus
Compositor: JRI Graphic Communications
Printer/binder: Port City Press

Library of Congress Cataloging-in-Publication Data
Infection protocols for obstetrics and gynecology / edited by
Philip B. Mead and W. David Hagar; prepared by the members of
the Infectious Diseases Society for Obstetrics and Gynecology.
    p. cm.
  Includes bibliographical references and index.
  1. Generative organs, Female—Infections—Handbooks, manuals, etc.
2. Communicable diseases in pregnancy—Handbooks, manuals, etc.
I. Mead, Philip B., 1937- . II. Hagar, W. David (William David),
1946- . III. Infectious Diseases Society for Obstetrics and Gynecology.
  [DNLM: 1. Genital Diseases, Female—therapy. 2. Gynecology—
methods. 3. Obstetrics—methods. 4. Pregnancy complications,
Infectious—therapy. WQ 100 143]
RG218.I52   1992
618—dc20
DNLM/DLC
for Library of Congress   92-48224 CIP

ISBN 1-880080-02-8

To Ann and Linda

Contents

INFECTION PROTOCOLS IN THE GYNECOLOGIC PATIENT

VAGINITIS AND CERVICITIS

SEXUALLY TRANSMITTED DISEASES

Lower tract

Upper tract

Contributors

H. Hugh Allen, MD, Professor of Obstetrics and Gynecology, University of Western Ontario, London, Ont., Canada

Marvin S. Amstey, MD, Professor of Obstetrics and Gynecology, University of Rochester School of Medicine and Dentistry, and Chief of Obstetrics and Gynecology, Highland Hospital, Rochester, N.Y.

Joseph J. Apuzzio, MD, Professor of Obstetrics and Gynecology, University of Medicine and Dentistry of New Jersey, New Jersey Medical School, Newark, N.J.

David A. Baker, MD, Director, Division of Infectious Diseases, Department of Obstetrics and Gynecology, School of Medicine, State University of New York at Stony Brook, Stony Brook, N.Y.

Roger Bawdon, PhD, Associate Professor of Obstetrics and Gynecology, University of Texas Southwestern Medical Center, Dallas, Tex.

Alan B. Berkeley, MD, Associate Professor of Obstetrics and Gynecology, Cornell University Medical College, and Director of Gynecology, New York Hospital, New York, N.Y.

Jorge D. Blanco, MD, Professor and Vice Chairman, Department of Obstetrics and Gynecology and Reproductive Sciences, University of Texas Medical School at Houston, Houston, Tex.

J. R. Bobitt, MD, Associate Professor, Department of Obstetrics and Gynecology, University of North Carolina, Chapel Hill, N.C.

Noelle Bowdler, MD, Associate Professor, Department of Obstetrics and Gynecology, University of Iowa College of Medicine, Iowa City, Iowa

David Charles, MD, consultant in obstetrics and gynecology, Powys, Wales, United Kingdom

Susan M. Cox, MD, Associate Professor and Director of Maternal-Fetal Medicine, Department of Obstetrics and Gynecology, Albert B. Chandler Medical Center, University of Kentucky College of Medicine, Lexington, Ky.

William R. Crombleholme, MD, Professor and Vice Chairman for Clinical Affairs, Department of Obstetrics, Gynecology, and Reproductive Sciences, University of Pittsburgh School of Medicine, Pittsburgh, Pa.

F. Gary Cunningham, MD, Professor and Chairman of Obstetrics and Gynecology, University of Texas Health Science Center at Dallas, Dallas, Tex.

Mara J. Dinsmoor, MD, Assistant Professor of Obstetrics and Gynecology, Medical College of Virginia, Richmond, Va.

Patrick Duff, MD, Professor of Obstetrics and Gynecology, Division of Maternal-Fetal Medicine, University of Florida College of Medicine, Gainesville, Fla.

David A. Eschenbach, MD, Chief, Division of Gynecology, University of Washington School of Medicine, Seattle, Wash.

Sebastian Faro, MD, PhD, Professor and Vice Chairman, Department of Obstetrics and Gynecology, Baylor College of Medicine, Houston, Tex.

Rudolph P. Galask, MD, Professor, Department of Obstetrics and Gynecology, University of Iowa College of Medicine, Iowa City, Iowa

Stanley A. Gall, MD, Professor and Chairman of Obstetrics and Gynecology, University of Louisville School of Medicine, Louisville, Ky.

Sheldon M. Gelbart, PhD, Director, Ob-Gyn Research Laboratory, Department of Obstetrics and Gynecology, University of Wisconsin, Sinai Samaritan Medical Center, Milwaukee, Wisc.

Ronald S. Gibbs, MD, Professor and Chairman, Department of Obstetrics and Gynecology, University of Colorado Health Sciences Center, Denver, Colo.

Mark Gibson, MD, Professor and Chairman, Department of Obstetrics and Gynecology, West Virginia University School of Medicine, Morgantown, W. Va.

Larry C. Gilstrap III, MD, Professor of Obstetrics and Gynecology, University of Texas Southwestern Medical Center, Dallas, Tex.

Bernard Gonik, MD, Associate Professor of Obstetrics and Gynecology, University of Texas Medical School at Houston, Houston, Tex.

Michael G. Gravett, MD, Assistant Professor of Obstetrics and Gynecology, Oregon Health Sciences University, and Director of Ob-Gyn Infectious Disease, Emanuel Hospital and Health Center, Portland, Ore.

John H. Grossman III, MD, PhD, Professor of Obstetrics and Gynecology and Microbiology, and Director, Division of Maternal-Fetal Medicine, George Washington University Medical Center, Washington, D.C.

W. David Hager, MD, Professor of Obstetrics and Gynecology, Albert B. Chandler Medical Center, University of Kentucky College of Medicine, Lexington, Ky.

James H. Harger, MD, Professor of Obstetrics and Gynecology, University of Pittsburgh School of Medicine, Pittsburgh, Pa.

David L. Hemsell, MD, Director, Division of Gynecology, University of Texas Southwestern Medical Center, Dallas, Tex.

Gale B. Hill, PhD, Associate Professor of Obstetrics and Gynecology, and Microbiology and Immunology, Duke University Medical Center, Durham, N.C.

Michael K. Hill, MD, Clinical Assistant Professor of Medicine, Section of Infectious Diseases, School of Medicine in New Orleans, Louisiana State University Medical Center, New Orleans, La.

Hans A. Hirsch, MD, Professor of Obstetrics and Gynecology, Universitäts-Frauenklinik, Tübingen, Germany

Udo B. Hoyme, MD, Professor of Obstetrics and Gynecology, Zentrum für Frauenheilkunde, Universitätsklinikum Essen, Essen, Germany

Mahmoud A. Ismail, MD, Associate Professor, Department of Obstetrics and Gynecology, University of Chicago, Pritzker School of Medicine, Chicago, Ill.

A. Karen Kreutner, MD, is in the private practice of obstetrics and gynecology in Charleston, S.C.

Daniel V. Landers, MD, Assistant Professor of Obstetrics, Gynecology, and Reproductive Sciences, University of California, San Francisco, and San Francisco General Hospital, San Francisco, Calif.

Bryan Larsen, PhD, Professor of Obstetrics and Gynecology, Marshall University School of Medicine, Huntington, W. Va.

John W. Larsen, Jr., MD, Professor of Obstetrics, Gynecology, and Genetics, George Washington University School of Medicine and Health Sciences, Washington, D.C.

William J. Ledger, MD, Chairman, Department of Obstetrics and Gynecology, Cornell University Medical College, New York, N.Y.

Thomas William Lowe, MD, Assistant Professor of Obstetrics and Gynecology, University of Texas Health Science Center at Dallas, Dallas, Tex.

Nancy E. Madinger, MD, Assistant Professor, Division of Infectious Diseases, Department of Medicine, University of Colorado Health Sciences Center, Denver, Colo.

Mark G. Martens, MD, Associate Professor of Obstetrics and Gynecology and Director, Division of Infectious Disease, University of Texas Medical Branch, Galveston, Tex.

William M. McCormack, MD, Professor of Medicine and of Obstetrics and Gynecology and Chief, Infectious Diseases Division, SUNY–Health Science Center at Brooklyn, Brooklyn, N.Y.

James A. McGregor, MD, Professor and Vice Chairman, Department of Obstetrics and Gynecology, University of Colorado Health Sciences Center, Denver, Colo.

S. Gene McNeeley, Jr., MD, Associate Professor of Obstetrics and Gynecology, Wayne State University Medical Center, and Chief, Division of Gynecology, Hutzel Hospital, Detroit, Mich.

Philip B. Mead, MD, Clinical Professor of Obstetrics and Gynecology, University of Vermont College of Medicine, and Hospital Epidemiologist, Medical Center Hospital of Vermont, Burlington, Vt.

R. David Miller, MD, Medical Director for Gynecology, Infertility, and Infections, Medical Specialists for Women, Tustin, Calif.

Howard L. Minkoff, MD, Professor of Obstetrics, Department of Obstetrics and Gynecology, SUNY–Health Science Center at Brooklyn, Brooklyn, N.Y.

Gilles R. G. Monif, MD, Professor of Obstetrics and Gynecology, Creighton University, Omaha, Neb.

Walter J. Morales, MD, PhD, Director of High-Risk Obstetrics, Orlando Regional Medical Center, Orlando, Fla.

James W. Orr, MD, Director of Gynecologic Oncology, Watson Clinic, Lakeland, Fla.

Newton G. Osborne, MD, PhD, Professor of Obstetrics and Gynecology, Creighton University, Omaha, Neb.

Jorma Paavonen, MD, Associate Professor of Obstetrics and Gynecology, University of Helsinki, Helsinki, Finland

Joseph G. Pastorek II, MD, Chief, Section of Infectious Disease, and Associate Professor, Department of Obstetrics and Gynecology, Louisiana State University Medical Center, New Orleans, La.

Charles V. Sanders, MD, Edgar Hull Professor and Chairman, Department of Medicine, Section of Infectious Diseases, School of Medicine in New Orleans, Louisiana State University Medical Center, New Orleans, La.

Richard H. Schwarz, MD, Professor, Department of Obstetrics and Gynecology, and Provost and Vice President for Clinical Affairs, SUNY–Health Science Center at Brooklyn, Brooklyn, N.Y.

N. J. Scaglione, NP, Ob-Gyn Nurse Practitioner and Gynecology Clinical Research Specialist, Department of Obstetrics and Gynecology, University of Wisconsin, Sinai Samaritan Medical Center, Milwaukee, Wisc.

John L. Sever, MD, PhD, Professor, Departments of Pediatrics, Obstetrics and Gynecology, and Microbiology and Immunology, George Washington University, Children's National Medical Center, Washington, D.C.

David E. Soper, MD, Associate Professor of Obstetrics and Gynecology, Medical College of Virginia, Virginia Commonwealth University, Richmond, Va.

Michael R. Spence, MD, MPH, Professor of Obstetrics and Gynecology, Hahnemann University School of Medicine, Philadelphia, Pa.

Rhoda S. Sperling, MD, Director, Division of Ob-Gyn Infectious Diseases, Department of Obstetrics, Gynecology, and Reproductive Science, Mount Sinai Medical Center, New York, N.Y.

Richard L. Sweet, MD, Professor and Chairman, Department of Obstetrics, Gynecology, and Reproductive Sciences, University of Pittsburgh School of Medicine, Pittsburgh, Pa.

Jessica L. Thomason, MD, Professor and Director, Division of Gynecology, and Chief, Section of Infectious Diseases, Department of Obstetrics and Gynecology, University of Wisconsin, Sinai Samaritan Medical Center, Milwaukee, Wisc.

Gael P. Wager, MD, MPH, Staff Perinatologist, Flagstaff Medical Center, Flagstaff, Ariz.

Peter C. Welch, MD, PhD, Chief of Medicine, Northern Westchester Hospital and Medical Center, Mount Kisco, N.Y.

George D. Wendel, Jr., MD, Associate Professor of Obstetrics and Gynecology, University of Texas Southwestern Medical Center, Dallas, Tex.

Sandra White, Clinical Studies Coordinator, Marshall University School of Medicine, Huntington, W. Va.

Christine L. Williams, MD, MPH, Professor of Pediatrics and Medicine, New York Medical College, Valhalla, N.Y.

Steven S. Witkin, PhD, Associate Professor of Immunology and Director, Immunology Division, Department of Obstetrics and Gynecology, Cornell University Medical College, New York, N.Y.

Pål Wölner-Hanssen, MD, DMS, Department of Obstetrics and Gynecology, University of Lund, Lund, Sweden

M. Lynn Yonekura, MD, Associate Professor of Obstetrics and Gynecology and Chief of Obstetrics/Maternal-Fetal Medicine, Harbor–UCLA Medical Center, Torrance, Calif.

Preface

This book is patterned after the popular *Protocols for High-Risk Pregnancies,* edited by John T. Queenan and John C. Hobbins. In 1982, these pioneers recognized that rapid advances in technology and new clinical knowledge had created a pressing need for guidelines in the work-up and management of high-risk pregnancies. They were farsighted enough to anticipate the current pressure for uniform standards to minimize unnecessary practice variation and complexity, and thereby increase the quality and efficiency of patient care. These same concerns—the almost unmanageable increase in the knowledge base and the demand for practical management guidelines—prompted the creation of this book of protocols for infectious disease problems in obstetrics and gynecology.

Several textbooks have taken an in-depth approach to the subject of ob-gyn infections. For this project, we asked the leaders in this field to provide the essentials on incidence, pathophysiology, etiology, diagnosis, treatment, and sequelae of the major disease entities encountered by the practicing physician. Each chapter was contributed by a member of the Infectious Diseases Society for Obstetrics and Gynecology. We believe this to be the first book authored by a medical society, which may explain the enthusiasm and intellectual synergism evident in the volume as a whole.

Protocols for Infections in Obstetrics and Gynecology contains sections on bacterial, viral, and parasitic diseases, as well as several chapters on areas of special interest to the clinician. We hope it will serve you as a ready reference to help you diagnose and manage these conditions. Suggested readings are provided at the end of each chapter for closer study.

We're grateful to John Queenan, MD, and to Barbara Pritchard and James Swan of *Contemporary Ob/Gyn* for their encouragement and assistance in preparing this book. We trust that you, the reader, will share our enthusiasm for the field of ob-gyn infections as you read these pages and will find this information helpful in caring for your patients.

Philip B. Mead, MD
Burlington, Vermont

W. David Hager, MD
Lexington, Kentucky

Infection Protocols in the Obstetric Patient

1
Intra-amniotic infection

By Jorge D. Blanco, MD

Background and incidence
Confusion exists over the definition of chorioamnionitis, also called amnionitis. To the clinician, it is the clinically evident infection of the fetus, amniotic cavity, and mother; to the pathologist, it is the leukocytic infiltration of the placenta. Since there may be histologic findings without evidence of clinical infection, the two entities are not synonymous. In this chapter, for the sake of clarity, I will use the term intra-amniotic infection for the clinical entity.

The infection occurs in approximately 0.5% to 1% of all pregnancies, and the rate may increase with prolonged periods of ruptured membranes (ROM). Although the majority of infected patients have ROM, the infection may also occur with intact membranes.

Etiology
In the patient with intact membranes, microorganisms such as *Listeria monocytogenes* can infect the fetus transplacentally by hematogenous spread from the mother. In patients with ROM, or those with intact membranes but in labor, the usual cause is ascending infection by organisms from the cervical microflora. The microbiology in these patients includes the usual genital tract pathogens, including anaerobes (especially the *Bacteroides* group and the peptostreptococci), the group B streptococci, and the aerobic gram-negative bacilli (especially *Escherichia coli*).

In the majority of patients, the etiology of intra-amniotic infection is polymicrobial. The role of the genital mycoplasmas is unclear, but they do not appear to be prominent in this infection. Likewise, the role, if any, of *Chlamydia trachomatis* is not well delineated.

Diagnosis

Diagnosis is often difficult because it is one of exclusion. The clinical signs and symptoms are neither sensitive nor specific. Common findings include ROM and fever. Maternal tachycardia, fetal tachycardia, uterine tenderness, and malodorous amniotic fluid are seen less often. Table 1 lists the recommended diagnostic criteria.

Certain laboratory tests also assist in the diagnosis. An elevated peripheral leukocyte count is common, but care should be exercised in interpreting the peripheral white blood cell count, since labor itself may commonly elevate levels. Urinalysis and culture will exclude a urinary tract infection. Cultures of the amniotic fluid are helpful in isolating the organisms involved in the infection. For culture, an amniocentesis specimen is ideal, but in many patients—especially those with ROM—this is difficult to obtain.

An adequate specimen may be acquired transcervically by means of an intrauterine pressure catheter. The first 3 to 5 mL aspirated through the catheter should be discarded, and the next 2 to 3 mL sent for culture. Because bacteria gain entry to the amniotic cavity after ROM and because labor itself may result in the finding of amniotic fluid leukocytes, Gram stain results should be interpreted with care. However, finding no leukocytes or bacteria can be useful in excluding intra-amniotic infection. Vaginal pool aspirates are of little use for culture or for the diagnosis of infection.

TABLE 1

Diagnostic criteria for intra-amniotic infection

Fever (≥37.8° C)

Rupture of membranes

Two or more of the following:
Maternal tachycardia
(pulse >100)
Fetal tachycardia (fetal heart tones >160)
Uterine tenderness
Malodorous amniotic fluid
Peripheral leukocytosis
(WBC >15,000)
No other site of infection

Source: Looff JD, Hager WD: Surg Gynecol 1984;158:161

Treatment

Management consists of prompt initiation of antibiotic therapy and progression to delivery. Giving antibiotics as soon as the diagnosis is made will limit the extent of infection in the mother and neonate. Because of this infection's polymicrobial etiology and its potential severity, potent broad-spectrum antibiotic agents are indicated.

Since large, comparative studies are not available, the majority of regimens are used on an empiric basis. There are studies that support the use of IV penicillin G, 5,000,000 U every 6 hours, combined with gentamicin, 1 to 1.5 mg/kg every 8 hours. Other studies support the use of ampicillin, 1 g IV every 6 hours, plus gentamicin, 1.5 mg/kg IV every 8 hours, which theoretically may have some benefit since the ratio of transplacental transmission is better for ampicillin than for penicillin. Neither of these combinations, however, provides adequate coverage for anaerobes such as *Bacteroides* sp. Therefore, patients undergoing cesarean section (C/S) should be given clindamycin, 900 mg IV every 8 hours, in addition to ampicillin and gentamicin. For patients who deliver vaginally, a penicillin–gentamicin or ampicillin–gentamicin regimen is adequate.

An alternative may be the use of a broad-spectrum third-generation cephalosporin or an extended-spectrum penicillin. Such agents have a good safety record, and many are well transmitted to the fetus. Most provide the required broad-spectrum coverage; however, there are few data on their efficacy in intra-amniotic infection.

The timing of antibiotic administration is as critical to success as which antibiotics are used. Several studies show clear neonatal benefits from immediate initiation of antibiotics. Delay in instituting therapy, even when delivery is imminent, may markedly increase perinatal morbidity and mortality. Equally important is prompt progression to delivery. Drainage of the uterine cavity is essential. While there is no arbitrary or absolute time limit after which the risks for mother and fetus increase, efforts to effect delivery should begin as soon as the diagnosis is made.

Intra-amniotic infection is not an indication for C/S. In fact, because of the lower maternal morbidity, a vaginal delivery is preferred. Many patients, however, will require C/S for obstetric indications. Duff and co-workers have found that these patients more frequently require oxytocin for induction of labor and more frequently have arrest of labor leading to cesarean section for failure to progress.

Sequelae

Although maternal morbidity is increased with intra-amniotic infection, maternal mortality is extremely rare. Patients treated aggressively with antibiotics and delivered promptly will usually do well. About 10% to 12% will have bacteremia, and 40% to 50% will need C/S because of unsatisfactory progression in labor.

With appropriate intrapartum and neonatal treatment, the infected term baby will do well. Up to 20% of these neonates may have pneumonia on chest x-ray, and 8% to 10% may have documented bacteremia. However, in several small studies the mortality rate for these babies was not increased. Unfortunately, outcomes for preterm infants are not as good. Perinatal mortality and morbidity are significantly higher for preterm neonates born to infected mothers than for those born to uninfected mothers. The combination of prematurity and intra-amniotic infection is ominous and the addition of respiratory distress syndrome may be devastating.

SUGGESTED READING

Duff P, Sanders R, Gibbs RS: The course of labor in term patients with chorioamnionitis. Am J Obstet Gynecolol 1983;147:391

Garite TJ, Freeman RK: Chorioamnionitis in preterm gestation. Obstet Gynecol 1982;59:539

Gibbs RS, Dinsmoor MJ, Newton ER, et al: A randomized trial of intrapartum versus immediate postpartum treatment of women with intra-amniotic infection. Obstet Gynecol 1988;72:823

Gibbs RS, Duff P: Progress in pathogenesis and management of clinical intra-amniotic infection. Am J Obstet Gynecol 1991;164:1317

Looff JD, Hager WD: Management of chorioamnionitis. Surg Gynecol Obstet 1984;158:161

Romero R, Oyarzun E, Avila C, et al: Diagnosis of intra-amniotic infection. Contemp Ob/Gyn 1989;34(May):99

Sperling RS, Newton ER, Gibbs RS: Intra-amniotic infection in low birthweight infants. J Infect Dis 1988;157:113

Yoder PR, Gibbs RS, Blanco JD, et al: The prospective, controlled study of maternal and perinatal outcome after intra-amniotic infection at term. Am J Obstet Gynecol 1983;145:695

2

Group B streptococcal infections

By J. R. Bobitt, MD

Background and incidence

Group B *Streptococcus* (GBS) was not recognized as an important human pathogen until the 1960s, when it emerged as a frequent cause of early-onset neonatal sepsis. This observation was the catalyst for widespread study over the next two decades. Early reports indicated neonatal infection is acquired during labor and delivery. Detection of pregnant carriers did not predict risk, however, since the ratio of maternal GBS carriage (up to 30%) to neonatal sepsis (3/1,000 live births) is 100 to 1. This low attack rate is believed to reflect activity of maternal protective antibodies. If this is so, vaccination may prevent neonatal sepsis, and that issue is currently being studied. The neonatal attack rate is inversely related to infant birthweight (Table 1).

There is concern that the spectrum of perinatal complications may extend beyond neonatal infections. An association of prolonged rupture of membranes and preterm labor with GBS colonization has been observed, but a causal relationship has not been established. A causal relationship between prolonged rupture of membranes/premature labor and GBS bacteriuria is believed to exist, however.

Pathophysiology

I. Early-onset GBS neonatal sepsis. This entity presents during the first 5 days of life, with a mean onset of 20 hours. The clinical picture is one of septic shock, pneumonia, and bacteremia, with 10% to 15% of infants also having meningitis. Mortality ranges from as low as 9% in term infants to as high as 66% in preterm babies.

Though GBS early neonatal sepsis is infrequent, its occurrence is of significant concern. In many instances, infection is unsuspected

TABLE 1

Neonatal attack rate of GBS infection

Infant birthweight (g)	Attack rate (per 1,000 live births)
1,000–1,500	18.8
1,501–2,000	7.7
2,001–2,500	4.8
>2,500	0.9

because the baby appears normal at birth and labor has not been complicated by either maternal fever or prolonged rupture of membranes. Subtle signs of sepsis then go unnoticed in the nursery, and early assessment and treatment are delayed. The problem is further complicated by the fulminant nature of GBS sepsis. Babies who appear normal at birth may develop apnea or shock and die within hours of delivery. Also, since many infections occur in preterm infants, signs and symptoms caused by infection have been misdiagnosed and attributed to respiratory distress syndrome. This recurring scenario contributes to the high mortality rate and emphasizes the need for preventive measures.

Antepartum prevention. Once it was recognized that GBS infection in newborns could be serious and that the organism was transmitted from the mother during labor, preventive strategy was directed at detecting the carrier population before onset of labor. This approach soon proved impractical, however, because some carrier populations reach 30%. Carriage may be transient or intermittent, and colonization often recurs after treatment. Sexual partners must be treated since this organism is sexually transmitted. In addition, treatment directed at women near term fails to protect those who deliver prematurely and whose culture status is unknown.

Intrapartum prevention. When prenatal detection and eradication of GBS in carriers was judged ineffective, interest turned to intrapartum chemoprophylaxis. Ampicillin administered to GBS carriers in labor reduced the incidence of GBS colonization in newborns. Similar treatment was subsequently shown to help prevent early GBS sepsis.

Although intrapartum antibiotic prophylaxis is effective, important questions remain unresolved. One is whether to detect carriers by doing screening cultures at approximately 26 weeks or by testing all patients on admission to labor and delivery. Since the presence of GBS in the genital tract is not constant, antepartum screening may not be optimal. In addition, there are logistic problems in screening all antepartum patients at 26 weeks, and unregistered patients are missed. Moreover, 8.5% of patients with negative screens may acquire the organism by the time of delivery, and one third of those with positive antepartum screens will lose the organism spontaneously by delivery.

Though screening on admission with rapid diagnostic techniques is appealing, the practicality of this method remains to be established. These new rapid antigen detection tests have a sensitivity of only 40% to 60%.

Another issue is choice of selection criteria for intrapartum antibiotic prophylaxis. No one suggests all colonized women should be treated, since less than one infant for every 100 colonized women is infected. Most agree prophylaxis should be restricted to those with additional risk factors. Whether risk is best predicted by clinical or microbiologic assessment is not known. However, the combination of prenatal GBS carriage and preterm labor or prolonged rupture of membranes has been effective for selecting patients at risk. With this strategy, described by Boyer and Gotoff, early neonatal sepsis may be reduced by 75% but only 4% of the obstetric population will require treatment.

A second strategy, suggested by Minkoff and Mead, involves treating all mothers presenting in preterm labor or with preterm premature rupture of membranes who are GBS carriers or of unknown status. A third approach is to use rapid diagnostic techniques rather than traditional cultures to identify GBS carriers. These new agglutination tests have been used antepartum and intrapartum to differentiate between light and heavy vaginal colonization. Giving penicillin intrapartum to heavily colonized patients has been shown by Tuppurainen and Hallman to reduce the incidence of early GBS sepsis.

Neonatal prevention. The administration of penicillin to newborns within 1 to 2 hours of birth is also effective in preventing GBS infections. When used to prevent gonococcal ophthalmia, penicillin also reduces the risk of early GBS sepsis. Unfortunately, this strategy is not consistently effective, perhaps because as many as two thirds of newborns with early-onset GBS neonatal sepsis have well-established infection at birth. It has also been shown ineffective in infants of birthweight less than 2,000 g.

II. Subclinical infection and preterm delivery. Unrecognized intrauterine infections may be involved in 20% to 30% of preterm births. The clinical manifestations of these silent infections are preterm labor and/or premature rupture of membranes rather than maternal fever. Although many microorganisms have been isolated from the amniotic fluid of women with these complications, GBS has received special attention. On many obstetric services, the initial assessment of women in preterm labor or with premature rupture of membranes includes cervical and vaginal cultures for GBS. Though detection of carriers will not prevent delivery, recognition may affect perinatal management. Since views on managing such patients vary, decisions about antibiotic prophylaxis for GBS-positive patients are best arrived at after consultation with appropriate subspecialists.

III. Urinary tract infection. GBS has been found in the urine of about 2% of pregnant women, and cultures from the vagina and cervix of these patients are usually positive. Such patients should have their bacteriuria eradicated with ampicillin because of the observed relationship between GBS bacteriuria and premature delivery, as well as to prevent the development of pyelonephritis.

IV. GBS puerperal infection. The morbidity associated with GBS postpartum endomyometritis appears to be greater than that caused by less virulent organisms. In addition to rapid onset of fever, tachycardia, and abdominal distension, 35% of patients develop bacteremia. Women who have these clinical findings after delivery warrant immediate antibiotic therapy. Delaying treatment to fulfill infection criteria based on postpartum febrile morbidity is not warranted.

Treatment

Ampicillin is the antibiotic most commonly recommended for preventing GBS neonatal sepsis because its pharmacokinetics in pregnancy has been well studied and it has been used empirically in treating chorioamnionitis. Erythromycin may be substituted in patients allergic to penicillin.

Intrapartum prophylaxis. Ampicillin dosage is 2 g IV, repeated every 4 to 6 hours until delivery for high-risk patients (those in preterm labor or with prolonged rupture of membranes) who are in labor and whose GBS culture is positive or pending. For patients not in labor or whose labor has been arrested, antibiotic therapy may be postponed until culture reports are available.

Preterm premature rupture of membranes. Women with preterm rupture of membranes who are GBS positive and who do not go into labor should also be treated with ampicillin, 500 mg every 6 hours orally for 1 to 2 weeks. Some authors recommend reculturing weekly, with retreatment if recolonization occurs. Others feel recolonization is so common that reculturing is unnecessary and suggest these patients simply be treated with IV ampicillin during subsequent labor.

Vaccine for prevention

Low levels of GBS antibodies in pregnancy have been found to increase susceptibility to maternal and neonatal infections. This observation suggests immunization during pregnancy would be an effective strategy for preventing GBS perinatal infections. Preliminary studies by Baker and co-workers of women vaccinated in the third trimester indicate that some patients respond with increased IgG and that corresponding increases are found in the newborn. Although preliminary results are encouraging, only 57% of susceptible women responded with increased antibody levels. More immunogenic vaccines must be developed before their clinical effectiveness can be determined.

Late-onset GBS neonatal sepsis

The epidemiology of late-onset infection is not as well defined as that of early-onset disease. The organisms that cause late-onset GBS infection in a particular infant may have been acquired from the mother at birth, in the nursery, or at home from the mother or other sources in the community. There can be no doubt that nosocomial transmission of GBS occurs, although the extent of nosocomial spread appears to vary greatly from hospital to hospital. Crowding and understaffing probably contribute to transmission of GBS as well as other nosocomial pathogens.

Since many babies in all nurseries are colonized with GBS and since nosocomial transmission has been a significant problem in only a few institutions, routine culturing of newborns to document colonization is not advocated. Morover, isolation or cohorting of colonized newborns is not recommended in the absence of an epidemic. Adherence to routine infection control procedures, particularly handwashing, is the most practical and least costly strategy for limiting the spread of GBS infection in the nursery.

SUGGESTED READING

Baker C, Bench M, Edwards M, et al: Immunization of pregnant women with a polysaccharide vaccine of group B streptococcus. N Engl J Med 1988;319:1180

Bobitt JR, Hayslip CC, Damato JD: Amniotic fluid infection as determined by transabdominal amniocentesis in patients with intact membranes in premature labor. Am J Obstet Gynecol 1981;140:947

Boyer KM, Gotoff SP: Prevention of early-onset neonatal group B streptococcal disease with selective intrapartum chemoprophylaxis. N Engl J Med 1986;314:1665

Gotoff SP, Boyer KM: Prevention of group B streptococcal early onset sepsis: 1989. Pediatr Infec Dis J 1989;8:268

Minkoff H, Mead P: An obstetric approach to the prevention of early-onset group B beta-hemolytic streptococcal sepsis. Am J Obstet Gynecol 1986;154:973

Tuppurainen N, Hallman M: Prevention of neonatal group B streptococcal disease: intrapartum detection and chemoprophylaxis of heavily colonized parturients. Obstet Gynecol 1989;73:583

3
Postpartum endometritis

By Philip B. Mead, MD

Background and incidence

Postpartum infection of the uterus, the most common cause of puerperal fever, is designated endometritis, endomyometritis, or endoparametritis, depending on the extent of disease. Cesarean delivery, particularly after labor or rupture of the membranes of any duration (nonelective C/S), is the dominant predictor of postpartum endometritis. After vaginal delivery, the reported incidence ranges from 0.9% to 3.9%, whereas after C/S it ranges from 10% on most private services to 50% or higher on large teaching services caring for indigent patients. Postulated secondary predictors of postcesarean endometritis include duration of labor or rupture of membranes, presence of bacterial vaginosis, number of vaginal examinations, and use of internal fetal monitoring.

Although prolonged membrane rupture, anemia, midforceps delivery, and maternal soft-tissue trauma are commonly mentioned as factors predisposing to endometritis after vaginal delivery, these events are not identified in the vast majority of patients who develop such infections. Probably they are relative risk factors.

Indigent patients are at substantially higher risk after either vaginal or abdominal delivery, although the reasons for this observation have never been clearly delineated.

Etiology

This polymicrobial infection is caused by a wide variety of bacteria. Group B streptococci, enterococci, other aerobic streptococci, *Gardnerella vaginalis*, *Escherichia coli*, *Bacteroides bivius*, other *Bacteroides* species, and peptostreptococci are the most common endometrial isolates that are encountered. Group B streptococci and

12

G vaginalis are the most common pathogens isolated from blood.

The isolation of *Ureaplasma urealyticum* and *Mycoplasma hominis* from the endometrium and blood suggests that these organisms can cause infection. Good clinical responses, however, have been obtained in patients who have had mycoplasmas cultured from their blood but who were treated with antibiotics not active against these organisms.

Chlamydia trachomatis is associated with a late form of endometritis occurring more than 2 days to 6 weeks postpartum among women who deliver vaginally. Group A ß-hemolytic streptococcal endometritis is rare and epidemiologically unique because it is caused by exogenous infection (usually in a caregiver), and is characterized by early onset and rapid progression with poor localization.

Diagnosis

The diagnosis is suggested by the development of fever, usually on the first or second postpartum day. Significant fever is defined as an oral temperature of 38.5°C (101.3°F) or higher in the first 24 hours after delivery or 38.0°C (100.4°F) or higher for at least 4 consecutive hours 24 or more hours after delivery. Other consistently associated findings are uterine tenderness, lower abdominal pain, and leukocytosis.

Objectives of management include establishing a diagnosis, obtaining appropriate specimens for culture, choosing and administering effective antimicrobials, and ascertaining and treating the cause of failure in those rare situations in which systemic antimicrobials fail to effect a rapid recovery. The following diagnostic techniques and plan of management are appropriate when endometritis is suspected:

(1) Be aware this infection is rare after uncomplicated vaginal delivery in a nonindigent patient. Rule out other causes of fever in such patients before accepting endometritis as the entity to be treated.

(2) Consider the differential diagnosis of early postpartum fever: urinary tract infection, pneumonia (especially if the patient underwent general anesthesia and is a smoker), appendicitis, viral syndrome, and noninfectious fever such as drug fever or breast engorgement.

(3) Perform a pelvic examination on an appropriate examining table. Using a sterile speculum, visualize the cervix, wipe it with sterile sponges or cotton balls to remove extraneous secretions, and obtain endocervical swabs for *C trachomatis* and *Neisseria gonorrhoeae* if indicated. Cleanse the cervix using povidone iodine–soaked gauze and obtain endometrial cultures using a sterile cotton-

tipped swab grasped with a sterile sponge forceps and inserted carefully into the endometrial cavity. Place the swab directly into an aerobic/anaerobic tube containing transport media and immediately send it to the microbiology laboratory. Double- or triple-lumen brush cultures or aspirates of amniotic fluid with a sterile cannula may also be used. Cultures or rapid antigen detection tests for *C trachomatis* should be obtained from patients with late-onset infection, or those at high risk for chlamydial colonization (for example, pregnant teenagers or women with a history of multiple sexual partners).

(4) Perform a bimanual examination to determine uterine size, consistency, and tenderness. You can also ascertain the presence of an adnexal mass or pelvic abscess at this time.

(5) Obtain a complete blood count and two sets of blood cultures. Blood is an important source for cultures from these women because 10% to 20% of such patients have a documentable bacteremia. Bacteremia does not predict the severity of clinical illness nor a prolonged clinical recovery. If pneumonia is a strong consideration, as it would be with auscultatory findings in a smoker who has undergone general anesthesia, perform a chest x-ray as well.

Treatment

Depending on the clinical course, findings of general systemic toxicity, and patterns of pulse and fever, patients can be classified as having mild/moderate or severe endometritis. Patients with severe endometritis but normal renal function can be treated with a regimen of clindamycin, 900 mg IV every 8 hours, plus gentamicin, given as a loading dose of 2.0 mg/kg IV followed by a maintenance dose of 1.5 mg/kg IV every 8 hours. Gentamicin and clindamycin are compatible in the same IV solution. An alternate regimen is imipenem, 500 mg IV every 6 hours.

Therapy for mild to moderate cases involves the use of one of the extended-spectrum cephalosporins or extended-spectrum penicillins (cefoxitin, 2.0 g IV every 6 hours; cefotetan, 2.0 g IV every 12 hours; piperacillin, 4.0 g IV every 6 hours; ampicillin/sulbactam, 3.0 g IV every 6 hours; mezlocillin, 4.0 g IV every 6 hours; or ticarcillin/clavulanic acid, 3.1 g IV every 4 to 6 hours). Continue parenteral therapy until the patient's temperature has remained below 37.5°C (99.5°F) for 24 to 48 hours, she is pain free, and the white blood cell count is normal. The use of oral antibiotics after discharge has been shown to be unnecessary.

Women with positive cultures for *C trachomatis* who have been treated with a ß-lactam antibiotic should receive erythromycin or doxycycline therapy for a full 10 days even if they have had an initial clinical response. (If they have received a clindamycin-containing regimen, which is effective for *C trachomatis*, they would need to complete 10 days of therapy with clindamycin, doxycycline, or erythromycin.)

Patients receiving aminoglycosides should have a serum creatinine determination every other day. Gentamicin maintenance doses after 24 hours of therapy should be adjusted to provide levels of 5 to 8 µg/mL 15 to 30 minutes after the end of a 30-minute infusion (the "peak" level), and less than 1 µg/mL immediately before the next dose (the "trough" level). Aztreonam, a monocyclic ß-lactam agent with a spectrum similar to gentamicin's, can be used as an alternative to gentamicin in patients with diminished renal function. The dose of aztreonam is 2 g IV every 6 to 8 hours.

Failure of antimicrobial therapy usually results from enterococcal superinfection or inadequate coverage of a multiresistant anaerobe. Enterococcal superinfection is suggested when patients fail to respond or relapse while on regimens that are not effective against enterococci (cephalosporins, clindamycin plus gentamicin), particularly when this organism is isolated in pure culture or heavy growth from an endometrial specimen. If enterococcal superinfection is suspected, use one of the following regimens: clindamycin or metronidazole plus ampicillin plus gentamicin; ampicillin/sulbactam; cefoxitin or cefotetan plus ampicillin; piperacillin; mezlocillin; or ticarcillin/clavulanic acid. Cases of antimicrobial failure due to lack of coverage of a multiresistant anaerobe often respond to a regimen containing metronidazole, clindamycin, or imipenem.

If fever persists, despite apparently appropriate antimicrobial therapy, search for a hidden abscess by bimanual examination and examination of the abdominal wound. You may use ultrasonography or computed tomography if the physical examination fails to reveal a suspected abscess. If these maneuvers reveal a pelvic or wound abscess, surgical drainage is usually necessary.

Patients in whom an abscess has been ruled out but who remain febrile with hectic fever spikes must be evaluated for the possibility of septic pelvic thrombophlebitis or puerperal ovarian vein thrombosis. Patients with septic pelvic thrombophlebitis have a plateau tachycardia and often a mild ileus, but otherwise may appear well despite the impressive fever pattern. Puerperal ovarian vein thrombosis typically presents with right paramedian pain developing on the second or third postpartum day. A tender mass is palpable just to the right of the uterine fundus in 50% of these patients. Treatment of either of these conditions with full IV heparin anticoagulation will usually result in lysis of the fever within 48 hours [see Chapter 64: Septic pelvic thrombophlebitis].

If group A ß-hemolytic streptococci are isolated from more than one patient over a brief time span, do the following:

- Notify local health authorities.
- Employ contact isolation of all infected patients for 24 hours after the start of effective therapy.
- Establish a cohort nursery system.
- Culture all involved professional and other hospital staff, and relieve from duty any who are colonized.
- Culture all newborns for group A streptococci.
- Consider stringent reduction of visitors.
- Stress rigid adherence to aseptic technique, especially handwashing.
- Save all positive group A streptococcal isolates for typing.

SUGGESTED READING

American College of Obstetricians and Gynecologists: Antimicrobial therapy for obstetric patients. ACOG Tech Bull 1988(June);No. 117

Hager WD, Pascuzzi M, Vernon M: Efficacy of oral antibiotics following parenteral antibiotics for serious infections in obstetrics and gynecology. Obstet Gynecol 1989;73:326

Hoyme UB, Kiviat N, Eschenbach DA: Microbiology and treatment of late postpartum endometritis. Obstet Gynecol 1986;68:226

Lev-Toaff AS, Baka JJ, Toaff ME, et al: Diagnostic imaging in puerperal febrile morbidity. Obstet Gynecol 1991;78:50

Martens MG, Faro S, Hammill HA, et al: Transcervical uterine cultures with a new endometrial suction curette: a comparison of three sampling methods in postpartum endometritis. Obstet Gynecol 1989;74:273

Watts DH, Eschenbach DA, Kenny GE: Early postpartum endometritis: the role of bacteria, genital mycoplasmas, and *Chlamydia trachomatis*. Obstet Gynecol 1989;73:52

4

Lower urinary tract infections in pregnancy

By S. Gene McNeeley, Jr., MD

Background and incidence

Urinary tract infection is one of the commonest medical complications occurring in pregnancy. The majority of these infections are asymptomatic and confined to the lower urinary tract. Untreated lower tract infections have been associated with preterm delivery and low birthweight. Of equal or greater importance is the development of pyelonephritis in the gravida and its serious complications, such as sepsis, renal dysfunction, and preterm labor in the mother and respiratory distress syndrome in the newborn.

Since the female urethra is close to the vagina and rectum, it may be colonized by a variety of pathogens. Bacteriuria occurs in approximately 1% of school-aged children and the incidence increases to 2% to 5% by the early teens. Approximately 5% to 7% of pregnant women have asymptomatic bacteriuria during pregnancy, but few women whose early pregnancy urine culture is negative will subsequently develop it. In contrast, among the 1% of pregnant women who develop cystitis (frequency, urgency, or dysuria with bacteriuria), recurrent asymptomatic bacteriuria is not uncommon. Either, left untreated, may result in upper tract infection. Recurrence after therapy, depending on the antibiotic prescribed and duration of therapy, occurs in 10% to 40% of women.

Etiology

The bacteria most often isolated from the urinary tract during pregnancy are *Escherichia coli*, *Klebsiella* sp, and *Enterobacter* sp. These organisms are responsible for approximately 90% of urinary tract infections, and of these *E coli* is the agent most frequently implicated. Bacterial characteristics associated with pathogenicity include ability to attach to human uroepithelial cells, resistance to the bactericidal effect of serum, the serotype identified, and hemolysin production. Isolates recovered from pregnant women with asymptomatic bacteriuria and acute cystitis are less likely to demonstrate these characteristics than isolates recovered from pregnant women with pyelonephritis.

Most infections in pregnant women are community acquired, and the pathogens recovered are susceptible to frequently prescribed antimicrobial agents. The notable exception is *E coli*, which is resistant to ampicillin and penicillin.

Diagnosis

Culture and susceptibility testing are the standard means of diagnosing and managing urinary tract infection during pregnancy. Bacteriuria is traditionally defined as the presence of more than 10^5 colony-forming units per milliliter (cfu/mL) of urine from two consecutive first-void midstream clean-catch urine specimens. Since most pregnant women are unable to provide a first-void specimen at routine prenatal visits, it has been suggested that the presence of more than 10^2 cfu/mL of a single pathogen from a non-first-void specimen signifies bacteriuria. The recovery of a single uropathogen by suprapubic aspiration or urethral catheterization indicates bacteriuria.

Because of the serious maternal complications of undetected bacteriuria and neonatal sequelae of preterm delivery, many feel nonculture tests, with their lower sensitivity, are not appropriate for bacteriuria screening during pregnancy. However, testing for leukocyte esterase and microbially produced nitrites with Chemstrip LN (Biodynamics, Indianapolis, Ind.) or similar products may be cost effective in specific settings. Likewise, the presence of at least one organism per oil-immersion field in a gram-stained centrifuged urine specimen detects bacteriuria at a level of 10^5 cfu/mL.

It is important to recognize that if a nonculture method detects evidence of bacteriuria, a urine specimen for culture and susceptibility testing should be obtained before treatment. This is particularly important in women with recurrent bacteriuria or upper urinary tract abnormalities such as renal calculi, settings where resistant bacteria are frequently encountered.

For women with acute urinary symptoms, appropriate testing for organisms associated with urethritis should be performed in addition to urine culture. Such testing should include culture for *Neisseria gonorrhoeae* and culture or antigen detection testing for *Chlamydia trachomatis*. Sexually transmitted infections should be treated as recommended for pregnancy by the Centers for Disease Control.

TABLE 1
Suggested treatment regimens for lower urinary tract infection

Indication	Regimen
Bacteriuria and acute cystitis	Nitrofurantoin macrocrystals, 50–100 mg q6–8h for 7 to 10 days;
	Amoxicillin, 500 mg q8h, for 7 to 10 days;
	Cephalexin, 250–500 mg q6h, for 7 to 10 days;
	Sulfisoxazole, 500 mg q6h, for 7 to 10 days
Long-term suppression	Nitrofurantoin, 50–100 mg at bedtime or 50 mg bid
	Cephalexin, 250–500 mg bid

Treatment

Appropriate management of lower urinary tract infections during pregnancy will prevent most upper tract infections and their sequelae. A variety of antibiotics can be prescribed to the pregnant patient, including nitrofurantoin macrocrystals, amoxicillin, oral cephalosporins, and sulfisoxazole (Table 1). The sulfonamides should be used with caution during the last trimester because of their potential for displacement of fetal bilirubin and subsequent kernicteris.

Nitrofurantoin and the sulfonamides may produce a fetal hemolytic anemia in the presence of glucose-6-phosphate dehydrogenase (G6PD) deficiency. Neither of these antibiotics should be administered during the last 4 weeks of pregnancy because of the risk of neonatal hyperbilirubinemia. There are no known fetal side effects from in utero amoxicillin or cephalosporin exposure.

Because of concerns about toxicity and teratogenicity, nitrofurantoin macrocrystals would be the treatment of choice for lower urinary tract infections during pregnancy. The high prevalence of resistance (35%) to ampicillin and related penicillins indicates these drugs should not be prescribed as first-line therapy on an empiric basis.

A 7- to 10-day course of therapy has been shown in many studies to be more effective than single-dose therapy for asymptomatic bacteriuria and acute cystitis during pregnancy. Three- and 5-day courses have also proven effective. Cephalosporins should not be used for single-dose treatment because of their consistently high failure rate (40%). Regardless of the regimen prescribed, a follow-up culture for test of cure is mandatory. Women with recurrent episodes of bacteriuria or cystitis should have long-term daily suppression with nitrofurantoin or possibly a cephalosporin.

SUGGESTED READING

Harris RE, Gilstrap LC: Cystitis during pregnancy: a distinct clinical entity. Obstet Gynecol 1981;57:578

Harris RE, Gilstrap LC, Pretty A: Single-dose antimicrobial therapy for asymptomatic bacteriuria during pregnancy. Obstet Gynecol 1982;59:546

Johnson JR, Stamm WE: Urinary tract infections in women: diagnosis and treatment. Ann Intern Med 1989;111:906

Stenqvist K, Sandberg T, Lidin-Janson G, et al: Virulence factors of *Escherichia coli* in urinary isolates from pregnant women. J Infect Dis 1987;156:870

5
Pyelonephritis in pregnancy

By Susan M. Cox, MD

Background and incidence

Antepartum pyelonephritis, the most common serious medical complication of pregnancy, is identified in 1% to 2% of all pregnancies. In the US in 1985, more than 85,000 pregnant women were hospitalized for this complication. The reported incidence of pyelonephritis has decreased over the past 20 years, however, largely because of widespread acceptance of screening for bacteriuria. Harris and Gilstrap reported a decrease from 4% to 0.8% during this time, attributing it to identification and eradication of bacteriuria, as well as frequent culture follow-up.

At Parkland Memorial Hospital, Dallas, 7% to 8% of pregnant women have had asymptomatic bacteriuria on routine screening. Before introduction of screening, nearly 3% of pregnancies were complicated by pyelonephritis, whereas afterwards incidence fell to 1%, owing to treatment of bacteriuria.

Most acute pyelonephritis occurs during the second and third trimesters. In a review of 656 obstetric patients with this condition, Gilstrap and co-workers identified 73% antepartum, 19% postpartum, and 8% intrapartum. Of the 482 antepartum cases, 9% were identified during the first trimester, and the remainder divided evenly between the second and third trimesters. Higher incidence later in pregnancy presumably is related to increasing urinary obstruction.

Etiology

Bacteria most commonly isolated from pregnant women with pyelonephritis are *Escherichia coli* (77%), *Klebsiella–Enterobacter* (15%), and *Proteus* sp (4%). In general, one should hospitalize pregnant women with pyelonephritis for close observation. They frequently have marked dehydration due to severe nausea, vomiting, and anorexia combined with fever. Careful monitoring is necessary to detect life-threatening complications, and close observation with frequent assessment of vital signs is mandatory.

Diagnosis

Signs and symptoms include fever, chills, nausea and vomiting, and costovertebral angle tenderness. Nearly 40% of women also complain of lower tract symptoms, such as urgency, frequency, and dysuria. Fever may reach 40°C (104°F) in many women and frequently has spikes. Among the 656 women cited above, 85% had a temperature of 38°C (100.4°F) or more, and 12% one of 40°C or more. Costovertebral tenderness was rightsided in 54%, bilateral in 27%, and leftsided in 16%.

Systemic signs and symptoms are the primary means of diagnosis. Confirmation is by a positive urine culture, which invariably yields more than 100,000 colonies/mL of a single organism. Cultures may be negative, however, because urinary tract infections tend to recur and women may take leftover medications when they feel initial symptoms. Even a single oral dose of an antibiotic may render the urine culture negative. Blood cultures are positive in approximately 15% of cases.

Treatment

Direct initial treatment toward restoration of the contracted blood volume. It is esssential that IV crystalloids—either physiologic saline or lactated Ringer's solution—be administered along with antimicrobial agents. Initially, give fluids rapidly in order to establish an hourly urinary output of at least 30 to 50 mL, while carefully monitoring pulmonary status for possible edema. As a rule, laboratory assessment should include a complete blood cell count, serum electrolyte and creatinine levels, and urine and blood cultures.

Although choice of an antimicrobial is empiric, prior in vitro sensitivities may be used to select therapy in women who have had a urinary tract infection (UTI) or asymptomatic bacteriuria during a previous pregnancy. In many institutions, ampicillin has long been used successfully to treat uncomplicated pyelonephritis. However, during the past decade studies of in vitro sensitivities have revealed that many uropathogens that cause community-acquired pyelonephritis resist ampicillin. Additionally, Duff reported therapeutic failures thought due to resistant organisms in 27% of 131 women treated with ampicillin alone.

Concern about increasing ampicillin resistance has prompted many investigators to add an aminoglycoside to their regimens. This action has aroused apprehension since 20% of infected women already have transient renal dysfunction resulting from the infection, and the aminoglycoside may compound this effect. Additionally, in pregnant women without renal dysfunction, therapeutic aminoglycoside levels are not easily obtained using standard formulas, resulting in underdosing. Synergistic nephrotoxicity from endotoxin and aminoglycoside is also of particular concern with such therapy.

One may use serial serum creatinine levels or peak and trough aminoglycoside concentrations to monitor dosing. For cost effectiveness, simplicity, and minimal side effects, therapy with a single agent deemed safe during pregnancy is preferable. Extended-spectrum penicillins are ideally suited for these women. The ureidopenicillins, mezlocillin and piperacillin, are broad-spectrum semisynthetic penicillinase-resistant penicillins of FDA category B (animal reproduction studies have not established a fetal risk) and thus relatively safe for use during pregnancy.

Cox and Cunningham recently treated more than 190 women with these penicillins. The cure rate exceeded 95%, with no adverse maternal or fetal outcomes traceable to the drugs. In only a small percentage of women was the addition of an aminoglycoside considered necessary. Guidelines for adding aminoglycoside include:

- a positive follow-up urine culture 24 hours after initiation of antibiotics;
- poor clinical response after 72 hours of therapy;
- evidence of continuing sepsis;
- previous screening cultures showing resistance to penicillin or cephalosporins; and
- recurrent disease.

Follow-up. With appropriate IV hydration and antimicrobial treatment, pregnant women with pyelonephritis usually experience rapid clinical improvement. Cunningham, Morris, and Mickal showed that 85% of women with pyelonephritis given ampicillin, cephalothin, or chloramphenicol were afebrile after 48 hours. We found recently that of 190 women given either piperacillin or mezlocillin, almost 80% were clinically well after 48 hours and only 4% required parenteral therapy more than 96 hours. Failure to improve within the first 2 to 3 days suggests a complication often associated with underlying obstruction, such as urolithiasis or an anatomic anomaly.

Women with pyelonephritis who fail to show rapid clinical improvement after therapy should be evaluated for urinary tract obstruction. In many cases, this failure is caused by urolithiasis, but some women will have serious sequelae without evidence of obstruction. Passage of a double-J ureteral stent ordinarily will relieve any obstruction identified. If the stent fails, surgical removal of the stones is usually followed by rapid resolution of infection.

A plain abdominal radiograph is indicated for women who remain febrile after 72 hours of appropriate therapy since nearly 90% of renal stones are radiopaque. Possible benefits far outweigh any harm to the fetus from radiation exposure. If the radiograph is negative, then intravenous pyelography (IVP), modified by the number of radiographs taken after contrast injection, usually provides adequate imaging of the collecting system, permitting detection of stones or structural anomalies.

In some women, there will be nonvisualization of the collecting tract with IVP, making further workup necessary. Retrograde pyelography may disclose an end-stage obstructed kidney with pyonephrosis as a cause of continuing sepsis. In these cases, calculi frequently coexist, and removal of the infected kidney may be lifesaving. An alternative technique is renal sonography to detect underlying lesions, such as pyelocaliceal dilation, urinary calculi, and intrarenal or perinephric abscess.

Acute pyelonephritis or frequent UTI during pregnancy may reflect a urinary tract abnormality. Indeed, as many as 37% of these women when nonpregnant will have either recurrent infection or radiographic urinary anomalies. All women who had pyelonephritis during pregnancy should have a urine culture 6 to 8 weeks after delivery to rule out asymptomatic infection. In an 8- to 13-year follow-up of 208 women with acute pyelonephritis, Gilstrap and co-workers treated 41% for one or more episodes of symptomatic UTI when not pregnant, and 38% of those with subsequent pregnancies had another infection during pregnancy. Fortunately, despite risks for frequent recurrences and the presence of urinary tract abnormalities, development of end-stage renal insufficiency is uncommon.

Sequelae

Acute pyelonephritis during pregnancy can be devastating for both mother and fetus. Approximately 25% of women with severe infection show clinical evidence of multiple organ-system derangement. These complications, which are more common in women who are clinically ill or "toxic," appear to be mediated by bacterial endotoxin or lipopolysaccharide (LPS).

Septic shock. Septic shock, fortunately, is rare, although up to 15% of women with severe antepartum pyelonephritis have bacteremia. One must differentiate hypotension and diminished perfusion as a consequence of endotoxemia from that caused by dehydration from nausea, vomiting, and fever. Although many dehydrated women have other evidence of endotoxemia, only a few show evident hypotension after fluid resuscitation. Generally, cardiac output is restored with aggressive IV fluid resuscitation. Vasopressor drugs are rarely required.

Renal dysfunction. In a prospective study of 220 women with antepartum pyelonephritis, Whalley and co-workers found 25% to have seriously diminished glomerular filtration rates, defined by creatinine clearance of less than 80 mL/min. Pragmatically, renal dysfunction is identified when serum creatinine concentration exceeds 1 mg/dL after hydration.

Renal dysfunction usually is transient and returns to normal within several days. It is believed these pathologic changes are mediated by LPS, known to be nephrotoxic. Management includes observation combined with continuous administration of IV fluids and antimicrobials and serial monitoring of serum creatinine levels. Select antimicrobials that have no nephrotoxicity or appropriately reduce dosage of those that do.

Hematologic changes. Although hematologic aberrations with acute pyelonephritis have been reported, they are seldom clinically important. There is abundant evidence that endotoxemia causes hemolysis, which may result in moderate to severe anemia, but erythrocyte transfusions are seldom indicated. Cox and Cunningham reported that 25% of pregnant women with pyelonephritis had anemia defined by a hematocrit of less than 30 vol%. However, Cavenee and co-workers did not find a decreased level of serum erythropoietin—the major regulator of erythropoiesis and produced by the kidney—in these women. Overt severe thrombocytopenia, an ominous finding, is uncommon.

Pulmonary injury. Perhaps 2% of women with severe antepartum pyelonephritis will develop some variety of respiratory insufficiency. Clinically, pulmonary injury is similar to that found in so-called adult respiratory distress syndrome. Fortunately, clinical manifestations are transient and respond to increased oxygen delivered by face mask. Occasionally, tracheal intubation with mechanical ventilation and positive end expiratory pressure is required.

Thus, in addition to close monitoring of blood pressure, pulse, and urinary output, attention to respiratory rate and development of dyspnea is needed. One should promptly investigate tachypnea by chest radiography and arterial blood gas analysis. Prompt recognition and appropriate respiratory therapy should prevent severe hypoxemia that may cause fetal death or preterm labor.

Pulmonary injury is due to endotoxin, which alters the permeability of the alveolar–capillary membrane, and frequently coexists with evidence of other organ injury, such as hematologic aberrations or renal dysfunction. This combination of symptoms is more likely in women with proven bacteremia or infections caused by *Klebsiella pneumoniae*.

Hypothalamic instability. In pregnant women with acute pyelonephritis, fever as high as 40°C (104°F) may be followed during the same day by hypothermia. This fluctuation is mediated by endotoxin effects. The LPS of bacterial endotoxin is a potent exogenous pyrogen, and very small quantities are capable of producing a febrile response. Increase in body temperature results from an alteration in the set-point of the hypothalamic thermoregulatory center.

SUGGESTED READING

Cavanee M, Cox S, Mason R, et al: Erythropoietin and pyelonephritis in pregnancy. Am J Obstet Gynecol 1991;164:287

Cox SM, Cunningham FG: Ureidopenicillin therapy for acute antepartum pyelonephritis. Curr Ther Res 1988;44:1029

Cox SM, Shelburne P, Mason R, et al: Mechanisms of hemolysis and anemia associated with acute antepartum pyelonephritis. Am J Obstet Gynecol 1990;164:587

Cunningham FG, Lucas MJ, Hankins GDV: Pulmonary injury complicating antepartum pyelonephritis. Am J Obstet Gynecol 1987;156:797

Cunningham FG, Morris GB, Mickal A: Acute pyelonephritis of pregnancy: a clinical review. Obstet Gynecol 1973;42:112

Duff P: Pyelonephritis in pregnancy. Clin Obstet Gynecol 1984;27:17

Gilstrap LC, Cunningham FG, Whalley PJ: Acute pyelonephritis in pregnancy: an anterospective study. Obstet Gynecol 1981;57:409

Gilstrap LC, Leveno KJ, Cunningham FG, et al: Renal infection and pregnancy outcome. Am J Obstet Gynecol 1981;141:709

Harris RE, Gilstrap LG: Prevention of recurrent pyelonephritis during pregnancy. Obstet Gynecol 1974;44:637

Whalley PJ, Cunningham FG, Martin FG: Transient renal dysfunction associated with acute pyelonephritis of pregnancy. Obstet Gynecol 1974;46:174

6
Mastitis

By W. David Hager, MD

PUERPERAL MASTITIS

Background and incidence

Inflammatory disorders of the breast have been recognized as causing problems among mothers as long as they have nursed their infants. In 1953, Gibberd categorized these inflammatory disorders as epidemic and nonepidemic (sporadic).

Epidemic mastitis is defined as an acute adenitis and cellulitis primarily involving the lactiferous apparatus of the breast, and often including nonadjacent lobes. Epidemic outbreaks are frequently associated with *Staphylococcus aureus* infections in the nursery.

Nonepidemic mastitis is defined as an acute puerperal cellulitis with extension to the periglandular connective tissue. The connective tissue infection results in a V-shaped area of involvement between lobes.

Thomsen and co-workers have divided nonepidemic mastitis into three categories—milk stasis, noninfectious inflammation, and acute mastitis—based on progression of disease. Milk stasis results from incomplete emptying of the breast and causes engorgement and pain. When stasis of milk is persistent and severe, noninfectious inflammation may follow with edema, erythema, pain, and tenderness. These conditions may each last for a few days and, if unresolved, lead to acute mastitis with edema, erythema, pain, myalgias, chills, fever, and tenderness.

In the past, acute mastitis was often epidemic, and associated with longer hospital stays, lack of antibiotics, and outbreaks of *S aureus* infection in nurseries. Today, it is more likely to be nonepidemic. Studies show that 7% to 11% of nursing mothers will develop inflammation or acute mastitis. The effect of avoiding nursery outbreaks is emphasized by a study from the former Soviet Union that showed a 30-fold decrease in acute mastitis when infants were allowed to room in with their mothers.

Etiology

The onset of symptoms and signs of acute puerperal mastitis often results from a vicious cycle of events. Bacteria from the infant's mouth or from the mother's skin may enter the breast through a cracked nipple. Infection may occur when these bacteria confront milk that remains in the breast when the organ fails to empty completely. Infection causes pain and tenderness that further impede emptying. Infection also causes engorgement, which prevents the infant from drawing the nipple and areola into its mouth completely. The result is nibbling and further cracking, which allows more bacteria to enter and infect.

There are not a large number of well-designed studies on the bacterial etiology of mastitis. Niebyl and co-workers isolated pathogenic bacteria from 53% of their patients who had nonepidemic mastitis. Of those with bacteria isolated, 37% had *S aureus* alone or in combination with other bacteria. Marshall and co-workers recovered *S aureus* from more than 50% of their patients with puerperal mastitis. Bacteria isolated in other reports include coagulase-negative *S aureus*, group A and group B ß-hemolytic streptococci, *Escherichia coli*, and *Bacteroides* species.

Several factors predispose the nursing mother to mastitis. Failure to empty the breast adequately is undoubtedly the most important one and must be reemphasized. Fissuring of nipples and bacterial inoculum from the infant's mouth or mother's skin have also been mentioned. Incorrect preparation and care of the nipples and improper positioning of the infant for nursing may increase chances of nipple fissuring. Lowered maternal immune defenses must also be considered, and may result from fatigue, stress, or improper nutrition.

Diagnosis

The diagnosis of acute puerperal mastitis is made on the basis of clinical symptoms and signs. The most frequent symptoms are malaise, myalgias, fever, chills, and pain. Signs of disease include edema, erythema, temperature elevation above 37.8°C (>100°F), and breast tenderness. The erythema is frequently found to occur in a V-shaped distribution. Engorgement of the breast from milk stasis is often bilateral and not associated with fever or erythema, whereas noninfectious inflammation and mastitis are more frequently unilateral.

Diagnosis is seldom based on culture results alone. If culturing is

TABLE 1

Classification of nonepidemic mastitis

Milk stasis

$<10^6$ leukocytes/mL milk

$<10^3$ bacteria/mL milk

Noninfectious inflammation

$>10^6$ leukocytes/mL milk

$<10^3$ bacteria/mL milk

Infectious mastitis

$>10^6$ leukocytes/mL milk

$>10^3$ bacteria/mL milk

Source: Thomsen AC, et al: Am J Obstet Gynecol 1984;149:492

done, the specimen should be obtained from expressed milk after discarding the first 2 to 3 mL. Differentiating milk stasis from noninfectious inflammation and infectious mastitis by quantitative evaluation of the mother's milk has been described by Thomsen and co-workers (Table 1). This classification is based on quantitative leukocyte counts and quantitative bacterial cultures (per milliliter of milk).

Treatment

The key to managing mastitis is early recognition of a potential problem. Infection may be prevented by effectively treating milk stasis with adequate breast emptying. Among patients with noninfectious inflammation, 79% had a poor outcome when the breast was not emptied regularly and adequately.

Since the site of infection in acute puerperal mastitis is extraductal, continued nursing is not detrimental to the baby. There are no data to indicate adverse effects on the infant from continued nursing. Weaning the infant from the breast during an acute infection has been shown to increase the risk of prolonged infection and of developing an abscess.

In addition to emptying the breasts, supportive measures include the use of moist heat to the involved breast, adequate hydration of the mother, and use of anti-inflammatory agents such as acetaminophen. If the pain is so severe that the mother cannot nurse, she may choose to use a breast pump or to express the milk while lying in a tub of warm water, with the breast floating comfortably.

Antibiotics are selected empirically. Devereux has shown that the response to treatment is best when antibiotics are begun in the first 24 hours of the course of disease. Thomsen's data indicate a good response in 15% of women with no treatment, in 51% of those who only emptied their breasts regularly, and in 96% of those who emptied their breasts regularly and received antibiotics orally.

Antibiotics that have been used effectively include penicillin, 500 mg orally every 6 hours; ampicillin, 500 mg orally every 6 hours; oxacillin, 500 mg orally every 6 hours; dicloxacillin, 500 mg orally every 6 hours; erythromycin base, 500 mg orally every 6 hours; and cephalosporins such as cephalexin, 500 mg orally every 6 hours, or cephradine, 500 mg orally every 6 hours. In order to provide coverage for staphylococci and streptococci, we have used an oral cephalosporin as our first-line agent, with good results.

Prevention
Any program for avoiding acute mastitis must stress regular emptying of the breasts, proper positioning of the infant for nursing, and appropriate nipple care. Although good data are lacking to confirm the protective benefit of nipple care, we have found vitamin E expressed directly onto the nipple and areola from capsules to be the best preparatory agent available. Lanolin creams tend to promote cracking and should not be used.

Sequelae
The most frequent immediate consequences of mastitis are persistent infection and development of an abscess. Devereux diagnosed an abscess in 11.1% of women treated for acute puerperal mastitis, while Marshall and co-workers found an abscess in 4.6% of their patients.

Cessation of nursing increases the risk of prolonged infection and abscess and should be discouraged. The milk of women with mastitis has been found to have increased sodium content, which may cause the infant to reject the breast. Milk from mastitis patients has been reported to be lower in lactose, fat, and total protein. Persistent rejection of the breast by an infant should alert the physician to investigate carcinoma of the breast.

When a breast abscess is diagnosed, the patient should stop nursing on that side and be treated with parenteral antibiotics such as cefazolin, 1 g IV every 6 to 8 hours; ampicillin, 1 g IV every 6 hours; or methicillin, 1 to 2 g every 6 to 8 hours. Anaerobic coverage should be provided with clindamycin, 900 mg every 8 hours, or metronidazole, 500 mg every 6 hours. If the response is not favorable within 48 to 72 hours, the physician should incise and drain the abscess, then give appropriate wound care. Careful follow-up must be done to evaluate for recurrent abscess.

Acute nonepidemic puerperal mastitis is a frequent cause of morbidity among recently pregnant women. Alertness to the possibility of infection, early diagnosis, and appropriate therapy, as outlined above, should result in successful outcome for most patients.

NONPUERPERAL MASTITIS

Background
Infection of the breast in nonpregnant women is an uncommon clinical problem. However, it is important to understand the presentation of this disease and its etiology because, untreated, it can lead to chronic sinus tract formation and severe abscesses.

The disease is characterized as a partial blockage of the lactiferous ducts by keratotic debris and squamous metaplasia of the epithelium lining the milk sinus.

Etiology
The etiology of nonpuerperal infection has been uncertain because of disagreement in the literature about which bacteria are causative. Most case reports have identified *S aureus* as the predominant microbial isolate. Recent data indicate that anaerobic cocci and bacilli are often isolated from breast secretions and from abscesses. Edmiston and co-workers have reported that peptostreptococci are the most common isolates among women with nonpuerperal mastitis. The literature would thus seem to confirm that the etiology frequently involves mixed aerobes and anaerobes when the process is chronic.

Predisposing factors. Unlike puerperal mastitis, in which bacteria that are introduced into cracked nipples and ascend to areas of milk stasis are an obvious predisposing factor, the factors that lead to nonpuerperal disease are less certain. Some authors have suggested that manipulative breast procedures or oral stimulation of the breast are possible inciting factors. It is also possible that cutaneous infections may invade nearby breast tissue.

Diagnosis
Nonpuerperal mastitis can present as acute, subacute, or chronic disease. Patients with acute disease present with complaints of pain and fever and are found to have edema and erythema of the involved breast, along with a firm, tender mass in the subareolar region. Patients with subacute disease present like those with acute disease but have a tender, fluctuant mass. Chronic disease presents after multiple, recurrent infections and leads to sinus tract formation, suppuration, and possibly a fluctuant mass, along with pain and edema.

Treatment
Women with acute nonpuerperal mastitis will usually respond to antibiotic therapy that combines a penicillinase-resistant penicillin with an agent such as metronidazole that provides anaerobic coverage (see doses for puerperal mastitis). Metronidazole should be

given in a dose of 500 mg orally every 8 hours. Another option would be giving a broad-spectrum antibiotic, such as one of the fluoroquinolones, in doses of 300 to 400 mg orally every 12 hours.

Subacute disease will usually require surgical drainage, along with broad-spectrum antimicrobial therapy. Chronic disease requires aggressive surgical excision and debridement, followed by extended antibiotic treatment.

Preventive measures, such as treating skin lesions aggressively and encouraging avoidance of oral breast stimulation may help to decrease the prevalence of disease.

SUGGESTED READING

Devereux WP: Acute puerperal mastitis: evaluation of its management. Am J Obstet Gynecol 1970;108:78

Edmiston CE, Walker AP, Krepel CJ, et al: The nonpuerperal breast infection: aerobic and anaerobic microbial recovery from acute and chronic disease. J Infect Dis 1990;162:695

Goldsmith HS: Milk rejection sign of breast cancer. Am J Surg 1974;127:280

Leach RD, Eykyn SJ, Phillips I, et al: Anaerobic subareolar breast abscess. Lancet 1979;1:35

Marshall BR, Hepper JK, Zirbel CC: Sporadic puerperal mastitis—an infection that need not interrupt lactation. JAMA 1975:233;1377

Niebyl JR, Spence MR, Parmley TH: Sporadic (nonepidemic) puerperal mastitis. J Reprod Med 1978;20(2):97

Puerperal mastitis. Editorial. Br Med J 1976;1:920

Thomsen AC, Espersen T, Maigaard S: Course and treatment of milk stasis, noninfectious inflammation of the breast, and infectious mastitis in nursing women. Am J Obstet Gynecol 1984;149:492

7

Chlamydial infections in pregnancy

By Jorma Paavonen, MD

Background

Chlamydia trachomatis was first isolated from the female genital tract in 1959. A tissue culture technique for isolation of *C trachomatis* was developed in 1965 and a microimmunofluorescence test for serotyping and seroepidemiologic studies was developed in 1970. The etiology of uncomplicated and complicated genital infections started to unfold in the late 1960s and early 1970s. By the late 1970s the wide spectrum of clinical manifestations of genital chlamydial infections had largely been recognized. In the 1980s rapid tests replaced cumbersome tissue culture in the detection of *C trachomatis*.

Genital chlamydial infections have now been recognized as a major public health problem. In clinical studies the research focus has turned from acute infections to chronic and subclinical manifestations of *C trachomatis* infection, such as chronic endometritis, tubal pregnancy, tubal factor infertility, and adverse pregnancy outcome.

Demographic factors associated with an increased risk for *C trachomatis* infection include young age, single marital status, use of oral contraceptives, recent history of a new sex partner, and risk-taking behavior in general. Studies have demonstrated a surprisingly high prevalence of asymptomatic *C trachomatis* infections in adolescents. Young women are particularly susceptible because of the presence of cervical ectopy that provides target cells for *C trachomatis*.

C trachomatis is the major cause of mucopurulent cervicitis and pelvic inflammatory disease (PID). Other clinical manifestations of chlamydial infection include acute urethral syndrome, acute bartholinitis, and proctitis.

The clinical spectrum of chlamydial PID ranges from endometritis to salpingitis, pelvic peritonitis, periappendicitis, and perihepatitis. Late manifestations of chlamydial PID include tubal infertility and tubal pregnancy.

The majority of patients with tubal factor infertility or tubal pregnancy have high serum antibody levels to *C trachomatis*, indicating past chlamydial infection. Nevertheless, fewer than half of all women with tubal factor infertility or tubal pregnancy and serum antichlamydial antibodies have a history of frank PID. This suggests genital chlamydial infections are often subclinical. Tubal factor infertility is frequently the first sign of genital chlamydial infection.

Pathophysiology

As the spectrum and incidence of many sexually transmitted diseases have grown, consequences during pregnancy have received more attention. Tubal pregnancy, spontaneous abortion, stillbirth, preterm premature rupture of the membranes and prematurity, congenital and perinatal infections, and puerperal infections represent adverse pregnancy outcomes associated with STDs. The association between *C trachomatis* and perinatal infections is well established. Many, but not all, studies have demonstrated an association between *C trachomatis* infection and adverse pregnancy outcome.

Perinatal infections. The newborn is a sensitive indicator of untreated chlamydial cervicitis in the mother. *C trachomatis* infection during pregnancy is associated with risks to both mothers and their infants. The clinical manifestations of neonatal chlamydial infection include conjunctivitis and pneumonitis [see Chapter 8].

C trachomatis was first identified in conjunctival scrapes of neonates with ophthalmia neonatorum in 1909, and neonatal inclusion conjunctivitis became a well-known entity by the 1940s. The association between *C trachomatis* and pneumonia in the newborn was first described in 1975, and confirmed in 1977. The attack rates of neonatal chlamydial disease have been well defined. Overall, approximately two thirds of infants exposed to *C trachomatis* during delivery will acquire the infection. Inclusion conjunctivitis will develop in one of three exposed infants, and pneumonia will develop in one of six. The incidence of these diseases in a given community thus depends on the prevalence of chlamydial cervicitis in pregnant women.

Clinical findings of inclusion conjunctivitis cover a spectrum from asymptomatic infection to severe purulent conjunctivitis. The symptoms usually appear between 1 and 2 weeks of age. The eyelids become edematous, with conjunctival erythema and discharge. Initially, there is infiltration of polymorphonuclear leukocytes followed by mononuclear cells. Chlamydial pneumonitis typically develops between 3 and 16 weeks of age with relatively mild symptoms, but one of four infants develops serious coughing, tachypnea, dyspnea, or even apnea, and may require hospitalization. Seroepidemiologic studies suggest that up to 40% of infant pneumonias in the first 6 months of life are associated with *C trachomatis*. Serum levels of IgG and IgM are usually elevated, and blood eosinophilia is commonly found.

The potential impact of *C trachomatis* on perinatal outcome is high, since the prevalence of asymptomatic infection is surprisingly high in young populations in particular. Prevalence figures up to 30% to 40% have been reported in adolescent prenatal clinics in the US. A cost–benefit analysis has indicated that if the maternal infection rate exceeds 6%, it is cost-effective to screen pregnant women for *C trachomatis* and treat those found to be infected to prevent vertical transmission to the infants.

Diagnosis

Slow and cumbersome tissue culture techniques have been largely replaced by more rapid and simple techniques. These include detection of chlamydial particles by immunofluorescence staining or immunoperoxidase staining, detection of chlamydial antigens by enzyme immunoassay, and detection of chlamydial nucleic acids by DNA hybridization techniques, most recently by enzymatic amplification of chlamydial target DNA [polymerase chain reaction (PCR)]. Although enzyme immunoassays are now most widely used, cross-reactions with other bacterial antigens can give false-positive results. Thus, the positive predictive value of these assays in a low-prevalence population can be surprisingly low although their performance in a high-prevalence population is usually satisfactory. Therefore, such tests should be used only if positive results can be confirmed by another test to demonstrate chlamydial elementary bodies. Recent results of diagnosing *C trachomatis* infection by examining first-voided urine for chlamydial antigen using enzyme immunoassays have been promising. Such use for testing men is an attractive alternative to urethral swabbing.

Treatment

Erythromycin, 500 mg four times daily for 10 to 14 days, eradicates *C trachomatis*. Shorter courses probably are inappropriate since *C trachomatis* is an intracellular microorganism and latent persistent infections are known to occur. Tetracycline should not be used in treating pregnant women.

If gastrointestinal intolerance to erythromycin develops, a smaller dose can be used (equivalent to 1 g of erythromycin base per day). Amoxicillin is a reasonable alternative to erythromycin, although the risk for late recurrences may be higher than with erythromycin.

Proper timing of screening and treatment for *C trachomatis* infection has not been adequately addressed. Early diagnosis and treatment would probably prevent complications related to preterm delivery, but might increase the likelihood of repeat infection from untreated male partners. There is no doubt that diagnosing and treating genital chlamydial infection during pregnancy has a profound effect on the incidence of perinatal chlamydial disease as well as on maternal postpartum infections.

Sequelae

C trachomatis is one of the numerous cervicovaginal microorganisms associated with adverse pregnancy outcome. (Others include group B *Streptococcus, Ureaplasma urealyticum, Mycoplasma hominis, Trichomonas vaginalis, Gardnerella vaginalis,* and *Neisseria gonorrhoeae.*) However, there is still conflicting evidence on the possible role of *C trachomatis* in adverse pregnancy outcomes, independent of coinfections.

Overall, after 1982, several major cohort or case–control studies have demonstrated an association between prematurity or low birthweight and culture-proven *C trachomatis* infection. Some studies have demonstrated such association only among women with *C trachomatis* infection who had serum IgM antichlamydial antibodies (suggesting an acute infection), whereas at least four studies have demonstrated no association between *C trachomatis* and adverse pregnancy outcome. In a landmark study by Gravett and co-workers at the University of Washington, cervical infection with *C trachomatis* was independently associated with preterm PROM, preterm labor, and low birthweight. Current data suggest that the relative risk for adverse pregnancy outcome among pregnant women with *C trachomatis* infection is modestly increased, and probably only among women with recent or acute infection as indicated by the presence of serum IgM antichlamydial antibodies.

Puerperal infections. Since *C trachomatis* is a leading cause of PID among nonpregnant women, it is not surprising that this organism is associated with postpartum endometritis and postabortion endometritis as well. Because of the slow growth cycle of *C trachomatis*, postpartum endometritis develops no sooner than 2 to 6 weeks after delivery. Several studies have consistently shown an association between *C trachomatis* infection and postpartum endometritis following vaginal delivery. Similarly, many studies have shown a link between *C trachomatis* and postabortion PID. Most, but not all, studies have demonstrated that antibiotic treatment for chlamydial infection antepartum (doxycycline or erythromycin) significantly decreases the occurrence of postabortion PID.

SUGGESTED READING

Crombleholme WR, Schachter J, Grossman M, et al: Amoxicillin therapy for *Chlamydia trachomatis* in pregnancy. Obstet Gynecol 1990;75:752

Gravett MG, Nelson HP, DeRouen T, et al: Independent associations of bacterial vaginosis and *Chlamydia trachomatis* infection with adverse pregnancy outcome. JAMA 1986;256:1899

Holmes KK, Mårdh P-A, Sparling PF, et al: *Sexually Transmitted Diseases*, ed 2. New York, McGraw-Hill, 1990, chaps 64 and 66.

Paavonen J, Wölner-Hanssen P: *Chlamydia trachomatis*: a major threat to reproduction. Human Reprod 1989;4:111

Pitegoff JG, Cathro DM: Chlamydial infections and other sexually transmitted diseases in adolescent pregnancy. Semin Adolesc Med 1986;2:215

Schachter J, Grossman M, Sweet RL, et al: Prospective study of perinatal transmission of *Chlamydia trachomatis*. JAMA 1986;255:3374

Thompson S, Lopez B, Wong K-H, et al: A prospective study of *Chlamydia* and mycoplasma infections during pregnancy: relation to pregnancy outcome and maternal morbidity, in Mårdh PA, Holmes KK, Oriel JD, et al (eds): *Chlamydial Infections*. New York, Elsevier Biomedical Press, 1982, p 155

8

Neonatal chlamydial infections

By William R. Crombleholme, MD

Background

At present, the most common sexually transmitted organism in the US is *Chlamydia trachomatis*. It is responsible for several distinct infectious illnesses in adults, including urethritis and epididymitis in men and cervicitis and salpingitis in women. Further, endocervical infection in women during pregnancy may lead to vertical transmission of the infection to their infants in the course of vaginal delivery [see Chapter 10: Ophthalmia neonatorum].

Incidence

The prevalence of cervical infections with *C trachomatis* among pregnant women is influenced by the population studied. Women who are younger, unmarried, nonwhite, and of lower socioeconomic status tend to have higher rates of infection. In reported series, prevalence has ranged from 2% to 26%, with an overall estimate of 6% to 8% of all pregnant women harboring the organism. More important, most of these women were asymptomatic.

Pathophysiology

Perinatally acquired *C trachomatis* causes two major infectious complications among infants: inclusion conjunctivitis and pneumonitis. Inclusion conjunctivitis is seen in 35% to 50% of infants born to untreated mothers with cervical *C trachomatis* infection. Clinical findings usually appear between the 5th and 12th day of life. Symptoms include a mucoid discharge that becomes more purulent, followed by edema of the eyelids with erythema of both the palpebral and bulbar conjunctivas. Chlamydial pneumonia is seen in 11% to 20% of infants born to untreated mothers. Onset of symptoms is often as early as 2 to 3 weeks of age, gradually worsening and prompting the diagnosis by 4 to 6 weeks of age. Symptoms include tachypnea with a staccato cough and rales, with the chest radiograph showing hyperexpansion with diffuse interstitial and patchy alveolar infiltrates. Treatment for both infections can be accomplished with a 2-week course of oral erythromycin. This offers the advantage of clearing all colonization sites, including the nasopharynx, which is not accomplished when only topical antibiotic therapy is used to treat conjunctivitis.

Diagnosis

Chlamydiae have a unique growth cycle and are therefore quite different from the other common agent causing endocervical infection, *Neisseria gonorrhoeae*. The infectious particle is called the elementary body and is the extracellular form. It is not metabolically active and is quite resistant to environmental influences. It attaches to the host cell and appears to induce phagocytosis to gain access to the host. In the host, it remains within the phagocytic vesicle but changes to a metabolically active and dividing form called the reticulate body.

The chlamydiae are thus obligate intracellular parasites. They are unable to synthesize high-energy compounds themselves and must use host cell substrates to synthesize their proteins, including RNA and DNA. For this reason, for purposes of identification, they can be grown only in tissue culture, not in artificial media. Alternatively, they can be identified by immunofluorescence staining of smears with monoclonal antibody or detection of chlamydial antigen by enzyme-linked immunoassay (ELISA). It is the introduction of these latter techniques particularly that has made the screening of pregnant women for *C trachomatis* more practical.

Treatment

Neonatal prophylaxis. Though oral antibiotics can treat the infection, it is far preferable to prevent the development of infection at the outset. Initial strategies for preventing inclusion conjunctivitis due to *C trachomatis* focused on newborn ocular prophylaxis. Prevention of gonococcal ophthalmia neonatorum by prophylactic instillation of silver nitrate drops had long been standard practice in almost all newborn nurseries. With recognition that in more currently studied populations *C trachomatis* was the most common organism causing neonatal conjunctivitis, attention was turned to ocular antibiotic preparations that would cover both *N gonorrhoeae* and *C trachomatis*. In 1980 Hammerschlag and co-workers suggested that 0.5% erythromycin ophthalmic ointment was effective in preventing chlamydial conjunctivitis and was known also to prevent gonococcal ophthalmia. Laga and co-workers in 1988 reported that 1% tetracycline ointment was also effective in preventing conjunctivitis from either *N gonorrhoeae* or *C trachomatis.*

Hammerschlag and co-workers later prospectively evaluated use of silver nitrate drops, erythromycin ointment, and tetracycline ointment for preventing neonatal conjunctivitis among infants born in a large urban hospital. The total incidence of gonococcal ophthalmia was low in this group of newborns (0.06%) and the prophylaxis failure with each regimen was comparable. The frequency of prophylaxis failure for each regimen was also comparable with respect to chlamydial conjunctivitis. However, the rate of failure was disturbingly high and not significantly different: 20% in the silver nitrate group, 14% in the erythromycin group, and 11% in the tetracycline group. The investigators concluded that ocular prophylaxis with any of the regimens was effective for gonococcal conjunctivitis but that chlamydial conjunctivitis would be prevented most effectively by the screening and treatment of pregnant women before delivery.

Maternal therapy. Two studies have addressed the issue of preventing vertical transmission of *C trachomatis* by screening and treating women during pregnancy. In 1986 Schachter and co-workers reported their experience using erythromycin ethylsuccinate, 400 mg four times daily for 7 days at 36 weeks' gestation. Mothers were followed with serial chlamydial cultures at the end of treatment, at delivery, and at routine postpartum examinations. Their partners were treated at the same time with tetracycline, 500 mg four times daily for 7 days.

The infants of treated mothers were followed for 1 year or until maternal antichlamydial antibody had disappeared. At routine visits, or if infants were seen because of illness, chlamydial cultures were obtained from the conjunctivas, nasopharynx, and rectum. As Table 1 shows, 92% (98/107) of women who completed a course of therapy and had tests of cure were successfully cleared of their chlamydial infection. Among infants with complete follow-up, vertical transmission was prevented in 93% (55/59), with no evidence of chlamydial infection by culture and/or antichlamydial serology. However, 6.6% of treated women experienced gastrointestinal side effects so severe that half of them stopped their therapy.

The latter observation led the same investigators to seek an alternative regimen for women intolerant of, or allergic to, erythromycin. They compared a regimen of amoxicillin, 500 mg three times daily for 7 days, with erythromycin base, 500 mg four times daily for 7 days. Maternal and infant follow-up was completed as in the initial study with erythromycin ethylsuccinate. Of women treated with amoxi-

TABLE 1
Treatment outcomes during pregnancy

Patients enrolled (total)	Erythromycin ethylsuccinate (n = 152)	Erythromycin base (n = 100)	Amoxicillin (n = 93)
Patients evaluable			
Mothers with negative cervical cultures	98/107 (92.0%)	55/58 (94.8%)	63/64 (98.4%)
Infants with negative cultures or serologies	55/59 (93.2%)	32/36 (88.8%)	37/39 (94.9%)
Side effects	10/152 (6.6%)	15/100 (15.0%)	8/93 (8.6%)
Stopped therapy	5/152 (3.3%)	13/100 (13.0%)	2/93 (2.2%)

cillin, 98% (63/64) had eradication of their chlamydial infection compared with 95% (55/58) of women treated with erythromycin base (Table 1). Vertical transmission was prevented in 95% (37/39) of infants whose mothers were treated with amoxicillin compared with 89% (32/36) of infants in the erythromycin base group. Of eight patients (8.6%) in the amoxicillin group who experienced side effects, only two stopped their therapy. In contrast, of 15 patients (15%) in the erythromycin group with side effects, 13 discontinued therapy. The authors conclude that amoxicillin may be an acceptable alternative in pregnancy when erythromycin treatment is not feasible.

SUGGESTED READING

Crombleholme W, Schachter J, Grossman M, et al: Amoxicillin therapy for *Chlamydia trachomatis* in pregnancy. Obstet Gynecol 1990;75:752

Hammerschlag MR, Chandler JW, Alexander ER, et al: Erythromycin ointment for ocular prophylaxis of neonatal chlamydial infection. JAMA 1980;244:2291

Hammerschlag M, Cummings C, Roblin P, et al: Efficacy of neonatal ocular prophylaxis for the prevention of chlamydial and gonococcal conjunctivitis. N Engl J Med 1989;320:769

Harrison HR, Alexander ER: *Chlamydia trachomatis* infections of the infant, in Holmes KK, Mårdh PA, Sparling PF, et al (eds): *Sexually Transmitted Diseases*. New York, McGraw-Hill, 1990, pp 811-820

Laga M, Plummer F, Piot P, et al: Prophylaxis of gonococcal and chlamydial ophthalmia neonatorum. N Engl J Med 1988; 318:653

Schachter J, Sweet R, Grossman M, et al: Experience with the routine use of erythromycin for chlamydial infections in pregnancy. N Engl J Med 1986;314:276

9

Gonococcal infections in pregnancy

By Walter J. Morales, MD, PhD

Background and incidence

Neisseria gonorrhoeae infection is the most common sexually transmitted disease in the US, with 1 million new cases reported annually and another 1 million estimated. The causative organism, a gram-negative diplococcus, may infect the epithelium of the genitourinary tract as well as the rectum, pharynx, or eye. A localized acute infection may give rise to a bacteremia and disseminated disease. In men, *N gonorrhoeae* can infect the urethra after an incubation period of 5 to 7 days. The risk of transmission from an infected male to an unprotected female partner is about 70%.

Depending on the socioeconomic status of the population studied, the incidence of gonococcal infection in pregnancy ranges from 0.5% to 10% and results in a broad spectrum of maternal and neonatal disease. In addition, colonized pregnant patients have been reported in some studies to have an increased risk of preterm birth and premature rupture of membranes, underscoring the continued need to diagnose gonococcal disease in pregnancy properly and to provide effective therapy.

Diagnosis

Clinical diagnosis. Gonococcal infection in women is frequently asymptomatic. However, genitourinary infection may result in dysuria and purulent discharge after a 1- to 3-week incubation period. On examination, the cervix may be erythematous and friable, with a mucopurulent discharge. Frequently, the findings are minimal. Pus may be expressed from the urethra, Skene's ducts, or Bartholin's glands. Ascending infection is very rare in pregnancy, but tends to appear in the first trimester when it does occur.

Untreated gonococcal infection may progress to disseminated disease. This serious complication follows an initial bacteremic phase characterized by a pustular dermatitis. During this first stage of disseminated disease, blood cultures are positive for *N gonorrhoeae* in half of the patients. Cultures from the pustules are positive in only one fifth of cases. Lesions are frequently located in the periphery of the arms and eventually resolve without residual scarring. Typically, lesions have necrotic centers and hemorrhagic bases caused by gonococcal emboli. In addition to bacteremia, patients with disseminated gonococcal infection often have a low-grade fever, myalgias, and migratory polyarthralgia. The bacteremia may lead to endocarditis, pericarditis, and meningitis.

Disseminated gonococcal infection (DGI) can also take the form of an acute febrile illness associated with a severe arthritis. In these cases, purulent synovial effusion may cause significant pain and limit range of motion. The skin overlying the joint—usually the knees, ankles, or wrists—is warm to touch and erythematous. Aspiration of the purulent effusion permits identification of the organism, although blood cultures are usually negative.

Laboratory diagnosis. A Gram stain of the purulent material from the genitourinary tract exudate can provide rapid identification of *N gonorrhoeae*. Smears are positive on microscopic examination in 90% of infected men but only 60% of infected women. Detection of the gonococcal antigen by an enzyme immunoassay (Gonozyme, Abbott Laboratories, North Chicago, Ill.) has been described. This test is highly specific (97%) but only about 60% sensitive. While its sensitivity improves with increasing numbers of colony-forming units/plate, this test should not be employed for diagnostic confirmation of clinical infection or for widespread screening of a low-prevalence asymptomatic population.

The laboratory diagnosis of *N gonorrhoeae* is best accomplished by isolating the organism on a selective medium such as Thayer-Martin broth. Some colonies may appear as early as 24 hours after incubation; most appear by 48 hours.

Perinatal implications. In the first trimester of pregnancy, patients with untreated endocervical gonococcal infection are at increased risk for endometritis after elective abortion or chorionic villus sampling. Therefore, proper documentation of a negative culture is required before carrying out either procedure.

Acute salpingitis in pregnancy is extremely rare and very difficult to diagnose; if it does occur, it does so most frequently during the first trimester and is associated with substantial fetal wastage. Acute salpingitis should be considered in the differential diagnosis of appendicitis in the febrile patient with abdominal or pelvic tenderness, particularly in those who are at risk for sexually transmitted disease and who have a mucopurulent discharge. Correct diagnosis will permit proper antibiotic therapy, sparing the patient the risk of unnecessary abdominal surgery.

While subclinical lower genital tract infection has been strongly correlated with prematurity, the specific role of gonococcal infection is uncertain. Earlier reports failed to correct for the potentially detrimental contributions of chlamydial and group B streptococcal infection to preterm birth and may have overestimated the importance of gonococcal infection. However, recent studies by Elliot and co-workers and Alget and co-workers have once more associated *N gonorrhoeae* with preterm delivery. In addition, women with gonococcal endocervical infection are at high risk for concomitant cervical chlamydial infection, itself associated with preterm birth. *N gonorrhoeae* has also been isolated in the amniotic fluid of patients with intact membranes who ultimately developed clinical amnionitis.

Other recent studies have failed to confirm a direct relationship between gonococcal infection and preterm birth. Nevertheless, all patients in idiopathic preterm labor and certainly those with ruptured membranes should be cultured and treated if positive. *N gonorrhoeae* endocervical infection has been identified by several studies as a risk factor for postpartum endomyometritis. Therefore, the practice of routine antenatal culture for this organism should continue in all at-risk patients.

Finally, maternal endocervical colonization with *N gonorrhoeae* can lead to vertical transmission to the newborn, with a risk of conjunctivitis of 30% to 40% [see Chapter 10: Ophthalmia neonatorum]. Although there has been an increase in the detection of penicillinase-producing *N gonorrhoeae* (PPNG), no evidence exists other than requiring alternative neonatal therapy that the emergence of the new strain has affected the risk of vertical transmission. While neonatal sepsis caused by this organism is a rare event, it has been reported by Hammerschlag and co-workers.

Treatment

Culture for *N gonorrhoeae* and tests for chlamydial infection and syphilis should be done at the first prenatal visit. For women at high risk of sexually transmitted disease, culture and testing should be repeated late in the third trimester.

The recommended regimen for pregnant women with gonococcal infection is a single dose of ceftriaxone, 250 mg IM, plus erythromycin base, 500 mg orally four times daily for 7 days. Women allergic to penicillin should be given a single dose of spectinomycin, 2 g IM, followed by erythromycin. Cervical and rectal cultures for *N*

TABLE 1

**Recommended treatment schedule
for gonorrhea in pregnancy**

Type of infection	Regimen
Anogenital	Ceftriaxone, 250 mg IM or Spectinomycin, 2.0 g IM **plus** Erythromycin base, 500 mg four times daily for 7 days
Disseminated (7 days treatment)	Ceftriaxone, 1.0 g IV or IM daily or Ceftizoxime, 1.0 g IV every 8 hours or Cefotaxime, 1.0 g IV every 8 hours or Spectinomycin, 2.0 g IM every 12 hours

Source: Centers for Disease Control: MMWR 1989;38(S-8):21-25.

gonorrhoeae should be done 4 to 7 days after treatment is completed.

Pregnant women with gonorrhea should also be treated for chlamydial infection if tests for *C trachomatis* are positive. They should be treated for chlamydial infection presumptively if such tests are not available. Treatment with tetracyclines, including doxycycline, or fluoroquinolones is contraindicated in pregnancy because of the possibility of adverse effects on the fetus.

Patients with DGI should be hospitalized and examined for clinical signs of endocarditis or meningitis. The recommended regimen for DGI is ceftriaxone, 1 g IM or IV every 24 hours; ceftizoxime, 1 g IV every 8 hours; or cefotaxime, 1 g IV every 8 hours. DGI patients allergic to penicillin should be treated with spectinomycin, 2 g IM every 12 hours. If the infecting organism is proven to be penicillin sensitive, the patient may be switched to ampicillin, 1 g IV every 6 hours. Women being treated for DGI should be tested for genital chlamydial infection or treated empirically for such infection if testing is not available.

Patients with uncomplicated DGI may be discharged 24 to 48

hours after symptoms resolve and may complete treatment (total of 1 week of antibiotic therapy) with an oral regimen of cefuroxime axetil, 500 mg twice daily, or amoxicillin, 500 mg, with clavulanic acid three times a day. Ciprofloxacin should not be used in pregnancy.

Gonococcal meningitis and endocarditis require high-dose therapy with ceftriaxone, 1 to 2 g IV every 12 hours, or an antibiotic effective against the strain causing the disease. Optimal duration of therapy is unknown, but most authorities advise treating gonococcal meningitis for 10 to 14 days and gonococcal endocarditis for at least 4 weeks.

Women with gonococcal meningitis, endocarditis, or nephritis and those with recurrent DGI should be evaluated for complement deficiencies. Complicated DGI should managed in consultation with an expert.

Prophylaxis for the newborn against ophthalmia neonatorum has been changed from the use of silver nitrate to use of either erythromycin or tetracycline [see Chapter 10].

SUGGESTED READING

Alexander E: Gonorrhea in the newborn. Ann NY Acad Sci 1988;549:180

Alger LS, Lovchik JC, Hebel JR, et al: The association of *Chlamydia trachomatis, Neisseria gonorrhoeae*, and group B streptococci with preterm rupture of membranes and pregnancy outcome. Am J Obstet Gynecol 1988;159:397

Amstey MS, Steadman KT: Symptomatic gonorrhea and pregnancy. J Am Vener Dis Assoc 1976;3:14

Blanchard AC, Pastorek JG: Pelvic inflammatory disease during pregnancy. South Med J 1987;80:1363

Christmas JT, Wendel GD, Bawdon RE, et al: Concomitant infection with *Neisseria gonorrhoeae* and *Chlamydia trachomatis* in pregnancy. Obstet Gynecol 1989;74:295

Elliott B, Brunham RC, Laga M, et al: Maternal gonococcal infection as a preventable risk factor for low birth weight. J Infect Dis 1990;161:531

Hammerschlag M, Cummings C, Roblin P, et al: Efficacy of neonatal ocular prophylaxis for the prevention of chlamydial and gonococcal conjunctivitis. N Engl J Med 1989;320:769

Lieberman RW, Wheelock JB: The diagnosis of gonorrhea in a low prevalence female population: enzyme immunoassay versus culture. Obstet Gynecol 1987;68:743

Mason PR, Katzenstein DA, Chimbira TH, et al: Vaginal flora of women admitted to hospital with signs of sepsis following normal delivery, cesarean section or abortion. The Puerperal Sepsis Study Group. Cent Afr J Med 1989;35:344

Smith LG, Summers PR, Miles RW, et al: Gonococcal chorioamnionitis associated with sepsis: a case report. Am J Obstet Gynecol 1989;160:573

Thomason JL, Gelbart SM, Sobieski VJ, et al: Effectiveness of Gonozyme for detection of gonorrhoeae in low risk pregnant and gynecologic populations. J Sex Transm Dis 1989;16:28

10
Ophthalmia neonatorum

By Mara J. Dinsmoor, MD

Background and incidence

We define ophthalmia neonatorum (ON) as the occurrence of conjunctivitis within the first month of life. The association between maternal vaginal discharge and neonatal conjunctivitis was first noted in the mid-1700s, and by 1881 ON was seen in up to 10% of infants. With the advent of silver nitrate prophylaxis and the subsequent discovery of antibiotics, blindness due to ON has become increasingly rare, the incidence dropping 100-fold in this century alone.

The incidence of ON parallels that of maternal gonorrhea and chlamydial infections. Overall, there are approximately three to ten cases for every 1,000 live births, although some prospective studies report incidences of chlamydial conjunctivitis alone of up to 63 cases for every 1,000 births.

Chemical conjunctivitis, characterized by conjunctival edema, hyperemia, and watery discharge, occurs in up to 90% of infants after prophylactic instillation of topical 1% silver nitrate. It typically appears within a few hours and is always sterile (Table 1).

Although the proportion of ON due to infectious agents remains fairly constant, the relative proportion of specific pathogens varies among institutions. This variation may be due to changes in prevalence of maternal infection and differences in prenatal surveillance for and treatment of sexually transmitted diseases. Differences in microbiology may also arise from variations in ocular prophylactic regimens and diagnostic techniques used.

Etiology

Chlamydia trachomatis has become recognized as an important etio-

47

TABLE 1
Causes of ophthalmia neonatorum

Source	Approximate frequency	Time of onset
Chemical conjunctivitis	7%	6–24 hours
Chlamydia trachomatis	3%–13%	5–14 days
Escherichia coli	5%–9%	5–21 days
Haemophilus sp	5%	5–21 days
Herpes simplex virus	Rare	2–14 days
Neisseria gonorrhoeae	3%	2–5 days
Staphylococcus aureus	5%–30%	5–21 days
Streptococcus viridans	4%–16%	5–21 days

logic agent, especially after use of silver nitrate prophylaxis, which is not effective against it. Approximately 20% to 40% of newborns exposed intrapartum to *C trachomatis* will develop ON, usually within 5 to 10 days after delivery. The overall incidence has been estimated to be eight in every 1,000 births. Characteristically, a large amount of mucopurulent exudate is present, with frequent pseudomembrane formation. The lower portion of the eye is more often involved than the upper.

Staphylococcus aureus and other bacteria cause a milder conjunctivitis rarely associated with corneal involvement. Other organisms frequently implicated are *Staphylococcus epidermidis*, *Haemophilus influenzae*, *Escherichia coli*, and α-hemolytic streptococci. Mixed infections can also occur.

Between 30% and 50% of newborns of women with gonococcal cervicitis will develop gonococcal conjunctivitis. The incidence appears to be increased following premature rupture of membranes and in premature infants. Gonococcal ophthalmia, typically seen as a bilateral, purulent conjunctivitis within the first week of life, occurs in approximately one of 2,000 live births.

Ocular involvement with herpes simplex virus (HSV) occurs in

15% to 20% of newborns infected with herpes. The eye is the only affected organ in approximately 4% of infected newborns. Ocular herpes infection usually appears within the first 2 weeks of life.

Diagnosis

Conjunctivitis developing after the first day of life, persisting for more than 3 days, or progressing is uncharacteristic of chemical conjunctivitis. Diagnostic evaluation should be done in all such cases. Although the type and timing of symptoms can be useful, such information is not diagnostic.

Gram stain of the exudate may reveal gram-negative intracellular diplococci (suggesting gonococcal infection), gram-positive cocci (*S aureus*), or gram-negative bacilli (*H influenzae*). The presence of multinucleated giant cells detected by Papanicolaou's stain is characteristic of a herpes infection. It is also useful to perform cultures of the exudate, including specific ones (chocolate or Thayer-Martin agar) for *Neisseria gonorrhoeae*. Cultures of the oropharynx and anus should be done if *N gonorrhoeae* infection is suspected.

If available, have cultures for *C trachomatis* and HSV performed. Because of low sensitivity, Giemsa stains of conjunctival scrapings should not be relied on alone to eliminate chlamydial infection as a possible cause of ON. However, positive findings may be used to guide early treatment. An immunofluorescence or enzyme-linked immunoassay (ELISA) performed on conjunctival scrapings is an acceptable alternative.

Treatment

Chlamydial conjunctivitis requires systemic treatment with erythromycin for 2 weeks. Although topical erythromycin ointment will effectively cure the conjunctivitis, nasopharyngeal carriage persists, putting the infant at risk for development of chlamydial pneumonia. Oral erythromycin regimens fail approximately 20% of the time, at which point IV treatment is recommended.

Treat all infants born to women with known cervical gonorrhea prophylactically with a single dose of ceftriaxone. Treatment for gonococcal ON consists of IV penicillin G or ceftriaxone for 7 days combined with irrigation of the eye with saline or ophthalmic solutions. Isolate infants with a diagnosis of gonococcal ophthalmia for the first 24 hours of treatment, as it is very contagious. In areas where penicillin-resistant strains of gonorrhea are common, treatment with ceftriaxone is advisable. Examine and treat the mother and her partner(s) when diagnosis of either chlamydial or gonococcal conjunctivitis is made.

Treatment of ON due to HSV infection consists of isolation and use of topical antiviral agents such as trifluorothimidine or adenine arabi-noside. Strongly consider evaluation for systemic involvement and initiation of systemic antiviral therapy, as ocular involvement may precede manifestations of systemic disease.

ON due to gram-negative bacilli may be treated with gentamicin ophthalmic ointment four times daily for 1 week. When pseudo-monal infections are suspected, institute parenteral antibiotics as well. One may treat infections due to gram-positive cocci or "non-specific" inflammation with erythromycin ophthalmic ointment four times daily for 1 week.

Sequelae
Undertreated or untreated bacterial conjunctivitis may result in sep-ticemia, nasolacrimal duct obstruction, corneal ulceration, or blind-ness. ON due to *S aureus* may be complicated by development of corneal ulcers or infiltrates, hypopyon (puslike fluid in the anterior chamber), endophthalmitis, and exfoliative dermatitis. Although untreated ON due to *C trachomatis* usually will resolve sponta-neously and rarely results in visual loss, it can lead to conjunctival scarring and pannus formation (neovascularization of the cornea). It may also give rise to colonization of the upper respiratory tract, lead-ing ultimately to chlamydial pneumonia. Early treatment will prevent ocular sequelae. ON secondary to herpes infection may bring on keratitis, cataracts, chorioretinitis, or optic neuritis.

Prevention
Introduced as prophylaxis against gonococcal ON in 1881, silver nitrate drops remained standard in the US until the 1970s, when concern arose about their effectiveness in preventing chlamydial conjunctivitis. Recent studies have found that both 0.5% erythro-mycin and 1% tetracycline ointment are as effective as silver nitrate drops in preventing gonococcal conjunctivitis, the most serious pathogen in terms of long-term sequelae. Results are conflicting, however, in their relative effectiveness in preventing chlamydial disease.

Relative costs of the different prophylactic regimens, along with local disease prevalence, thus become important factors in deciding on a prophylactic regimen. All three regimens have been approved by the American Academy of Pediatrics.

Because no regimen has been proved totally effective in prevent-ing either gonococcal or chlamydial conjunctivitis, further measures are needed. As noted by Hammerschlag and co-workers, most cases of gonococcal ON occur in infants born to women receiving no pre-natal care. Thus, diagnosis and treatment of maternal genital infections with *C trachomatis* and *N gonorrhoeae* before delivery remain of utmost importance.

SUGGESTED READING

American Academy of Pediatrics: *Report of the Committee on Infectious Diseases*, ed 21. Elk Grove Village, Ill., American Academy of Pediatrics, 1988

Hammerschlag MR, Cummings C, Roblin PM, et al: Efficacy of neonatal ocular prophylaxis for the prevention of chlamydial and gonococcal conjunctivitis. N Engl J Med 1989;320:769

Jarvin VN, Levine R, Asbell PA: Ophthalmia neonatorum: study of a decade of experience at the Mount Sinai Hospital. Br J Ophthalmol 1987;71:295

Prentice MJ, Hutchinson GR, Taylor-Robinson D: A microbiological study of neonatal conjunctivae and conjunctivitis. Br J Ophthalmol 1977;61:601

Sandstrom KI, Bell TA, Chandler JW, et al: Diagnosis of neonatal purulent conjunctivitis caused by *Chlamydia trachomatis* and other organisms, in Mårdh PA, Holmes KK, Oriel JD, et al (eds): *Chlamydial Infections*. New York, Elsevier Biomedical Press, 1982

11

Syphilis in pregnancy

By Larry C. Gilstrap III, MD, and George D. Wendel, Jr., MD

Background and incidence

The exact incidence of syphilis complicating pregnancy is unknown. However, it is known that incidence of primary and secondary syphilis in the general population has increased significantly in the United States over the past few years. The current rate of approximately 14 to 15 cases per 100,000 persons is the highest since 1950. Along with this increase in syphilis in the general population has come an increase in the number of cases occurring during pregnancy. A fourfold rise in the number of cases of congenital syphilis has also been reported in recent years in the US.

The increase in early syphilis in pregnant women is no doubt related to the increase in illicit drug use reported in different areas of the country and the concomitant exchange of sex for drugs. Many of these drug users receive little to no prenatal care, which in turn leads to an increased risk of having an infant with congenital syphilis.

Pathophysiology

Pregnancy itself does not affect the course of syphilis. However, syphilis may cause premature birth, stillbirths, and neonatal morbidity and mortality.

One of the most important consequences of maternal syphilis is congenital syphilis in the infant. Spirochetes readily cross the placenta to produce chronic infection in the fetus, although clinical disease is generally not evident before 18 weeks' gestation. The most common clinical findings in newborns with congenital syphilis are hepatosplenomegaly, osteochondritis or periostitis, jaundice or hyperbilirubinemia, petechiae, purpura, lymphadenopathy, and ascites or hydrops (Table 1).

TABLE 1
Findings in newborns with congenital syphilis

Clinical

Hepatosplenomegaly
Osteochondritis/periostitis
Lymphadenopathy
Jaundice
Ascites/edema/hydrops
Petechiae/purpura

Laboratory

Reactive serologic test in blood/CSF
Anemia/thrombocytopenia
Hyperbilirubinemia
Abnormal liver function tests
Elevated CSF cell count/protein

Newborns may also manifest rhinitis ("snuffles"), pneumonia alba, myocarditis, or nephrosis. The placenta may be involved as well, and characteristically is very large and "waxy" in appearance. Microscopic examination of the placenta frequently will reveal focal villitis, immature villi, and endarteritis.

Diagnosis

The diagnosis of syphilis in the pregnant woman is essentially the same as for the nonpregnant patient. For pregnant women with primary syphilis, identification of *Treponema pallidum* by dark-field examination of material taken from a chancre is confirmatory. However, since the majority of pregnant women with syphilis do not have lesions when they present for prenatal care, the diagnosis of antepartum syphilis is frequently made by serologic testing. Currently available are nontreponemal tests such as the Venereal Disease Research Laboratory (VDRL) or rapid plasma reagin (RPR) tests, as well as specific treponemal tests such as the microhemagglutination assay for antibodies to *T pallidum* (MHA-TP) and the fluorescent treponemal antibody absorption test (FTA-ABS). All pregnant women with syphilis should be carefully examined for the presence of other sexually transmitted diseases, including HIV infection.

The diagnosis of congenital syphilis is based primarily on clinical findings, suspicious history, and positive serologic tests. For the asymptomatic baby without clinical stigmata of syphilis, the diagnosis is much more difficult. Maternal IgG antibody readily crosses the placenta and may cause the newborn's serologic test to be positive. All newborns with suspected syphilis should have a lumbar puncture for cerebrospinal fluid analysis and radiographic studies of the bones, which will reveal significant changes in metaphyseal bone in approximately 95% of infected infants.

Confirmation of congenital syphilis in a stillborn infant may prove extremely difficult, especially in the severely macerated infant. Staining the fetal tissue to identify spirochetes, doing x-ray studies to look for osteochondritis, and evaluating the placenta may prove helpful.

Treatment
Treatment is the same for pregnant and nonpregnant women and consists primarily of long-acting benzathine penicillin G in doses appropriate for the stage of infection. According to the Centers for Disease Control's 1989 guidelines, patients with early syphilis (primary, secondary, and early latent syphilis of less than 1 year's duration) should receive a single IM dose of 2.4 million U of benzathine penicillin G. After treatment of early disease, more than 60% of these women will have the Jarisch-Herxheimer reaction. For pregnant women with late latent syphilis of more than 1 year's duration or of unknown duration or with cardiovascular syphilis, benzathine penicillin G, 2.4 million U IM, should be given weekly for three doses (7.2 million U total). Pregnant patients should be warned to watch for decreases in fetal activity and for signs of preterm labor. Pregnant women with neurosyphilis should receive aqueous crystalline penicillin G, 12 to 24 million U daily at an IV dosage of 2 to 4 million U every 4 hours for 10 to 14 days. An outpatient program of IM procaine penicillin, 2 to 4 million U daily, plus 500 mg of oral probenecid four times a day for a total of 10 to 14 days, may also be utilized. Because the efficacy of these regimens has not been prospectively studied in the pregnant patient and because of potential serious adverse fetal effects, it is important to follow all such pregnant women with monthly serologic tests and clinical examinations to detect both therapeutic failures and recurrent disease.

Treatment before 20 weeks is uniformly effective in preventing congenital syphilis, barring reinfection. Treatment failures occur in 1% to 2% of patients because of advanced, irreversible fetal infection. These failures are seen more frequently with maternal secondary syphilis or treatment in the late second or third trimesters.

The pregnant woman with syphilis who is allergic to penicillin presents a therapeutic challenge. The CDC-recommended alternate regimens for the nonpregnant patient—erythromycin, tetracycline, and doxycycline—all present special problems for the pregnant patient. Although erythromycin offers a high cure rate for adults with early syphilis, it may not treat the fetus adequately. Erythromycin is therefore not included in the CDC's 1989 recommendations. Tetracycline and doxycycline are also not recommended for use in pregnancy by the CDC. Although effective in the nonpregnant patients, it is well documented that tetracycline may discolor the deciduous teeth in the fetus.

The 1989 CDC guidelines suggest skin testing and referral for penicillin desensitization for the pregnant patient proven to be allergic to penicillin. Desensitization can be accomplished either orally or IV. Patients who undergo successful desensitization and treatment with penicillin will again require desensitization if penicillin must be used in the future. Although the tetracyclines are not currently recommended for use during pregnancy, they have not been shown to be teratogenic and may be considered as an alternative for the penicillin-allergic pregnant patient in whom penicillin desensitization is not practical or readily available. Informed consent must be obtained from such patients, since use of tetracycline during pregnancy may cause permanent discoloration or enamel hypoplasia in the infant's teeth.

Treatment of the newborn with congenital syphilis should consist of 100,000 to 150,000 U/kg of aqueous crystalline penicillin G, given daily at 50,000 U/kg every 8 to 12 hours, or 50,000 U/kg of procaine penicillin, given IM once daily for 10 to 14 days.

Prevention

The mainstay of prevention for congenital syphilis is early detection and appropriate treatment and follow-up. All pregnant women should have serologic testing for syphilis at their first prenatal visit and again in the third trimester of pregnancy. The CDC currently recommends that all seropositive pregnant women should be considered infected and treated unless a history of adequate treatment is obtained and confirmed with serologic antibody titers. Finally, all syphilis patients should be counseled about the risks of HIV infection and be encouraged to be tested for HIV antibody.

SUGGESTED READING

Centers for Disease Control: 1989 sexually transmitted diseases treatment guidelines. MMWR 1989;38(S-8):5

Centers for Disease Control: Syphilis and congenital syphilis—United States, 1985-1988. MMWR 1988;37:486.

Hira SK, Bhat GJ, Patel JB, et al: Early congenital syphilis: clinicoradiologic features in 202 patients. Sex Transm Dis 1985;12:177

Wendel GD: Gestational and congenital syphilis. Clin Perinatol 1988;15:287

Wendel GD, Gilstrap LC: Syphilis during pregnancy, in Gilstrap LC, Faro S (eds): *Infections in Obstetrics*. New York, Alan R Liss, 1989

Zenker PN, Rolfs RT: Treatment of syphilis, 1989. Rev Infec Dis 1990;12(suppl 6):S590

12

Lyme disease in pregnancy

By Christine L. Williams, MD, MPH, and
Peter C. Welch, MD, PhD

Background and incidence

Lyme disease is a multisystem, inflammatory disease characterized clinically by a distinctive primary skin lesion, erythema chronicum migrans (ECM). In many cases arthritis, arthralgia, and neurologic or cardiac manifestations are also present. The disease is caused by a spirochete, *Borrelia burgdorferi,* which is transmitted to man through the bite of a deer tick, usually *Ixodes dammini.*

The incidence of Lyme disease has been increasing dramatically since it was first described in the United States in 1976. In 1989, 8,803 cases were reported to the Centers for Disease Control (CDC), compared with 461 in 1981. Individuals of all ages are affected, but the majority of cases occur in children and young adults because of their greater exposure to ticks outdoors. Ninety percent of all cases have occurred along the Northeastern coastal belt, especially in areas of Connecticut and New York close to Long Island Sound. Peak onset of ECM rash occurs during the months of June, July, and August when the nymphal tick is most abundant.

The exact incidence of Lyme disease during pregnancy is unknown, although serosurveys suggest about 1% of pregnant women have serologic evidence of prior Lyme disease infection at the time of their first prenatal visit.

Pathophysiology

Lyme disease frequently occurs in stages, beginning with flu-like symptoms a week to a month after the tick bite. ECM, the characteristic expanding bull's-eye skin lesion, is the most commonly reported symptom and is seen in up to 80% of cases. More severe cardiac, neurologic, musculoskeletal, and arthritic symptoms may follow in the second stage of the disease, which usually occurs within weeks to months after the initial infection. The third stage involves chronic recurring symptoms of arthritis and/or neurologic impairment, which can continue for months to years after infection. Fewer than half of those affected by Lyme disease can recall having been bitten by a tick, probably because the nymphal tick responsible for transmitting most infection is about the size of the head of a straight pin.

In the limited number of cases reported, symptoms of Lyme disease during pregnancy have been similar to those of nonpregnant women, with ECM skin rash and arthritis most commonly reported. Maternal Lyme disease may lead to infection of the fetus with *B burgdorferi*. The first documented case of maternal–fetal transmission of the Lyme disease spirochete, described by Schlesinger and co-workers in 1985, involved a woman who had symptoms in the first trimester of pregnancy. The disease was not diagnosed and was not treated. At 35 weeks' gestation, the woman gave birth to a 3,000-g male infant who rapidly developed heart failure and died at 39 hours of life. Autopsy revealed significant multiple congenital heart defects. Spirochetes morphologically compatable with *B burgdorferi* were seen in stained sections of spleen, renal tubules, and bone marrow. The mother had antibody to *B burgdorferi* and negative serology for syphilis.

Several other cases of maternal–fetal transmission of Lyme disease, often resulting in stillbirth or neonatal death, have also been reported. These reports provide evidence that *B burgdorferi* may be transmitted transplacentally and that this infection may be severe enough to cause death of the fetus during intrauterine life or in the neonatal period.

The CDC has reported adverse outcomes for 5 of 19 women (26%) diagnosed with Lyme disease during pregnancy. Adverse outcomes included intrauterine fetal death, prematurity, syndactyly, cortical blindness with developmental delay, and rash. All of the adverse outcomes were different, and none could definitely be attributed to Lyme disease infection. However, 14 of the women in this study had normal babies. There have been other reports, summarized by Luger, of Lyme disease during pregnancy in which the resulting newborn was normal at birth. A preliminary report of a study at the Marshfield Clinic in Wisconsin also showed no significant association between positive Lyme disease serology and spontaneous miscarriage in a group of healthy women followed throughout pregnancy.

In a pilot study of 463 infants, Williams and co-workers obtained a cord blood sample from each at birth, as well as a hospital discharge summary and a questionnaire filled out by the mother. At 6-month follow-up, incidence rates for major and minor congenital malformations were not significantly greater in infants with antibody to *B burgdorferi* than in seronegative babies. In addition, malformation rates were no higher in babies born in a hospital in the middle of an area endemic for Lyme disease than in those born in a hospital in a county with no cases.

Diagnosis

The diagnosis of Lyme disease must often be made on the basis of the clinical presentation alone, since serologic ELISA and immuno-fluorescent antibody (IFA) tests may be negative more than half the time during the first (rash) stage of the disease. Antibiotic treatment early in the course of the disease may blunt the antibody response so that seroconversion may not occur.

Difficult management decisions face the clinician responsible for the prenatal care of women in Lyme disease–endemic areas, and even in areas where only a few cases have been reported. A woman may contract the disease while traveling through an endemic area. Exposure can run the gamut in a pregnant woman from deer tick bites before or during pregnancy, treated prophylactically or not, to actual Lyme disease before or during pregnancy, treated or not treated. Serologic tests may be negative in the face of overwhelming clinical evidence of present or past Lyme disease, and may be positive in the absence of any history of either Lyme disease or a deer tick bite.

Both the ELISA and IFA serologic tests for *B burgdorferi* are relatively insensitive during the early stage of Lyme disease, characterized by the ECM rash but also often accompanied by flu-like symptoms. Fifty percent or fewer patients will be seropositive during this stage. Treatment is given immediately to prevent more serious disease. By destroying the spirochete, however, such treatment may also blunt the antibody response so that seroconversion may not occur. The physician may therefore be faced with lack of serologic confirmation of his or her diagnosis.

Patients who present with arthritic, neurologic, or cardiac manifestations of Lyme disease are more likely to have serologic evidence of infection. During pregnancy, therefore, the usual Lyme disease diagnostic problems become magnified because of added concern for the health of the fetus.

Treatment

Tick bites. Prophylactic treatment of tick bites during pregnancy is now widely practiced. Even though the risk of Lyme disease after a documented tick bite is probably less than 5%, most physicians would choose to treat the bite to avoid even the slight chance of clinical infection. A 3-week course of amoxicillin, 500 mg three times daily, or penicillin V, 500 mg four times daily, is commonly recommended. Tetracycline and doxycycline are not used because of the potential for discoloring the teeth of the child. Erythromycin, 250 to 500 mg four times daily, is less effective but is prescribed for women allergic to penicillin. High doses of erythromycin, however, commonly produce gastrointestinal side effects.

Lyme disease. For Lyme disease that has onset during pregnancy, treatment varies from oral antibiotics for rash and flu-like early-stage disease to IV antibiotics for later arthritic or neurologic stages. Some recommend universal IV therapy for all stages of Lyme disease during pregnancy. Oral therapy again most commonly consists of amoxicillin, 500 mg three times daily, or penicillin V, 500 mg four times daily, given for 3 or more weeks. Intravenous therapy consists of penicillin G, 20 million U per day divided into doses given every 4 hours, for 2 to 3 weeks. Alternatively, ceftriaxone given IV at 2 g per day for 14 to 21 days is preferred by some because it may be given on an outpatient basis once a day.

If a woman's history suggests she had Lyme disease before becoming pregnant, management during pregnancy will depend on current symptoms, current serologic status (both IgG and IgM antibody), and a review of antibiotic treatment received in the past. If there is a question of persistent disease, consultation with an infectious disease specialist may be needed to determine whether additional follow-up and treatment are indicated.

Serologic tests for syphilis should be run on all sera positive for antibody to *B burgdorferi* since there is some cross-reactivity between *B burgdorferi* and *Treponema pallidum*. Patients with Lyme disease, however, are more likely to have a negative VDRL or RPR test with a positive fluorescent treponemal antibody (FTA) test result. Patients positive for rheumatoid factor may also have a false-positive Lyme titer, particularly IgM. Serologic tests for Lyme disease will be positive in cases of infection with other less common borreliae or treponemes. Under usual clinical circumstances, however, this possibility would be a minor consideration.

If Lyme disease is suspected as the cause of a miscarriage, stillbirth, or neonatal death, attempts may be made to culture the spirochete from the placenta or from infant organs. In addition, fixed tissues may be prepared with special stains to look for spirochetes, which may be present in very small numbers. Maternal sera and infant cord blood should be tested for antibody to *B burgdorferi*.

The decision to further treat a newborn infant whose mother had Lyme disease during pregnancy usually depends on:

■ the status of the mother;

- the timing, adequacy, and duration of the mother's treatment with antibiotics;
- whether treatment was oral or intravenous;
- the status of the infant at birth; and
- the serologic status of mother and infant. (The latter may not be of immediate help since results of tests done at birth or soon after may not be available at the time one needs to make a clinical decision about treatment.)

If there is any suggestion that the mother was treated inadequately, and especially if the infant shows any clinical signs of neonatal infection, the infant should be treated with IV penicillin using the CDC's suggested regimen for congenital syphilis: 100,000–150,000 U/kg (body weight) of aqueous crystalline penicillin G daily, administered as 50,000 U/kg IV every 8 to 12 hours for 10 to 14 days. Alternatively, procaine penicillin may be given at a dosage of 50,000 U/kg/day IM for 10 to 14 days.

If the baby and mother are well, further treatment of the baby is probably not indicated. In other instances where both mother and baby are well but there are some minor concerns about some aspects of the mother's case management, physicians have elected to treat the infant with a course of oral amoxicillin on an outpatient basis. In these cases, if the IgM Lyme antibody is negative and the baby remains well, no further treatment need be given. The IgG titer, acquired passively during gestation, will frequently be positive in babies whose mothers have had Lyme disease. This antibody will gradually disappear during the first year of life.

Prevention
Women in Lyme disease–endemic areas who are pregnant or trying to get pregnant should avoid areas infested with deer ticks. Lyme disease is usually transmitted by the immature ticks and less often by the larger adult tick. Because nymphs are most abundant in the summer months, special care must be taken at this time. Ticks tend to "quest" on tall grass, especially along pathways. Keeping grass cut low, dressing with long white pants tucked into socks, and daily personal inspection for ticks will help avoid problems, since ticks usually have to feed for 24 hours or more to transmit disease.

Tick repellents should be used with caution because repeated skin applications have been associated with convulsions in children. Use during pregnancy should be based on assessment of both risks and benefits and avoided or minimized, as with exposure to any toxic product. If temporary protection is essential, spraying the repellent on clothing alone is advised.

SUGGESTED READING

Centers for Disease Control: Lyme disease surveillance—United States, 1989-1990. MMWR 1991;40:417

Centers for Disease Control: Update: Lyme disease—United States. MMWR 1984;33:268

Luger S: Active Lyme borreliosis in pregnancy—outcomes of six cases with stage 1, stage 2, and stage 3 disease. Abstract. IV International Conference on Lyme Borreliosis. Stockholm, Sweden, June 18-21, 1990

MacDonald AB: Human fetal borreliosis, toxemia of pregnancy and fetal death. Zentralbl Bakteriol Hyg 1986; A263:189

MacDonald AB, Benach JL, Burgdorfer W: Stillbirth following maternal Lyme disease. NY State J Med 1987;87:615

Markowitz LE, Steere AC, Benach JL, et al: Lyme disease during pregnancy. JAMA 1987;255:3394

Schlesinger PA, Duray PH, Burke BA, Steere AC, et al: Maternal-fetal transmission of the Lyme disease spirochete, *Borrelia burgdorferi.* Ann Intern Med 1985;103:67

Weber K, Bratzke H, Neubert U, et al: *Borrelia burgdorferi* in a newborn despite oral penicillin for Lyme borreliosis during pregnancy. Pediatr Infect Dis 1988;7:286

Williams CL, Benach JL, Curran AC, et al: Lyme disease during pregnancy: a cord blood serosurvey. Ann NY Acad Sci 1988;539:504

13
Listeria infections in pregnancy

By M. Lynn Yonekura, MD, and Philip B. Mead, MD

Background and incidence

Listeria monocytogenes has been recognized as a cause of human disease since 1929, and presently causes 1,700 cases of meningitis and sepsis in the United States each year, with a mortality rate of 33%. Listeriosis primarily affects pregnant women, neonates, the elderly, and individuals with immune system dysfunction. Neonatal disease was first described in 1936, and maternal and fetal infections account for about 50% of reported cases. Although most maternal infections are mild, *Listeria* infection in pregnancy may result in abortion, preterm labor, and fetal infection, with reported rates of neonatal mortality ranging from 7% to more than 50%.

Pathophysiology

Several epidemics of listeriosis in the 1980s as well as a substantial portion of sporadic cases were caused by food-borne organisms. Thus, while listeriosis is less common than infections due to other food-borne pathogens, *L monocytogenes* causes more deaths in the US than any other food-borne pathogen. The median incubation period is 31 days (range 11 to 70 days). Prodromal symptoms include fever, myalgias, headache, diarrhea, nausea, and vomiting.

The pathogenesis of fetal *Listeria* infection starts with maternal hematogenous infection, which leads to placental infection and results in fetal septicemia and multiorgan involvement. Amniotic fluid becomes infected as the agent is excreted in fetal urine. Aspiration and swallowing of infected amniotic fluid then leads to respiratory and gastrointestinal tract involvement.

Variend and Blumenthal have reported two cases that lend support to this proposed transplacental route of infection, one involving early-onset neonatal listeriosis following elective cesarean section at term and the other involving vaginal birth of twins (with twin A uninfected and twin B seropositive for *Listeria*). Alternatively, an ascending route of infection associated with rectovaginal colonization by *L monocytogenes* may account for some fetal infections.

Nosocomial transmission of listeriosis between newborns has been reported on two occasions.

Etiology

L monocytogenes is a small, aerobic, non–spore-forming, gram-positive rod that is ß-hemolytic on blood agar. Major serotypes causing infection are 1/2a, 1/2b, 4a, and 4b. *L monocytogenes* is widely distributed in the environment and in animals. Food-borne outbreaks have been traced to soft cheeses, milk, raw vegetables, and paté. Sporadic cases have been caused by the ingestion of undercooked chicken, unheated hot dogs, and foods purchased from store delicatessen counters. Asymptomatic fecal and vaginal carriage occurs in humans and may account for a few sporadic cases.

Both early- and late-onset forms of neonatal listeriosis occur, much as in group B streptococcal infection. The early type presents within 2 days of birth with signs of septicemia and pneumonia, and is felt to derive from transplacental infection. Early-onset disease is most commonly associated with serotypes 1b and 4b. The late form of the disease appears after the 5th day of life and usually presents as meningitis. Late-onset neonatal listeriosis is associated with serotype 4b and is believed to result from infection acquired during or after delivery.

Diagnosis

Maternal infection with *L monocytogenes* is often asymptomatic, but patients may present with a flu-like syndrome characterized by chills, fever, and back pain, occasionally mimicking a pyelonephritis. Although diarrhea is commonly believed to be a symptom of listeriosis, it was not reported by any pregnant patients in a recent outbreak. Most infected gravidas present with fever, active preterm labor, and brown-stained amniotic fluid that is frequently mistaken for meconium. Intrapartum fetal monitoring commonly shows nonspecific abnormalities consistent with intrauterine infection—for example, fetal tachycardia, decreased variability, and absence of accelerations.

Infants with early-onset disease characteristically are preterm but of appropriate weight for gestational age. Typically, they will have respiratory distress at birth and evidence of congenital pneumonia. Some will have a fleeting, salmon-colored maculopapular rash.

Treatment

Maternal listeriosis should be suspected in a pregnant woman with a flu-like syndrome, especially if she has back pain and premature labor. Blood cultures, which are often positive, and rectovaginal cultures and Gram stains should be performed as part of the evaluation of such a patient. Amniocentesis specimens for Gram stain and culture have also been utilized for diagnosis. Antimicrobial therapy with IV ampicillin plus gentamicin is essential for infection diagnosed during pregnancy, since it may prevent fetal infection and its consequences. In penicillin-allergic patients, use of trimethoprim/sulfamethoxazole or erythromycin has been successful.

Congenital listeriosis should be considered in the differential diagnosis of a depressed preterm infant after a labor complicated by fetal distress and meconium- or brown-stained amniotic fluid. Gram stains of amniotic fluid and of the newborn's gastric aspirate, cerebrospinal fluid, or skin lesions should be performed. Gram stain of a fecal smear from an infected newborn may show the organism in profusion. The findings of gram-positive rods or coccobacillary forms should prompt a presumptive diagnosis of listeriosis. Inform the microbiologist that *Listeria* infection is a concern, since *L monocytogenes* can easily be mistaken for diphtheroids and ignored.

Presumptive diagnosis of *Listeria* infection by Gram stain demands immediate institution of therapy; awaiting confirmation by culture may result in fatal delay. The optimal therapeutic regimen for the infected newborn is unknown, but initial therapy with ampicillin plus gentamicin is recommended because this combination is highly effective in animal models of *Listeria* infection.

Sequelae

In a recent report of listeriosis identified at perinatal autopsy, gross pathologic lesions were encountered in only one of seven cases and consisted of a skin rash and small hepatic abscesses. Microscopic lesions in six cases consisted of rare, localized microabscesses and granuloma-like lesions. One patient had no gross or microscopic findings. Placental lesions, consisting of chorioamnionitis and villitis, were found in all cases, while three of five examined cords showed acute funisitis.

Although fetal or neonatal infection with *L monocytogenes* is known to have high fatality, long-term morbidity is unclear. Some studies have found an increased incidence of developmental delays among *Listeria*-infected infants who weighed less than 1,250 g and who required assisted ventilation. Others have reported neurodevelopmental handicaps, hydrocephalus, ptosis, and strabismus. In contrast, one author found no evidence of neurodevelopmental sequelae in six of eight survivors, and concluded that sequelae for neonatal early-onset listeriosis were uncommon if meningitis was not present. Because meningitis is not characteristic for early-onset disease, the outcome may be generally good. The prognosis for late-onset neonatal sepsis and meningitis has not been extensively studied.

Prevention

In order to prevent listeriosis, all individuals should:

- thoroughly cook raw food from animal sources, whether meat, poultry, or fish;
- avoid raw milk and other unpasteurized dairy products;
- wash raw vegetables thoroughly before eating them;
- wash hands, knives, and cutting boards after handling uncooked foods.

Moreover, pregnant women and immunocompromised individuals should:

- avoid soft cheeses such as Brie, feta, and Camembert, as well as Mexican-style and blue-veined cheeses;
- avoid refrigerated, ready-to-eat meats such as paté, frankfurters, and sandwich meats;
- thoroughly reheat leftovers until piping hot ($\geq 165°F$) and eat them within 2 days.

In addition, they should avoid potentially infective materials, such as animal manure or aborted animal fetuses on farms.

SUGGESTED READING

Bortolussi R, Seelinger HPR: Listeriosis, in Remington JS, Klein JO (eds): *Infectious Diseases of the Fetus and Newborn Infant*, ed 3. Philadelphia, WB Saunders, 1990, chap 24, p 812

Cruikshank DP, Warenski JC: First-trimester maternal *Listeria moncytogenes* sepsis and chorioamnionitis with normal neonatal outcome. Obstet Gynecol 1989;73:469

Farber JM, Peterkin PI, Carter AO, et al: Neonatal listeriosis due to cross-infection confirmed by isoenzyme typing and DNA fingerprinting. J Infect Dis 1991;163:927

Kalstone C: Successful antepartum treatment of listeriosis. Am J Obstet Gynecol 1991;164:57

Liner RI: Intrauterine *Listeria* infection: prenatal diagnosis by biophysical assessment and amniocentesis. Am J Obstet Gynecol 1990;163:1596

Linnan MJ, Mascola L, Lou XD, et al: Epidemic listeriosis associated with Mexican-style cheese. N Engl J Med 1988;319:823

Schuchat A, Swaminathan B, Broome CV: Epidemiology of human listeriosis. Clin Microbiol Rev 1991;4:169

Teberg AJ, Yonekura ML, Salminen C, et al: Clinical manifestations of epidemic neonatal listeriosis. Pediatr Infect Dis J 1987;6:817

Variend S, Blumenthal I: Neonatal listeriosis. Postgrad Med J 1975;55:99

14
Tuberculosis in pregnancy

By Charles V. Sanders, MD, and Michael K. Hill, MD

Background and incidence

Congenital and neonatally acquired tuberculosis are frequently underdiagnosed, resulting in delayed treatment and a mortality rate approaching 50%. Most fatal cases are diagnosed at autopsy. In contrast, if the diagnosis is suspected early and appropriate treatment initiated, prospects for recovery are excellent.

Although tuberculosis in pregnancy and neonatal and congenital tuberculosis are rare, recent statistics suggest that these incidences will be increasing. Higher birth rates in women at risk, coupled with the AIDS epidemic, are the chief underlying factors. Among risk factors are poor living conditions, crowded housing, poor nutrition, and lack of adequate prenatal care.

Pathophysiology

Opinions about the influence of pregnancy on the prognosis for tuberculosis have varied widely. Good data are now available that suggest no increased risk of progression for women in pregnancy or postpartum as compared with nonpregnant women of the same age.

The most common manifestation of disease in pregnancy includes asymptomatic purified protein derivative (PPD) skin test conversions and pulmonary tuberculosis. Less common entities are peritonitis, meningitis, mastitis, and paraplegia secondary to spinal osteomyelitis (Pott's disease).

Fetal ingestion or aspiration of infected amniotic fluid (AF) and hematogenous infection have been proposed as modes of congenital infection. The liver or regional lymph nodes are the most frequent sites of involvement, owing to direct seeding from the umbilical vein. Disease may spread to the lungs by direct transplacental transport of organisms through the ductus venosus branch of the umbilical vein or aspiration of infected AF Although the liver and lungs are the primary organs affected, there is usually diffuse hematogenous seeding involving the bone marrow, bone, gastrointestinal tract, adrenal glands, spleen, kidneys, abdominal lymph nodes, and skin.

Lymphohematogenous spread or smoldering endometritis during pregnancy are frequently responsible for transmitting infection to the newborn at delivery. Untreated mothers with active pulmonary tuberculosis may infect their infants through close postpartum physical contact.

Diagnosis

Current recommendations are that pregnant patients considered to be at high risk for tuberculosis should be skin tested. These include any with signs or symptoms suggesting either tuberculosis or a history of exposure to it, as well as all HIV-positive patients. In addition, pregnant women who have had a gastrectomy or who work in a hospital, nursing home, or prison should be considered for screening. Finally, patients from high-risk ethnic groups such as Asian refugees and recent Haitian immigrants should be tested routinely.

Although there has been some controversy regarding the validity of PPD testing during pregnancy, there is now overwhelming evidence that such testing is valid at all times. A positive reaction requires further investigation for active disease. Obtain a chest roentgenogram with abdominal shielding. Also submit sputum specimens for smear and culture, along with appropriate biopsy specimens if there is evidence of extrapulmonary disease.

In all respects, clinical manifestations of active tuberculosis in pregnancy resemble those seen in nonpregnant patients. No substantial evidence suggests that extrapulmonary disease occurs more often.

Infants with congenital tuberculosis usually do not manifest signs of disease for several days to weeks after delivery. In most cases, signs are nonspecific and include fever, failure to thrive, lymphadenopathy, abdominal distension, hepatomegaly, and splenomegaly. Eventually, extensive progressive infiltrates will appear on the chest roentgenogram, and about half will show a miliary pattern (Table 1).

Diagnosis of congenital or neonatal tuberculosis is difficult. The PPD skin test is almost always initially negative, although it frequently becomes positive 6 weeks to 4 months later. Positive smear and culture results can frequently be obtained from liver biopsy specimens, spinal fluid, urine, bone marrow, middle ear fluid, tracheal aspirates, and biopsies of skin lesions or peripheral lymph nodes. Although direct smears from gastric aspirates are unreliable, culture

TABLE 1
Prediagnosis signs and symptoms in 26 cases of congenital tuberculosis

Sign or symptom	No. of cases
Respiratory distress	20
Fever	16
Hepatic and/or splenic enlargement Hepatosplenomegaly (11) Splenomegaly (4) Hepatomegaly (1)	16
Poor feeding	12
Lethargy and/or irritability	11
Lymphadenopathy	9
Other findings Abdominal distension Failure to thrive Ear discharge Skin lesions Jaundice Seizures	 7 5 4 3 2 1

Source: Hageman J, Shulman S, Schreiber M, et al: Congenital tuberculosis: Critical reappraisal of clinical findings and diagnostic procedures. Pediatrics 1980;66:980

of early morning aspirates may be highly productive.

Treatment

Exactly as in nonpregnant patients, therapy with two drugs in standard doses should be used for 9 months. Extensive experience has been accumulated with isoniazid in pregnancy. Although isoniazid crosses the placenta, there seem to be no teratogenic effects. Likewise, ethambutol appears to be safe, as there has been no relationship between its use during pregnancy and fetal abnormalities, including optic deformities. Although rifampin crosses the placenta and theoretically could cause fetal damage because of its ability to

TABLE 2
Treatment of tuberculosis in pregnancy

Condition	Regimen
Active disease	Isoniazid (INH), 300 mg daily, plus rifampin, 600 mg daily, or ethambutol, 2.5 g daily, for minimum of 9 months
Positive purified protein derivative (PPD) skin test (recent seroconversion, no evidence of active disease)	INH, 300 mg after first trimester for 6 to 9 months
Positive PPD (no evidence of active disease)	INH, 300 mg after delivery for 6 to 9 months
Neonatal prophylaxis	INH, 10 mg/kg daily for 3 months, recheck purified protein derivative skin test at 3 months, continue treatment

inhibit DNA-dependent RNA polymerase production, no such damage has been proven.

Streptomycin has, in some cases, been associated with severe, irreversible bilateral hearing loss and marked vestibular abnormalities in infants exposed to it in utero. Therefore, it is contraindicated in pregnancy. Capreomycin and kanamycin, which could have the same potential toxicity as streptomycin, are also contraindicated. As little is known about the effects of pyrazinamide in pregnancy, it is wise to avoid its use as well. Teratogenic effects have been linked to ethionamide. Also avoid cycloserine because of its central nervous system side effects.

Give pregnant women with active tuberculosis isoniazid and rifampin daily. Ethambutol should be added if there is potential isoniazid resistance. If sensitivities prove all drugs to be effective, treatment may be administered twice weekly after the first 1 to 2 months of therapy (Table 2). Always give 50 mg of pyridoxine daily with isoniazid.

Duration of therapy must be 9 months. In most cases, this time is needed because usually only two active drugs are administered. It may be necessary to consider therapeutic abortion if the mother is infected with a multi-drug-resistant organism and requires treatment with potentially teratogenic medications.

The consensus is that unless the infant is receiving antituberculous therapy, it is safe for a mother undergoing therapy to breast-feed. Infants receive less than 20% of the mother's isoniazid dose and less than 11% of other antituberculous drugs in breast milk.

Treatment of congenital or neonatally acquired tuberculosis should begin as soon as a presumptive diagnosis has been made and appropriate smears and cultures obtained. Start with daily isoniazid and rifampin. If there is possibility of a drug-resistant organism, treatment with four drugs is recommended. Streptomycin appears to be safe in young children. Isoniazid, rifampin, streptomycin, and pyrazinamide are recommended for cases involving potentially drug-resistant organisms. If possible, avoid giving ethambutol to young children and infants because of the potential for retrobulbar neuritis and inability to check visual acuity in these cases.

When drug susceptibility results are available, treatment can continue with two bactericidal drugs administered twice weekly. A total of 6 months of treatment is adequate if pyrazinamide, isoniazid, and rifampin are given daily for the first 2 months. Otherwise, treatment should be for 9 months.

Pregnant women under age 35 who are PPD-positive but without evidence of active tuberculosis should have 6 months of isoniazid prophylaxis starting immediately postpartum. If PPD conversion has occurred within the last 1 to 2 years, start isoniazid prophylaxis during the second trimester of pregnancy, regardless of the woman's age.

Infants born to mothers on antituberculous therapy and having negative sputum cultures at the time of delivery are unlikely to develop tuberculosis. One should skin-test the infant at birth and after 3 months. When the mother has positive sputum cultures, examine the infant thoroughly for tuberculosis. If there is no evidence of it, initiate isoniazid prophylaxis (assuming the mother's isolate was not isoniazid resistant). Bacille Calmette-Guérin vaccination may be an effective alternative to isoniazid prophylaxis in situations where compliance might be a problem.

Prevention

Give preventive therapy to pregnant women who have recently converted their PPD skin test and are at high risk of developing progressive disease. Starting treatment after the first trimester of pregnancy is preferable. On the other hand, treatment of active disease should be started as soon as a diagnosis of tuberculosis is made. Isoniazid, rifampin, and ethambutol, the preferred agents, are considered safe. Mothers taking antituberculous drugs can nurse safely provided the infant is not also receiving antituberculous therapy.

SUGGESTED READING

Bate TWP, Sinclair RE, Robinson MJ: Neonatal tuberculosis. Arch Dis Child 1986;61:512

de March P: Tuberculosis and pregnancy. Five- to ten-year review of 215 patients in their fertile age. Chest 1975;68:800

Jacobs RF, Abernathy RS: Management of tuberculosis in pregnancy and the newborn. Clin Perinatol 1988;15:305

Kendig EL Jr: The place of BCG vaccine in the management of infants born of tuberculous mothers. N Engl J Med 1969;281:520

Nemir RL, O'Hare D: Congenital tuberculosis. Review and diagnostic guidelines. Am J Dis Child 1985;139:284

Rieder HL, Cauthern GM, Kelly GD, et al: Tuberculosis in the United States. JAMA 1989;262:385

Scheinhorn DJ, Angelillo VA: Antituberculous therapy in pregnancy. West J Med 1977;127:195

15

Postabortal infections

By A. Karen Kreutner, MD

Background and incidence

Postabortal infection encompasses a wide range of conditions, from simple febrile morbidity associated with uterine tenderness to pelvic inflammatory disease with abscess. Septic pelvic thrombophlebitis, bacteremia, and septic shock are possible sequelae.

Data reported to the Centers for Disease Control's Abortion Surveillance Program (1980) revealed the following complication rates among 42,548 women undergoing abortion: pelvic infection, 1%; infection and hemorrhage, 0.7%; and fever, 2%.

Etiology

Postabortal infections are polymicrobial in nature. Causative organisms include *Chlamydia trachomatis*, *Neisseria gonorrhoeae*, group B ß-hemolytic streptococci, *Escherichia coli*, and *Staphylococcus aureus*, as well as anaerobes such as *Bacteroides* sp and peptostreptococci. The organisms associated with bacterial vaginosis have also been implicated.

Pathophysiology

Infection after abortion is an ascending process, and it occurs more commonly in the presence of retained products of conception or operative trauma. Perforation of the uterus, with or without bowel injury, may be followed by severe infection. Risk factors include greater duration of pregnancy, technical difficulties, and presence of unsuspected sexually transmitted diseases.

Diagnosis

Symptoms include fever, chills, abdominal pain, and vaginal bleeding, often with the passage of placental tissue. Postabortal infection generally has its onset within 4 days of the procedure.

Physical findings include an elevated temperature, tachycardia, and tachypnea. In the presence of bacteremia, low blood pressure or frank shock may occur, and the patient may be agitated or disoriented. Pelvic examination reveals a sanguinopurulent discharge and uterine tenderness, with or without adnexal and parametrial tenderness or fluctuance. It is important to look for cervical and vaginal lacerations, especially in a suspected illegal abortion.

Septic abortion due to *Clostridium perfringens* infection has a characteristic clinical picture. In the severe case, massive intravascular hemolysis very rapidly produces jaundice, mahogany-colored urine, and severe anemia. This hemolysis frequently leads to acute renal failure secondary to lower-nephron nephrosis. Although critically ill, these patients may appear composed and unconcerned about their illness. The pulse is often disproportionately higher than the fever.

Laboratory diagnostic evaluation for patients with more than early endometritis should include complete blood count, urinalysis, culture and Gram stain of cervical material, blood cultures, anteroposterior x-ray of the abdomen or pelvis, and upright chest x-ray.

Treatment

Simple endometritis can be treated with an oral regimen of doxycycline, 100 mg twice daily for 7 to 10 days. Clinical follow-up within 72 hours of initiating therapy must be arranged. Persistent bleeding or signs of infection require curettage to empty the uterus.

Patients with more serious infection should be admitted to the hospital for surgical removal of infected tissue and appropriate parenteral antibiotic therapy. After diagnostic procedures have been carried out, including pelvic ultrasound scans to confirm the presence of retained tissue, broad-spectrum antibiotic therapy with cefoxitin, cefotetan, ampicillin/sulbactam, or clindamycin plus gentamicin should be initiated. For the patient with septic shock, clindamycin plus ampicillin, plus either gentamicin or aztreonam, is advisable. In the rare case of clostridial postabortal sepsis, the regimen should include high-dose penicillin.

Surgical drainage is essential. In most cases, the infection can be controlled by prompt curettage of the retained products of conception shortly after admission. When the uterus is too large to allow suction curettage, oxytocin administration is often successful. Use of prostaglandin suppositories is contraindicated in the presence of acute pelvic infection. Concurrent laparoscopy may be needed when curetting a uterus perforated at the time of the abortion.

Indications for laparotomy and hysterectomy include failure to respond to curettage and appropriate medical therapy, perforation and infection with suspected bowel injury, pelvic and adnexal abscess, and gas gangrene (clostridial necrotizing myometritis).

Isolation of *C perfringens* does not mandate hysterectomy. Initial treatment should be with high-dose parenteral penicillin, curettage, and supportive therapy with intensive cardiovascular monitoring. Laparotomy is indicated if there is deterioration or no response.

Sequelae

Prognosis for even severe postabortal sepsis is good. The Centers for Disease Control reports that, since 1980, the death-to-case ratio for all abortions has been less than 1/100,000. From 1978 to 1985 there were only five reported deaths from illegal abortion.

Reproductive potential after an infected abortion may be compromised by Asherman's syndrome, pelvic adhesions, or incompetent cervix. Tubal infertility is a concern after postabortal infections caused by *N gonorrhoeae* or *C trachomatis*.

Prevention

Avoidance of unwanted pregnancies by making contraceptives available is the most important preventive measure. Screening for sexually transmitted diseases before performing elective abortion is optimal but often impractical.

The literature suggests that prophylactic antibiotics may be effective in reducing infectious morbidity when used routinely for first-trimester elective suction curettage abortion. Data are not available to support designation of an optimal regimen, but oral doxycycline has been used successfully. In some regimens, antibiotic prophylaxis is instituted after the procedure to minimize the common side effects of nausea and vomiting.

SUGGESTED READING

Grimes DA, Schulz KF: Morbidity and mortality from second-trimester abortions. J Reprod Med 1985;30:505

Grimes DA, Schulz KF, Cates W: Prophylactic antibiotics for curettage abortion. Am J Obstet Gynecol 1984;150:689

Levallois P, Rioux JE: Prophylactic antibiotics for suction curettage abortion: Results of a clinical controlled trial. Am J Obstet Gynecol 1985;158:100

16
Immunization in pregnancy

By Marvin S. Amstey, MD

Background

Vaccination of pregnant women is an uncommon preventive therapy. Few do it enough to understand the agents, doses, responses, or risks involved (Tables 1 and 2). Therefore, it would not be helpful to discuss the use of all the immunizing agents in pregnancy. For those interested, summaries are available elsewhere.

On the other hand, need for active and passive immunization in pregnancy is becoming greater as travel expands and transportation improves, leading to more rapid dissemination of infectious agents. The following discussion will be confined to a few generalizations, with specifics limited to products likely to be used more frequently.

Active immunization

The accepted criterion for the need for active immunization is susceptibility to the infection, or absence of antibodies. Since routine antibody testing is not done except for rubella and hepatitis B, susceptibility information is often unknown. Therefore, a history and record of previous vaccinations is important. Most women of child-bearing age in the United States should be immune to measles, mumps, polio, rubella, tetanus, pertussis, and diphtheria because of state requirements for school admissions. However, one should assume immunity to tetanus and diphtheria only if the last booster injection of vaccine was given less than 10 years ago.

In general, the most conservative statement on the subject—"avoid vaccination in pregnancy with any live bacterial or viral product"—is a safe guideline. While this interdiction was applied in the past to all immunizing products, it should not now include nonviable bacteria, bacterial products, inactivated viruses, or toxoids. In fact, it

TABLE 1
Vaccines available for active immunization

Live bacteria
Bacillus Calmette-Guérin
Tularemia

Killed bacteria or product
Cholera
Haemophilus influenzae
Meningococcus
Pertussis
Plague
Pneumococcus
Rocky Mountain spotted
fever *(Rickettsia)*
Typhoid
Typhus

Live virus
Mumps
Polio
Rabies
Rubella
Rubeola (measles)

Killed virus
Hepatitis B
Influenza
Polio

Toxoid
Anthrax
Diphtheria
Tetanus

is proper management to update a pregnant patient's tetanus immunization, which should be boosted every 10 years.

A theoretic fear voiced in some quarters is that introducing an antigen such as a vaccine product into the mother will make the fetus tolerant, and therefore unable to form an antibody. While this kind of tolerance can be found in some animals, it has never been seen in humans. In fact, a trial of maternal vaccination with *Haemophilus influenzae*, type b, provided newborns with high antibody levels. Vaccination of these infants at 18 months of age led to the expected boost in antibodies noted for infants of nonvaccinated mothers.

Tetanus
The most commonly used vaccine for active immunization—whether a patient is pregnant or not—is tetanus. If someone has never been vaccinated, or more than 10 years has elapsed since vaccination, the adult formulation of tetanus–diphtheria, consisting of the adsorbed toxoids of these bacteria, is the product of choice.

Primary vaccination is given as two doses, a month apart, followed by a third dose at 6 to 12 months after the second. The booster dose

TABLE 2
Passive immunization materials

Condition	Immunoglobulin or serum
Botulism	Antitoxin (horse serum)
Diphtheria	Antitoxin (horse serum)
Hepatitis A and measles	Pooled human IgG
Hepatitis B	Human hepatitis B hyperimmune IgG
Rabies	Human antirabies hyperimmune IgG
Snakebite (coral and crotalid snakes)	Antivenin (horse serum)
Tetanus	Human antitetanus hyperimmune IgG
Varicella-zoster	Human antivaricella-zoster hyperimmune IgG

is a single 0.5-mL injection every 10 years.

Vaccination should be part of good prenatal care. It's well known that this therapy prevents neonatal tetanus, which, although very rare in the US, is an important cause of neonatal mortality in the developing world. A 90% reduction in mortality from neonatal tetanus in Sri Lanka from 1978 to 1983 was effected by immunizing all pregnant women with tetanus toxoid.

Hepatitis B
Perhaps the second most common reason for vaccination in pregnancy is the need either for primary immunization with hepatitis B because of family, sexual, or work exposure to this virus or for continuing a series of hepatitis B injections begun before conception. Although this vaccine (or, for that matter, any vaccine) is not approved by the Food and Drug Administration for use in pregnancy, its benefits outweigh any potential risk. It is good medical practice to offer it or continue its use in women at high risk of contracting the disease.

There has been no reported harm from hepatitis B vaccine in pregnancy. The vaccine is administered as two 1-mL IM injections

2 months apart, with a third dose given 6 months after the second.

Influenza

While it is not routinely indicated in pregnancy, influenza vaccine should be given even to pregnant women at high risk for serious illness if they contract influenza. Women who have chronic cardiac or pulmonary disease or chronic metabolic disease, such as diabetes, should receive the most current formulation of influenza vaccine that is available for the "flu" season.

Physicians should consult local public health officials to learn which variety of influenza vaccine is recommended. Type B influenza virus is always the same strain, but type A influenza virus changes its antigenic makeup frequently, making last year's strain (and vaccine) less effective than the current one.

Typhoid and other vaccines

There is little call for typhoid vaccine, particularly in pregnancy, unless someone is traveling to an endemic area or is involved in a natural disaster affecting the water supply. In such situations, it is safe to give typhoid vaccine either as a primary series of two injections, 4 weeks apart, or as a single booster dose if primary vaccination has been within 5 years.

All other available vaccines are used so infrequently in pregnancy that one needs to contact public health officials for proper product and dose. It is self-evident that exposure to a life-threatening disease, even in pregnancy, warrants making an exception and even using live vaccines, such as those for rabies or yellow fever.

The Centers for Disease Control maintains a registry of women who receive live virus vaccines 3 months before or after conception. Physicians are urged to report such cases to the CDC [404-329-3091] so that pregnancy can be followed prospectively.

This registry has allowed the CDC to inform the medical community about such things as inadvertent rubella vaccination during pregnancy. It has enabled us to learn, for example, that administering live, but attenuated, rubella virus vaccine, thought to be a potential tragedy, actually poses very little to no risk to the developing fetus.

Passive immunization

There is no contraindication to using any immunoglobulin or serum in pregnancy. The danger of serum sickness from using horse serum in a pregnant woman is the same as for a nonpregnant woman and calls for the same precautions. Passive immunity is accomplished with heterologous antibody, which is metabolized with a finite half-life. Therefore, protection is limited, usually to 30 days.

It is necessary to use passive immunization when a woman is exposed to an infectious agent or toxin and time doesn't allow her to develop her own antibody by active immunization. For example, splashing of hepatitis B–contaminated blood in an eye requires passive immunization in order for antibodies to be available immediately. This measure must be followed by active immunization to provide long-lasting immunity.

Future developments

In addition to protecting the mother, immunization in pregnancy may also protect the newborn against infectious agents likely to cause serious harm soon after birth or in the first few months of life. Examples are group B streptococcal infection and invasive *H influenzae*. Maternal vaccination in these instances may confer passive immunity on the fetus and newborn because immunoglobulin G antibodies produced by the mother will cross the placenta.

The Vaccine Act passed by Congress in 1986 requires physicians to maintain accurate records, including lot numbers, of any vaccinations with diphtheria–pertussis–tetanus, oral polio, measles–mumps–rubella, and *H influenzae*, type b, vaccines. The Vaccine Act also requires reporting any untoward reactions to public health officials. While these four vaccines have no place in obstetrics at this point (with the possible exception of *H influenzae*, type b), this requirement should apply to all immunizing agents. Other recommendations regarding adult immunization are available from the CDC.

SUGGESTED READING

ACIP: General recommendations on immunization. MMWR 1989;38:205

American College of Obstetricians and Gynecologists: Immunization in pregnancy. ACOG Tech Bull 1991 (October); No. 160

Amstey MS: Vaccination in pregnancy. Clin Obstet Gynecol 1983;10:13

Amstey MS, Insel R, Munoz J, et al: Fetal-neonatal passive immunization against *Hemophilus influenzae*, type b. Am J Obstet Gynecol 1985;153:607

Amstey MS, Insel RA, Pichichero ME: Neonatal passive immunization by maternal vaccination. Obstet Gynecol 1984;63:105

Baker C, Rench M, Edwards M, et al: Immunization of pregnant women with a polysaccharide vaccine of group B streptococcus. N Engl J Med 1988;319:1180

Ramalingaswami V: Importance of vaccines in child survival. Rev Inf Dis 1989;II(suppl 3):S498

17

HIV infection in pregnancy

By Howard L. Minkoff, MD

Background

National serosurveys of human immunodeficiency virus (HIV) infection have suggested that in 1990 5,500 women with HIV infection would give birth. Since prenatal care providers are among the only clinicians being urged (by the Centers for Disease Control and the American College of Obstetricians and Gynecologists) to offer HIV tests routinely as part of the management of asymptomatic women, these physicians must be prepared to give ongoing care to those identified as HIV infected. This care should include post-test counseling, as well as antepartum, intrapartum, and postpartum care.

Post-test counseling

Post-test counseling of the HIV-positive woman is a delicate, time-consuming process that the obstetrician will be hard pressed to carry out unaided. It is best to be prepared for this task and to be familiar with individual and institutional resources that can be called upon to assist.

The counseling must cover the social as well as the medical and obstetric consequences of being HIV infected. The counselor must first be sure the woman understands the distinction between being diagnosed as having acquired immunodeficiency syndrome (AIDS) and being asymptomatically infected with HIV. The modes of spread of the virus and techniques needed to avoid infecting others should be stressed. It is important early in the counseling process to have the woman identify support people in whom she can confide and who can assist during these difficult times. Beyond these individuals and medical personnel having a need to know her serostatus, the patient should be cautioned not to give out her serostatus, as instances of discrimination against HIV-positive individuals are common.

Recent advances allow the clinician to be somewhat more encouraging in describing the medical aspects of HIV disease. New treatments for opportunistic infections, new antiviral regimens, and new prophylactic therapies have substantially increased disease-free intervals for the HIV infected. In one report, the majority of HIV-positive hemophiliacs were clinically asymptomatic 8 years after seroconversion. Counseling should emphasize the need to avoid reexposure to virus and to maintain good general health. It should also stress the importance of being under the long-term care of clinicians versed in the special needs of HIV-infected individuals.

The relevant obstetric data that should be shared with these women include the effects of the virus on their pregnancy and their offspring, and the effect of pregnancy on their disease. In Western countries, short-term pregnancy outcomes have not been found to be substantially altered by HIV infection. In these areas, when seropositive women are matched with seronegative women from the same risk groups, factors such as smoking, drinking, and drug use are more important determinants of short-term outcome than is HIV infection. The data from Africa differ in that HIV-infected mothers do have poorer outcomes. The difference between Western and African experience may reflect the higher percentage of clinically ill women in Africa.

Rates of HIV transmission from mother to child have generally been in the 25% to 35% range. The risk of transmission has been reported to increase with more advanced maternal disease (lower CD4 counts), prematurity, breast-feeding, previous affected sibling, and absence of maternal antibody to the gp120 portion of the virus. There are currently no practical tools available for prenatal diagnosis of fetal infection.

Although concerns have been raised that pregnancy might accelerate the course of HIV disease, empiric data are lacking. Small studies comparing the natural history of HIV infection in pregnant and nonpregnant women have not shown a substantial difference between the groups. There may be a slightly greater rate of decline of CD4 cells during pregnancy. A low CD4 cell level has been shown to carry the same ominous prognosis—higher risk of developing an opportunistic infection—in both pregnant and nonpregnant women. In all circumstances, consideration of prophylactic agents is warranted in the setting of low CD4 counts.

Antepartum management
When presented with the aforementioned facts and offered all reproductive options, including abortion, the large majority of infected

pregnant women have thus far chosen to maintain their pregnancies. Prenatal care of these women involves provision of social support as well as medical surveillance and obstetric care.

The cornerstone of medical surveillance is the absolute CD4 cell count. Women whose counts stay above 500/mm³ have been reported to have no HIV-related complications during pregnancy. Conversely, those whose CD4 levels drop below 500/mm³ are at greater risk of developing opportunistic infections. It is therefore prudent to keep a close eye on patients with low CD4 levels and to consider giving zidovudine (AZT) if the count falls below 500/mm³ and pentamidine if the absolute count falls below 200/mm³ or the percentage of CD4 cells falls below 20%. Other surveillance steps include obtaining baseline toxoplasmosis titers and screening for sexually transmitted diseases (syphilis, gonorrhea, *Chlamydia* infection, and hepatitis B infection).

HIV-infected women should also have Mantoux testing to exclude tuberculosis and should receive pneumococcal vaccine to reduce the risk of pneumonia. In research settings, other tests, such as those for β_2 microglobulin and neopterin levels, can be employed to help assess an individual's risk of disease progression.

Perhaps the most important role of the CD4 count is to alert the clinician to the patient's susceptibility to opportunistic infections. It signals the need for shortening the interval between visits, educating patients about the potential insidious first signs of infection, and responding quickly to subtle symptoms. If an opportunistic infection is diagnosed, it should be treated aggressively, in consultation with an expert in infectious diseases. In general, the threat to a mother's life in these circumstances is so grave that fetal considerations should not lead to a choice of suboptimal therapies.

Intrapartum management

The intrapartum management of a parturient is not markedly altered by serostatus. Obstetric manipulations such as cesarean delivery have not been clearly linked to improvement in neonatal HIV status. Nosocomial inoculation of the fetus through scalp sampling or placement of interval scalp electrodes should be avoided. Beyond that, management of labor should be standard, and efforts on behalf of the fetus should not be influenced by maternal serostatus.

Assiduous adherence to universal precautions is the obstetrician's best protection against acquiring HIV infection during the intrapartum period. HIV testing for protection is an impractical alternative for the following reasons:

■ the need to care for unregistered (and therefore untested) patients;

■ the existence of a virus-positive antibody-negative period (window phase) beyond the capability of current tests;

■ the emergence of viral strains (HTLV I, II, IV, V) for which testing is not routinely available.

With universal precautions properly applied, risks should be extremely low. All secretions should be treated as though infected. Surgeons should utilize goggles, double gloving, and waterproof gowns. Mouth suction should not be performed. Impenetrable needle disposal units should be easily accessible in all patient care areas.

Postpartum management

The immediate postpartum course is not markedly altered by HIV serostatus. Patients in areas of the world where safe alternatives to breast milk are readily available should be advised not to breast-feed. Although the data on breast milk transmission suggest that the risk may be high only at the time of maternal seroconversion, there is sufficient evidence to warrant the advice to bottle-feed. Mother and child may bond, however, with staff observing universal precautions for handling of both.

In the immediate postpartum period there may be a transient rise in CD4 counts. The inexorable progression of the disease, however, is not altered. It is crucial, therefore, that HIV-infected women and their children be discharged into the care of physicians who are prepared to provide close follow-up, including provision of antiviral and prophylactic therapies.

SUGGESTED READING

Biggar RJ, Pahava S, Minkoff HL, et al: Immunosuppression in pregnant women infected with human immunodeficiency virus. Am J Obstet Gynecol 1989;161:1239

Goedert J, Mendez H, Drummond JE, et al: Maternal-to-infant transmission of human immunodeficiency virus type 1: association with prematurity or low anti-gp120. Lancet 1989;2:1351

Minkoff HL: AIDS in obstetrics. Editorial. Clin Obstet Gynecol 1989;32:421

Minkoff HL: Care of pregnant women infected with human immunodeficiency virus. JAMA 1987;258:2714

Mok JQ, Giaquinto C, DeRossi A, et al: Infants born to mothers seropositive for human immunodeficiency virus. Lancet 1987;1:1164

Ryder R, Nsa W, Hassib SE, et al: Perinatal transmission of the human immunodeficiency virus type 1 to infants of seropositive women in Zaire. N Engl J Med 1989;320:1637

18

Herpes simplex virus infection in pregnancy

By Ronald S. Gibbs, MD

Background and incidence

The exact incidence of genital herpes simplex virus (HSV) infections in pregnancy is unknown. Estimates of 0.5% to 1.0% have been made. It appears that the vast majority (90% to 95%) are recurrent episodes. The others are either primary genital herpes infections or nonprimary first-episode genital herpes infections.

In pregnant women who have primary genital HSV infection there is a high rate of genital viral shedding and of complications, mainly when the primary infection occurs in the third trimester. But in women who have nonprimary first-episode genital herpes or recurrent genital HSV infection during pregnancy, the rate of asymptomatic viral shedding from the genital tract is much lower (approximately 1% on any given day) and the likelihood of fetal neonatal complications is much lower also.

[For the pathophysiology of genital herpes infection, see Chapter 43.]

Diagnosis

Viral isolation in tissue culture remains the standard against which all other diagnostic procedures have been compared. It is fortunate that HSV is hardy and tolerates transport well, and that most positive cultures are available in 3 to 7 days. Most laboratories report a final negative culture at 7 to 10 days.

A number of rapid diagnostic techniques have become available. These include the Papanicolaou smear, the fluorescein conjugated monoclonal antibody test, and the enzyme-linked immunosorbent assay (ELISA). The Pap smear is an insensitive test producing negative results in up to 50% of women who have lesions. The monoclonal antibody and ELISA tests appear fairly reliable in populations with a high prevalence of positive cultures. However, in lower-prevalence populations these rapid tests all have major limitations.

Treatment

Pregnant women who have recurrent episodes should in general be managed symptomatically. Although oral acyclovir has been demonstrated to be of value in severe recurrent episodes in nonpregnant adults, acyclovir is currently not recommended for recurrent episodes in pregnancy nor as suppressive therapy near term.

For women who have primary episodes during pregnancy, current CDC recommendations include the use of systemic acyclovir for life-threatening maternal HSV infection, such as encephalitis, pneumonitis, or hepatitis, even though the safety of acyclovir in pregnancy has not been clearly established.

For women who have primary HSV infections in pregnancy with marked constitutional symptoms and extensive lesions (but without encephalitis, pneumonitis, or hepatitis), the use of acyclovir must be decided on the basis of benefits versus potential risks. There is no evidence that acyclovir given in primary episodes decreases fetal–neonatal complications.

For women who have recurrent genital herpes infections during pregnancy, clinicians used to do weekly cultures and perform a cesarean delivery if the patient had either cultural or clinical evidence of recurrent infection at or near the time of delivery. However, in view of major studies demonstrating the failure of antepartum HSV cultures to predict culture status at delivery, management recommendations have been revised. Current recommendations for pregnant women with a history of recurrent genital herpes infections are summarized as follows:

(1) Weekly prenatal cultures should be abandoned.

(2) In the absence of genital herpetic lesions, vaginal delivery should be expected (unless, of course, other indications for cesarean section are present).

(3) In order to identify potentially exposed neonates, a culture for herpesvirus may be obtained from either the mother on the day of delivery or from the neonate.

(4) Isolation is not necessary for the mother.

It is recognized that with such a policy, there is a small risk (approximately 1/1,000) of neonatal infection. In women with herpetic lesions of the genital tract, when either labor or membrane rupture occurs, cesarean delivery can reduce the risk of neonatal herpes virus infection. Ideally, cesarean section should be performed before or within 4 to 6 hours of membrane rupture, but cesarean delivery may be of benefit in preventing neonatal herpes regardless of duration of membrane rupture.

In women with genital herpetic lesions at or near term, but before labor or membrane rupture, cultures collected at 3- to 5-day intervals may be performed to assure the absence of virus at the time of birth and to increase the likelihood of vaginal delivery. In the event that rapid diagnostic tests with sensitivity and specificity equivalent to herpes cultures become available, the stated policy will need revision.

Management of HSV infection in late pregnancy in women who have had a primary genital herpes episode during pregnancy is more problematic. In view of the high risk of premature birth, growth retardation, or neonatal death, appropriate surveillance measures for these complications ought to be instituted. Beyond that, measures such as amniocentesis with culture of amniotic fluid, prenatal lower genital tract cultures, or suppressive use of acyclovir all remain experimental.

For women who have recurrent HSV lesions in areas remote from the genital tract, one study has demonstrated that the cervical viral shedding rate in 47 patients was 2.1% when the "remote" lesions were in the perianal, buttock, thigh, and back areas. Because of this low rate of asymptomatic genital shedding in patients with such recurrent remote lesions, it is generally felt that vaginal delivery may be carried out safely, provided these lesions can be excluded from the field of vaginal delivery by drapes.

Postpartum care

Women do not need isolation if they have a history of recurrent episodes of genital HSV infection in pregnancy but do not have lesions or symptoms at the time of the delivery and the postpartum period. For women who have active, genital lesions at the time of delivery, most authorities feel that the mother may be permitted to handle and breast-feed the baby provided she follows strict handwashing measures and prevents contact with infected lesions or secretions.

Mothers who have active genital infection with herpes should be placed on drainage/secretion precautions after delivery. Use of acyclovir in the puerperium should be as in other nonpregnant adults.

SUGGESTED READING

Arvin AM, Hensleigh PA, Prober CG, et al: Failure of antepartum maternal cultures to predict the infant's risk of exposure to herpes simplex virus at delivery. N Engl J Med 1986;315:796

Brown ZA, Vontver LA, Benedetti TJ, et al: Genital herpes in pregnancy: risk factors associated with recurrences and asymptomatic viral shedding. Am J Obstet Gynecol 1985;153:24

Centers for Disease Control: 1989 sexually transmitted diseases treatment guidelines: MMWR 1989;38(S-8):17

Gibbs RS, Amstey MS, Sweet RL, et al: Management of genital herpes infection in pregnancy. Editorial. Obstet Gynecol 1988;71:779

Harger JH, Pazin GJ, Armstrong JA, et al: Characteristics and management of pregnancy in women with genital herpes simplex virus infection. Am J Obstet Gynecol 1983;145:784

Prober CG, Sullender VM, Yasukawa LL, et al: Low risk of herpes simplex virus infection in neonates exposed to the virus at the time of vaginal delivery to mothers with recurrent genital herpes simplex virus infections. N Engl J Med 1987;316:240

Wittek AE, Yeager AS, Au DS, et al: Asymptomatic shedding of herpes simplex virus for the cervix and lesion site during pregnancy. Am J Dis Child 1984;138:439

19
Cytomegalovirus infection in pregnancy

By John W. Larsen, Jr., MD

Background and incidence

Cytomegaloviruses belong to the herpesvirus family, members of which are well known for their ability to persist in the body after initial infection. The name reflects the characteristic cytopathology, with infected cells enlarged and containing intranuclear and cytoplasmic inclusions.

Cytomegalovirus (CMV) infection is the most frequent congenital viral disease in the United States. Primary infection of the mother occurs in 1% to 2% of pregnancies, setting up the possibility of transplacental viral transmission. While most fetuses infected by this route are not severely damaged, those with severe disease may have manifestations that include microcephaly, mental retardation, deafness, and chorioretinitis.

CMV infections have been demonstrated to be common in all population groups. When represented as lifetime data, the great majority of humans are infected at some time during their lives. If the mother is shedding virus at the time of parturition, the baby frequently acquires the infection during the first weeks to months of life. Child-to-child transmission in day-care centers is common, perhaps reflecting the high frequency of oral behavior in such groups. The frequency of serologic evidence of infection among children in group care settings can reach 80% to 95%. High rates of seropositivity seem to be correlated with conditions of crowding and close personal contact.

Overall in the US, fewer than 20% of preschool children show antibody to CMV. The frequency of antibody positivity in women increases to about 60% by childbearing age. Women in middle- or upper-income groups are more likely to be susceptible to infection than those of low-income groups because of the higher rate of CMV infection associated with low socioeconomic status.

Primary infection with CMV during pregnancy occurs in 1% to 2% of women. These are the women at highest risk of having a child affected by CMV. Transplacental transmission of the virus from mother to fetus will occur in approximately 30% to 40% of primary CMV infections. Of these infected infants, approximately 10% to 15% will have clinically apparent disease, which may range from mild to severe manifestations. While it has been suggested in some studies that there may be a higher pregnancy loss rate among this group, this is not well substantiated. Of the 85% to 90% of infected infants who are asymptomatic at birth, 5% to 15% will ultimately develop clinical sequelae of infection.

Women known to be seropositive before conception can also transmit CMV transplacentally to their fetuses. The rate of this kind of transfer is low (less than 1%), and infected infants in this group have extremely low likelihood of developing clinically important disease.

Diagnosis

Mother. Almost all maternal infections are asymptomatic. Uncommonly, there may be a mononucleosis-like syndrome in which there will be a negative heterophil test. Because there is not a symptom trail to follow in adults, the diagnosis depends on laboratory testing.

The definitive method for establishing the diagnosis of CMV infection is virus isolation. In the past, virus isolation has often required several weeks. Newer technology using cell tissue culture vials, centrifugation, and monoclonal antibodies has permitted results to be available in a few days. Virus can be isolated from virtually any body fluid, including saliva, blood, urine, breast milk, semen, and spinal fluid. Cultures of maternal urine and endocervical swabs taken during pregnancy have not proved useful for predicting which fetuses will become severely affected by CMV.

The serologic tests of antibody status can be useful in determining susceptibility to CMV infection as well as detecting which patients have become acutely infected during pregnancy. The most reliable method for establishing acute CMV infection during pregnancy is to be able to demonstrate seroconversion. This requires a prior serologic specimen that was seronegative. A CMV-specific IgM test may also be useful. In a woman suspected of having acquired CMV because of mild symptomatology or known exposure, a positive CMV-specific IgM test can support the diagnosis of acute infection.

However, the results of CMV IgM testing must be interpreted with caution. Only 75% to 80% of patients with primary infections will have a positive result, and about 10% of women with recurrent infections will have a positive test. False-positive CMV IgM tests also occur, caused by the presence of rheumatoid factor or antinuclear antibodies. Cross-reactive tests with the Epstein-Barr virus antibody have been reported as well.

Routine CMV antibody screening is not recommended for asymptomatic pregnant women. Recent evidence supports the use of viral culture of amniotic fluid as an adjunct procedure when performed as part of the antenatal evaluation of suspected fetal CMV infection.

Child. Severe CMV infection is detected at birth in 1/10,000 to 1/20,000 babies. A newborn who is severely affected will have evidence of damage to multiple organ systems. Brain damage may be manifested as microcephaly more often than hydrocephaly. Early in the course of infection, ventriculomegaly may be detected in utero by ultrasound. As CMV disease progresses, the fetal head may become microcephalic. Infection of the brain may also result in cerebral calcification that can be noted antenatally or postnatally.

Damage to the eye can include chorioretinitis and, less commonly, microphthalmia. While sensorineural hearing loss is one of the most common manifestations of CMV disease, it is difficult to detect at birth. A rash characterized as small petechiae may be present at birth or, more often, shortly after. The rash may be purpuric in some cases and associated with thrombocytopenia. Abdominal findings include hydrops, hepatosplenomegaly, and inguinal hernia. Fetal growth retardation may be expected in approximately 40% of severely infected fetuses.

In contrast with the dramatic manifestations of the rare cases of symptomatic severe cytomegalic inclusion disease, approximately 90% of infants infected with CMV are asymptomatic at birth. While these infants may have a 5% risk of developing hearing impairment in the first few years of life, this is not usually detectable at birth. The overall risk for clinical sequelae in this asymptomatic but infected group is approximately 5% to 15%. Manifestations that may be found in addition to hearing impairment are microcephaly, mental retardation, motor dysfunction, chorioretinitis, and dental defects.

The best method for documenting infection in either symptomatic or asymptomatic newborns is virus isolation. Appropriate specimens for testing include samples of urine, nasopharyngeal and conjunctival secretions, and spinal fluid. To confirm that congenital CMV infection of the child has occurred, a positive culture should be obtained within the first 2 weeks of life. Subsequent perinatal infection of the child can be due to exposure to virus in the maternal birth canal at the time of delivery, breast milk, blood transfusion, or other environmental sources. While the great majority of perinatal CMV infections remain asymptomatic, there are others in which there is pneumonitis and clinical evidence of multiorgan infection.

Serologic testing for CMV can be used as well. Caution must be used in interpretation of results and in application of the testing. Maternal IgG antibody against CMV will be transferred across the placenta to the fetus and be present in similar concentration to that found in the mother. While CMV-specific IgM produced by the fetus may be helpful in many cases, false positives, false negatives, and high cost have precluded use of this test as a routine clinical screening device for congenital CMV.

Treatment

Since the great majority of CMV infections are asymptomatic in adults, there is generally no treatment other than rest that might be advised during pregnancy. It is possible that an unusual immunosuppressed patient who might also have severe CMV disease might be treated with antiviral chemotherapy, such as acyclovir.

When a pregnant woman has been diagnosed as having a CMV infection during pregnancy, she should be counseled about the implications of this infection for her fetus. It is important to base the counseling on appropriate statistics. Risk for fetal damage is substantially, although not absolutely, confined to cases in which there has been primary infection of the mother during pregnancy. If the pregnant woman has a recurrent infection, she can be given the substantial reassurance that the likelihood of transmission of the virus to her fetus is less than 1%. Among pregnant women with primary CMV infection, 30% to 40% will transmit the infection to the fetus and 10% to 15% of these will have clinically apparent disease. Ultrasound scanning may provide some help in detecting those with the most severe manifestations, such as hydrocephaly, microcephaly, growth retardation, or hydrops. A normal ultrasound examination does not guarantee a normal outcome. While invasive testing of the fetal compartment by amniocentesis or cordocentesis is technically possible, its clinical utility has not been proven and use should therefore be considered investigational.

Various investigators of the effect of gestational age on transmission in utero have demonstrated that the viral transmission across the placenta occurs in first, second, and third trimesters. Preliminary evidence indicates that primary infection early in pregnancy produces the worst outcome. Following appropriate counseling, some women will seek pregnancy termination based on the information presented. Since there is no treatment for CMV infection of the fetus during pregnancy, physicians who manage these patients should have in place a process for diagnosis, plus specialized newborn care at the time of birth. For those who are shown to be infected but asymptomatic as newborns, there should be follow-up monitoring for hearing problems and developmental delays.

Prevention

Since CMV infections are transmitted by close contact, the mainstays of prevention in medical settings are handwashing and use of latex gloves. For household and day-care settings, these preventive measures would be regarded as unusual even though theoretically possible. Since it has been shown that hospital workers in high-risk settings such as dialysis units can limit their acquisition of CMV infections by use of latex gloves and handwashing, however, this approach could be extended to the pregnant serosusceptible woman who works in a day-care setting or has a young child at home. While application of contact precautions in a household setting may be nearly impossible, it is the only remedy that can be offered for a highly concerned patient seeking some advice regarding partial protection.

Since saliva, semen, urine, and blood have all been shown to contain infectious CMV particles, the virus is sexually transmitted. Higher rates of CMV shedding have been reported from sexually transmitted disease clinics than from other settings. Reasonable but unproven strategies are adhering to a mutually monogamous sexual relationship and using condoms when a sexual partner is known to be infected with CMV. The use of street drugs or shared needles should be considered risk factors for CMV transmission.

CMV can be transmitted to the infant by breast milk. This is rarely a problem for a term infant being breast-fed by its own mother. There may be circumstances that would lead to a recommendation that breast milk donors for premature infants be screened for CMV infection in order to reduce a risk to the premature infant population. Since blood transfusion can transmit CMV infection, efforts to reduce this risk for fetal or newborn transfusions have included use of seronegative donors, deglycerolized frozen red blood cells, and blood filtration.

Long-term prevention may be ultimately be achieved through use of vaccine. Vaccines for CMV are currently investigational.

SUGGESTED READING

Fadel HE, Ruedrich DA: Intrauterine resolution of nonimmune hydrops associated with cytomegalovirus infection. Obstet Gynecol 1988;71:1003

Gilbert GL, Hayes K, Hudson IL, et al: Prevention of transfusion-acquired cytomegalovirus infection in infants by blood filtration to remove leukocytes. Lancet 1989;1:1228

Grose C, Weiner CP: Prenatal diagnosis of congenital cytomegalovirus infection: two decades later. Am J Obstet Gynecol 1990;163:447

Sever JL, Larsen JW, Grossman JH: *Handbook of Perinatal Infections.* Boston, Little, Brown & Co., 1989, pp 38-44

Stagno S: Cytomegalovirus, in Remington JS, Klein JO (eds): *Infectious Diseases of the Fetus and Newborn Infant*. Philadelphia, WB Saunders, 1990, pp 241-281

Stagno S, Pass RF, Cloud G, et al: Primary cytomegalovirus infection in pregnancy. Incidence, transmission to fetus, and clinical outcome. JAMA 1986;256:1904

Stagno S, Whitley RJ: Herpesvirus infections of pregnancy. N Engl J Med 1985;313:1270

20
Varicella-zoster infection in pregnancy

By James A. McGregor, MD, and Nancy E. Madinger, MD

Background and incidence

Varicella-zoster virus (VZV) is a herpesvirus that causes two common clinical infections: varicella (chickenpox) and herpes zoster (shingles). While primary infection (varicella) during pregnancy is rare, it is associated with significant maternal morbidity and occasional mortality. Disease consequences may also be severe for the fetus or neonate if infected. Reactivation of latent VZV is manifest as herpes zoster, but this form poses little risk to mother or fetus.

Varicella is a nearly universal disease of children in industrialized countries. In these areas, only 2% of cases occur in the 15-to-49 age group, and incidence among pregnant women is about 5/10,000. By contrast, in tropical and subtropical countries, varicella is more frequently a disease of reproductive-aged adults. Women who spent their childhood in these regions are a population potentially susceptible to varicella during pregnancy. Prenatal serologic surveys have found 95% of US-born women to be immune compared with only 84% of those born in subtropical countries.

VZV is highly contagious, with peak incidence in winter and spring. Attack rates for both pregnant and nonpregnant susceptible women with household contacts approach 90%. Exposures other than household, such as nosocomial, school, or playmate contacts, are less likely to result in infection. Pregnancy does not predispose a woman to acquiring the infection.

Pathophysiology

Primary infection occurs through respiratory inhalation of virus particles. Direct contact with varicella or zoster lesions can also transmit virus. An initial transient and asymptomatic viremia ensues, with viral propagation into the reticuloendothelial system. An incubation period of 10 to 21 days (mean 14 days) is followed by a second viremia, with dissemination to skin and viscera. Clinical evidence of infection appears within 24 to 48 hours of the second viremia. Virus may therefore be transmitted to unsuspecting close contacts 1 or 2 days before the characteristic chickenpox rash is seen.

It has generally been accepted that one attack of viremia confers lifelong immunity to reinfection in the nonimmunocompromised patient. Virus-specific antibodies (IgA, IgM, IgG) rise rapidly during the first 5 days of clinically apparent infection and peak at 2 to 3 weeks. Thereafter, IgG persists at lower levels. Subclinical reinfection is known to occur, however, as shown by rising antibody titers. Rarely, some patients may experience clinically apparent but mild attacks in the face of demonstrated circulating antibody. Circulating antibody thus does not guarantee immunity, though it will ameliorate symptoms and probably prevent congenital infection.

Diagnosis

Before onset of rash, adults experience a prodrome of fever, malaise, myalgias, and headache. Lesions then appear in crops on the face, scalp, and trunk, with relative sparing of the extremities. Initially, lesions are maculopapular, but they progress rapidly to pruritic vesicles, pustules, and scabs. New crops appear for 3 to 4 days, and crusting is generally complete within a week. Characteristically, all stages of lesions will be present simultaneously. Infectivity persists until all of the vesicles become scabs; patients are therefore considered infectious from 2 days before the onset of rash until all lesions are crusted.

The overall mortality for varicella in normal adults is 50/100,000. Comparable data are not available for pregnant women.

Pneumonia is the most common complication of varicella in adults. Overall, hospitalization for pneumonia occurs in only 0.25% of cases of adult varicella, but for these cases mortality may be as high as 12% in nonpregnant and 35% in pregnant patients. Varicella pneumonia is a treacherous disease; cases range from asymptomatic illness to sudden death. Symptoms develop 1 to 6 days after the rash appears and may consist of cough, dyspnea, fever, pleuritic chest pain, and hemoptysis. Chest auscultation is often unremarkable, even in the face of severe pulmonary involvement. X-ray findings are not specific and appear as diffuse bilateral nodular infiltrates.

Pregnancy may place women at greater risk for varicella pneumonia, but case–fatality ratios for pregnant women with this disease remain poorly studied. Claims of rates above 40% based on literature reviews probably represent overreporting of severe cases. However, severe pneumonia and death are well documented. As with other severe illnesses during pregnancy, increased risk of preterm labor and delivery must be anticipated. Fetal distress and death during maternal pneumonia have been reported. Encephalitis is another serious, albeit rare, complication of varicella in the mother.

The varicella rash is so characteristic that diagnosis is usually based on physical examination alone. Other conditions to consider in the differential diagnosis of a varicella-like exanthem include disseminated zoster, disseminated herpes simplex, eczema vaccinatum, generalized vaccinia (cowpox), hand-foot-and-mouth disease, atypical measles, and rickettsialpox.

VZV may be identified in clinical specimens by means of a Tzanck preparation, although varicella, zoster, and herpes simplex infections are indistinguishable by this method. Culture or serologic tests are necessary for definitive identification. Seroconversion is diagnostic and can be detected by complement fixation (CF) assay, fluorescent-antibody-to-membrane-antigen (FAMA) testing, or enzyme immunoassay (EIA). However, seroconversion assays require acute and convalescent serum samples to be drawn 3 weeks apart. The presence of varicella-specific IgM, which remains in the blood for 4 to 5 weeks, is diagnostic.

Treatment

Three antiviral agents with activity against VZV are available: α-interferon, vidarabine, and acyclovir. None is FDA approved for use in pregnancy. Only acyclovir has been used with any frequency in pregnant women. The decision to treat a pregnant woman who has active varicella should be made on an individual basis. Treatment should be limited to women with visceral involvement, particularly pneumonia or encephalitis, as described by Haake and co-workers.

High-dose acyclovir therapy (12.4 mg/kg of body weight or 500 mg/m^2 IV every 8 hours) should begin within 72 hours of the onset of rash. Major side effects are local tissue irritation, transient elevation of hepatic transaminases, CNS toxicity, and renal dysfunction (crystalluria and azotemia).

Transplacental passage of acyclovir has been demonstrated, though drug levels in the fetus are unknown. Reports of acyclovir use in pregnancy for VZV and other indications have been favorable, with no maternal or fetal side effects noted. Antenatal use of acyclovir in an attempt to prevent or ameliorate congenital varicella syndrome or neonatal infection is of unproven benefit.

Prevention

The most effective method for preventing spread of VZV infection is isolation, but asymptomatic viral shedding often precludes this

approach. Ideally, persons exposed to VZV should have their susceptibility determined by either history or serology. If susceptible, the
exposed and presumably infected person should be isolated from at-
risk contacts from the 8th to 21st day after exposure. However, because isolation is often an impractical method of control, passive
immunization is more frequently employed for those at risk for vari-
cella-induced morbidity (pregnant women, immunocompromised
individuals).

Prevention or modification of maternal disease can be accomplished with passive immunization using several available products.
The most effective is varicella-zoster immune globulin (VZIG).
However, the limited supply and high cost of VZIG mandate that its
use be restricted to susceptible patients with a significant exposure to
the virus (household contact, close contact indoors for longer than
1 hour, or hospital contact through roommates or infected personnel).

Determining VZV susceptibility can be problematic. Up to half of
pregnant patients without detectable antibody may give a history of
varicella. Likewise, 80% of patients with a negative or uncertain
history are serologically immune. Most investigators agree that serologic screening of an exposed pregnant woman with a negative
history is an accurate method for determining the need for passive
immunization. Although costly, screening of all pregnant women
regardless of history has been recommended.

Routine prenatal testing could facilitate treatment when exposure
occurs to susceptible women, as well as help avoid "crisis" situations
on weekends with exposed pregnant women of unknown susceptibility. Serologic tests for detecting antibody against VZV are now
widely available and reliable in predicting immunity. FAMA (used
mainly in research laboratories) and EIA are comparable in sensitivity, specificity, and cost. Complement fixing (CF) antibody is short-
lived and not useful for determining immunity.

The efficacy of VZIG in preventing or attenuating maternal disease
has been well established (Figure 1). In a prospective study of pregnant women, 80% of seronegatives receiving VZIG within 96 hours
remained symptom free, whereas 89% of untreated controls developed illness. Susceptible pregnant women with a significant exposure to VZV should be given VZIG within 96 hours of exposure.
Laboratory determination of susceptibility will prevent unnecessary
administration of this costly preparation. A dose of 625 U should be
given IM as soon as possible, but no later than 96 hours postexpo-
sure.

There is no evidence VZIG administration will prevent intrauterine infection. VZIG should be used solely to prevent serious compli-

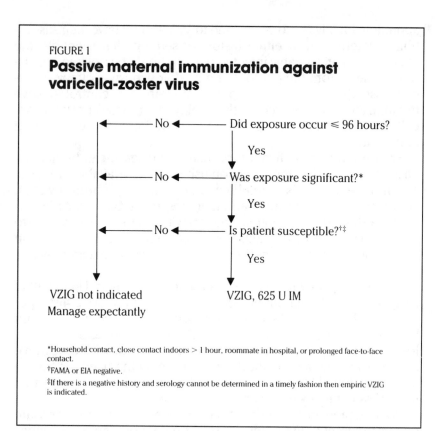

FIGURE 1
Passive maternal immunization against varicella-zoster virus

No ◄─── Did exposure occur ≤ 96 hours?

Yes

No ◄─── Was exposure significant?*

Yes

No ◄─── Is patient susceptible?†‡

Yes

VZIG not indicated
Manage expectantly

VZIG, 625 U IM

*Household contact, close contact indoors > 1 hour, roommate in hospital, or prolonged face-to-face contact.
†FAMA or EIA negative.
‡If there is a negative history and serology cannot be determined in a timely fashion then empiric VZIG is indicated.

cations in the mother; neonates exposed peripartum must be treated with VZIG after birth. VZIG is not effective treatment for maternal varicella.

Sequelae
Maternal varicella may lead to several possible outcomes for the fetus, largely dependent on its gestational age at the time of infection. In most cases, the fetus remains healthy without clinical or serologic evidence of illness. When intrauterine infection does occur, it may result in congenital varicella syndrome, neonatal varicella, or asymptomatic seroconversion.

Congenital varicella syndrome comprises abnormalities of the limbs, skin, eyes, and central nervous system, as well as mental retardation or even death. Specific sequelae include dermatologic scarring, hypoplasia of the extremities, paralysis, intestinal atresia, hydronephrosis, seizures, cortical atrophy, mental retardation, cataracts, and chorioretinitis. Of the fewer than 50 cases reported, most were associated with maternal infection occurring before 20 weeks' gestation. Reliable methods for diagnosing this syndrome are being sought. Ultrasound may detect microcephaly, limb deformities, and other abnormalities. Measurement of VZV-specific IgM in fetal blood obtained by cordocentesis has been used on a research basis. Asymptomatic intrauterine infection has been documented by persistence of antibody in infants. Both intrauterine and peripartum VZV infection predispose to development of childhood zoster.

Neonatal or perinatal varicella may result from maternal varicella occurring in the days preceding or following birth. The attack rate is 25% to 50% and the incubation period averages 11 days (range 1 to 16 days). Severity of infection is directly proportional to the presence of placentally acquired maternal antibody. Since maternal antibody is not transported across the placenta in sufficient quantities until the 5th day of maternal infection, neonates born 5 days or less from the onset of maternal disease receive no protective maternal antibody. Similarly, women who have onset of disease within 2 days following delivery were presumably viremic antepartum, so their infants will be born without antibody.

If possible, birth should be delayed until at least 5 days after the onset of the mother's illness. Administering VZIG to neonates born to mothers with onset of disease 5 days before to 2 days after delivery significantly reduces newborn complications, even though mortality is not entirely prevented and the attack rate may be unaltered. Although neonates born to mothers experiencing varicella more than 5 days before or more than 2 days after delivery are not at increased risk for complications, some experts recommend VZIG use in this setting.

Patients with varicella or zoster should be isolated and cared for only by immune employees. Isolation of the newborn from the varicella-infected mother is recommended. Although excretion of VZV into breast milk has not been demonstrated, to prevent neonatal exposure from direct maternal contact, breast-feeding during the active stage of varicella should be avoided unless the neonate is also affected.

SUGGESTED READING

Centers for Disease Control: Varicella-zoster immune globulin for the prevention of chickenpox. MMWR 1984;33:84

Feder HM: Treatment of adult chickenpox with oral acyclovir. Arch Intern Med 1990;150:2061

Gershon A: Chickenpox. Contemp Ob/Gyn 1988(Mar);31:41

Haake DA, Zakowski PC, Haake DL, et al: Early treatment with acyclovir for varicella pneumonia in otherwise healthy adults: retrospective controlled study and review. Rev Infect Dis 1990:12:788

Landsberger EJ, Hager WD, Grossman JH: Successful management of varicella pneumonia complicating pregnancy. J Reprod Med 1986;31:311

McGregor JA, Mark S, Crawford GP, et al: Varicella-zoster antibody testing in the care of pregnant women exposed to varicella. Am J Obstet Gynecol 1987;157:281

Miller E, Cradock-Watson JE, Ridehalgh MK: Outcome in newborn babies given anti-varicella-zoster immunoglobin after perinatal infection with varicella-zoster virus. Lancet 1989;2:371

Paryani SG, Arvin AM: Intrauterine infection with varicella-zoster virus after maternal varicella. N Engl J Med 1986;314:1542

Preblud SR, Cochi SL, Orenstein WA: Varicella-zoster infection in pregnancy. Letter. N Engl J Med 1986;315:1416

21
Parvovirus B19 infection in pregnancy

By Philip B. Mead, MD

Background and incidence

Parvovirus B19, a single-stranded DNA virus, was discovered in 1975 and first linked to human disease in 1981 when it was found in the blood of a child with sickle cell anemia in hypoplastic crisis. B19 can cause asymptomatic infection, and has been associated with five distinct clinical syndromes: erythema infectiosum (EI) or fifth disease; acute arthritis in adults; transient aplastic crisis (TAC) in patients with sickle cell disease or other chronic hemolytic states; chronic anemia in immunodeficient patients; and fetal hydrops.

Pathophysiology

The rash of EI and clinical manifestations of B19 arthritis are thought to be immune phenomena. The more serious hematologic manifestations of B19 infection result from selective infection and lysis of erythroid precursor cells with interruption of normal red cell production. In people with normal hematopoiesis, B19 infection produces a self-limited red cell aplasia that is clinically inapparent. In patients who have increased rates of red cell destruction or loss, and who depend on compensatory increases in red cell production to maintain stable red cell indices, B19 infection may lead to aplastic crisis.

The pathogenesis of B19 fetal hydrops appears to involve hematologic, hepatic, and cardiac factors. B19 infection of erythroid precursor cells causes arrest of red cell production. The fetus is particularly vulnerable because its red cell survival is short and its red cell volume is rapidly expanding. The resulting severe anemia causes high-output cardiac failure followed by generalized edema. Extramedullary erythropoiesis leads to hypoproteinemia and portal hypertension. B19 infection of myocardial cells has been observed, suggesting that direct damage to myocardial tissue may also contribute to heart failure in the fetus.

Epidemiology

B19 is transmitted effectively after close contact exposures, presumably by respiratory secretions. The virus can also be transmitted parenterally by transfusion of blood or blood products.

Patients with EI are likely to be most contagious prior to the onset of rash, and unlikely to remain contagious for more than a few days after the appearance of the rash. Patients with TAC appear to be infectious prior to the onset of clinical symptoms through the subsequent week.

Cases of EI occur sporadically and, as part of community outbreaks, are often associated with elementary or junior high schools. Community outbreaks are common from midwinter to early summer and often last for several months or until school recesses. The incubation period of EI is usually between 4 and 14 days but can be as long as 20 days.

The secondary attack rate for infection among susceptible household contacts of patients with EI is 50% to 90%. In school outbreaks, 10% to 60% of students may develop EI; 16% to 54% of susceptible teachers and other staff may develop serologic evidence of B19 infection. In one large school outbreak the minimal rate of B19 infection in susceptible personnel during the outbreak was 19%. In two studies, approximately 37% of susceptible health-care workers became infected with B19 after being exposed to children with TAC.

Diagnosis

Seroprevalence. The reported seroprevalence ranges from 2% to 15% in children 1 to 5 years old, 15% to 60% in children 5 to 19 years old, and 30% to 60% in adults. In one study of school personnel, previous B19 infection rates ranged from a low of 45% in nonteaching high-school staff to a high of 68% in day-care providers. Overall, 58% of school personnel had evidence of previous B19 infection.

The most sensitive test for detecting recent infection is the IgM antibody assay. B19 IgM antibody can be detected by ELISA or radioimmunoassay in approximately 90% of cases by the 3rd day after symptoms begin. The IgM antibody titer begins to fall 30 to 60 days after the onset of illness, but antibody can persist at a low level for 4 months or longer. B19 IgG antibody appears around the 7th day of illness and persists for years.

To summarize diagnostic serology: The absence of B19 IgM and IgG indicates no previous infection and a susceptible individual. The presence of only B19 IgG indicates previous infection and an immune individual, although the infection may have occurred as recently as 4 months earlier. The presence of only B19 IgM indicates a very recent infection, probably within the preceding 7 days, whereas the presence of both B19 IgM and IgG suggests recent exposure, from 7 days to 6 months previously. Physicians should be aware that the laboratory will report results of both B19 IgM and IgG antibody determinations. Therefore, only a single specimen taken between 4 days and 4 weeks after onset of symptoms is necessary for the serologic diagnosis of acute infection.

Fifth disease. Erythema infectiosum is often called fifth disease after an otherwise short-lived numerical classification system of childhood rashes devised around 1900. In children, EI is a mild exanthematous disease with few constitutional symptoms. After a brief prodrome of low-grade fever, facial erythema ("slapped cheek") develops, followed by a lacy reticular rash on the trunk and extremities.

Adults may have an extremity rash, but facial erythema is uncommon. Acute arthralgias and arthritis of the hands, knees, and wrists may occur as the sole manifestation of infection in adults. A flu-like illness is also common, as is numbness and tingling of the peripheral extremities. Approximately 25% of adults infected with B19 will have a non-rash illness, and 25% will be asymptomatic.

Sequelae of fifth disease and pregnancy

Hydrops fetalis and stillbirth were first reported in 1984 as having an association with B19 infection. Since then, more than 400 cases of B19 infection during pregnancy have been described. The results were as follows: normal seronegative newborns (most cases); normal seropositive newborns; and spontaneous abortion or stillbirth due to fetal hydrops. Cases of maternal infection and subsequent fetal death have occurred during each trimester. Stillbirth has occurred 1 to 16 weeks after maternal infection.

There is no evidence that the rate of congenital anomalies following B19 infection exceeds background rates. B19-associated congenital anomalies have not been reported among several hundred liveborn infants of B19-infected mothers. One aborted fetus born to a B19-infected woman had eye anomalies and histologic evidence of damage to multiple tissues. An anencephalic fetus has also been reported in a B19-infected woman, but the timing of the infection made it unlikely that B19 contributed to the defect.

Preliminary results from a study of 174 pregnant women in the United Kingdom suggest that the risk of fetal death attributable to B19 infection after documented maternal infection is less than 10%. Using this figure and the information on susceptibility and attack rates previously presented, one can estimate the risk of fetal death after maternal exposure to B19 as follows:

Mother exposed to a household member:

50% susceptible $\times$ 70% attack rate $\times$ 10% = 3.5%;

Teacher/staff exposed at school:

42% susceptible $\times$ 19% attack rate $\times$ 10% = 0.8%.

These assumptions are based on preliminary or imprecise data and await further refinement.

Management

For pregnant women with exposure to confirmed or probable cases of B19 infection, or with symptoms compatible with fifth disease, obtain B19 IgM and IgG antibody determinations on a single specimen taken between 4 days and 4 weeks after onset of symptoms, or approximately 2 weeks after exposure if there are no symptoms.

If maternal infection is documented by the presence of B19 IgM, monitor maternal serum α-fetoprotein (MsAFP) levels and perform serial ultrasound scans. At Medical Center Hospital of Vermont, we do these tests every 2 weeks until 20 weeks' gestation. A preliminary study and two additional case reports suggest that MsAFP levels become elevated when the fetus is affected and that this change occurs before fetal hydrops is detectable by ultrasound. Elevations in MsAFP have been discovered up to 6 weeks before fetal death and 4 weeks before abnormalities were apparent by ultrasound. In these preliminary reports, fetal loss did not occur when the MsAFP level remained within normal limits for gestational age. After the 20th gestational week, lack of normative data for MsAFP levels limits the continued use of this monitor.

Early ultrasound features of fetal hydrops include a dilated heart and ascites; generalized edema and pleural effusions are late signs. In the face of normal MsAFP levels, we continue ultrasonography every 1 to 2 weeks after 20 weeks' gestation until 16 weeks after maternal illness occurred. If MsAFP levels are elevated, begin weekly ultrasonography to diagnose fetal hydrops or ascites. If fetal hydrops or ascites is suggested by ultrasonography, consider cordocentesis to obtain the following studies: hematologic indices, fetal B19 IgM (which may be negative despite fetal infection), and B19 virus studies (by DNA hybridization and electron microscopy).

If nonimmune fetal hydrops due to B19 infection is documented by findings from cordocentesis, one must consider intervention, since all but one untreated case reported to date have resulted in fetal or neonatal death. Successful use of intrauterine transfusion has been reported in a small number of cases and represents the only currently available option for treating B19-associated nonimmune fetal hydrops. Prolonged bleeding from the punctured umbilical cord has been observed in two cases and was explained by an underlying thrombocytopenia. It may therefore be advisable to have fresh blood and platelets available at the time of intrauterine transfusion.

A single case of spontaneous resolution of B19 fetal hydrops has recently been reported by Morey and co-workers. In addition, the Centers for Disease Control is aware of four such cases occurring among eight well-documented cases of B19-associated fetal hydrops (personal communication: T. J. Torok, MD). Some of these cases have been submitted for publication. This information, suggesting at least a 50% rate of spontaneous resolution, is consistent with our knowledge of the pathophysiology of B19 hydrops and indicates that a cautious approach to intrauterine transfusion may need to be adopted.

Other considerations

Pathologists should study for possible B19 parvovirus infection any hydropic fetus with nonimmune hemolytic anemia, especially if hepatitis or nucleopathic changes in the erythroblasts are identified.

Pregnant health-care workers should avoid patients with EI until at least 24 hours after onset of rash, as well as patients likely to be viremic for their entire hospitalization. The latter are patients with hereditary or acquired chronic hemolytic anemias who develop aplastic crisis or are admitted with a fever of unknown origin.

No B19 vaccine for active immunization is available at this time. No studies of prophylaxis with commercially available immune globulin preparations have been conducted, and this use is not currently recommended by the CDC. The role of hyperimmune serum globulin in the prevention or modification of fetal B19 infection is presently undefined but seems worthy of investigation based on limited adult experience.

Finally, there are at present no Public Health Service guidelines for counseling pregnant women about the occupational risks of B19 infection. Serologic testing can document the natural immunity of the majority of school and day-care staff. The remaining susceptibles are left with the difficult choice between a less than 1% risk of fetal hydrops versus prolonged, recurrent, and unplanned absences from work during community outbreaks of fifth disease.

SUGGESTED READING

Bell LM, Naides SJ, Stoffman P, et al: Human parvovirus B19 infection among hospital staff members after contact with infected patients. N Engl J Med 1989;321:485

Centers for Disease Control: Risks associated with human parvovirus B19 infection. MMWR 1989;38(6):81

Gillespie SM, Cartter ML, Asch S, et al: Occupational risk of human parvovirus B19 infection for school and day-care personnel during an outbreak of erythema infectiosum. JAMA 1990;263:2061

Kurtzman G, Frickhofen N, Kimball J, et al: Pure red-cell aplasia of 10 years' duration due to persistent parvovirus B19 infection and its cure with immunoglobulin therapy. N Engl J Med 1989;321:519

Morey AL, Nicolini V, Welch CR, et al: Parvovirus B19 infection and transient fetal hydrops. Lancet 1991;337:496

Peters MT, Nicolaides KH: Cordocentesis for the diagnosis and treatment of human fetal parvovirus infection. Obstet Gynecol 1990;75:501

Pickering LK, Reves RR: Occupational risks for child-care providers and teachers. JAMA 1990;263:2096

22

Measles
in pregnancy

By Bryan Larsen, PhD, and Sandra White

Background and incidence
Measles (rubeola) is a highly contagious viral infection generally acquired during childhood. It may produce severe sequelae in adults, and death can result from complications such as pneumonia or encephalomyelitis.

Measles continues to be a major public health concern. The number of cases has been on the rise throughout the United States since 1988. In 1990 there were 27,672 cases with at least 89 suspected deaths, a 52% increase over the 18,193 cases reported for 1989.

Etiology
The measles virus is a member of the Paramyxoviridae family. It possesses a single-stranded RNA genome and a helical nucleocapsid covered with a lipoprotein envelope acquired as the nascent virions bud from the cell membrane. Both viral proteins and host membrane components are present on the envelope.

Diagnosis
The virus is spread among susceptible persons by direct or indirect contact with respiratory secretions, particularly aerosolized ones. An incubation period of 10 to 14 days is followed by fever, cough, rhinorrhea, conjunctivitis, and the pathognomonic Koplik's spots. These spots appear on the buccal mucosa just before the eruption of a maculopapular facial and upper body rash. The erythroderma later extends to the extremities. The temperature peaks at 38.9° to 40.6°C (102° to 105°F) on the second or third day of the rash and clinical improvement of symptoms follows.

Transmission of the virus occurs as early as 3 days before onset of symptoms and as late as 7 days after the rash appears. Immunity, conferred by natural infection, is considered lifelong.

Although the majority of measles cases are diagnosed by clinical presentation alone, laboratory confirmation can be obtained by cultivating the virus from patients' specimens or by serologic techniques. Viral neutralization tests, hemagglutination inhibition tests, and an enzyme-linked immunosorbent assay (ELISA) are currently available for serodiagnosis. Seroconversion, or a fourfold rise in serum antibody titers between acute and convalescent phases, confirms infection. A single specimen for the presence of measles-specific IgM antibody may be sufficient, but it must be remembered IgM antibody may not be detectable for the first day or two after the onset of rash and is usually undetectable 60 days after rash onset. Although serologic tests are specific, sensitive, and widely available, the time required to complete them and the reliability of clinical observation limits their comparative usefulness.

Complications

Complications are reported in nearly a quarter of cases, and include diarrhea (9%), otitis media (7%), pneumonia (6.5%), and encephalitis (0.1%). Direct measles virus infection of pulmonary parenchyma may result in Hecht's giant cell pneumonia. Moreover, the normal 8-day course of measles infection may be complicated by secondary pyogenic bacterial or viral infections of the upper and lower respiratory tracts. Adults who have tuberculosis may be adversely affected by measles, though little effect has been seen in children. Bacterial otitis media is a common mild complication.

Encephalomyelitis complicates between 50 and 400 of every 10,000 measles cases. Abrupt recurrence of fever, headache, lethargy, irritability, and confusion are characteristic. However, no relationship has been established between severity of the primary disease and risk of neurologic sequelae.

A rare but severe delayed complication, subacute sclerosing panencephalitis, may occur 5 to 7 years after the primary infection. This degenerative disease, characterized by mental deterioration and motor dysfunction, is limited primarily to children between 5 and 10 years of age. Its first signs may be personality change, intellectual decline, and inappropriate behavior. These may progress over years to seizures, coma, and death. Incidence among the unvaccinated is believed to range from 0.5 to 2.0 for every 100,000 cases.

The measles mortality rate is probably less than 0.1%, but measles infection is more likely to be fatal in infants less than 1 year of age. Recently, it has been suggested that vitamin A deficiency may predispose to increased measles complications and mortality.

Vaccines

Measles vaccines, both killed and live-attenuated, were introduced for general use in 1963. Since then, disease incidence has declined to relatively low levels.

The killed measles vaccine, which elicited only short-term protection and was linked to atypical measles syndrome, was withdrawn in 1967. The live-attenuated vaccine (Edmondston B strain) proved to be highly immunogenic but was associated with high adverse reaction rates unless given with antiserum. Other attentuated strains (Shwartz, Moraten) in general use by 1970 offered the advantage of fewer side effects in the immediate postvaccination period. These preparations are highly effective, stimulating production of protective antibodies in at least 95% of susceptible persons properly vaccinated.

The effectiveness of immunization, measured by antibody response and by protection afforded on subsequent exposure, ranges in various studies from 91% to 99% for adequately immunized children. As a result, persons so immunized have a high probability of protection. Most susceptible individuals in the population are either unvaccinated, improperly vaccinated, or were vaccinated at a time when a less effective preparation was in use.

Despite a constantly declining measles incidence since introduction of the measles vaccines, outbreaks still occur. New strategies for elimination are being considered by public health officials, particularly in urban areas where contact among contagious persons can cause rapid spread. Major outbreaks have occurred recently in the US among unvaccinated preschool-aged children as well as among vaccinated school- and college-aged populations.

In several inner-city areas, up to 88% of vaccine-eligible children between 16 months and 4 years of age have not been vaccinated. In school-aged children the vaccination level is above 98%. Primary vaccine failure accounts for part of this problem. Children vaccinated earlier than 15 months of age have higher attack rates than those vaccinated at older ages. The Advisory Committee on Immunization Practices has recently published a revised policy for measles vaccination. A routine two-dose measles vaccination schedule is now recommended (Table 1).

Although there are no reports of malformations among newborns whose mothers inadvertently received measles vaccine, pregnant women or women likely to become pregnant within 3 months after vaccination should not be given live attenuated-virus vaccines. However, children of pregnant women can be safely vaccinated without danger of transmitting the viruses to the mother.

Postpartum vaccination of a woman who is known to be suscepti-

TABLE 1
Recommendations for measles vaccination

Population	Dosage/documentation
Routine childhood schedule:	
Most areas	Two doses: first at 15 months; second at 4 to 6 years (entry to kindergarten or first grade)
High-risk areas	First dose at 12 months; second dose at 4 to 6 years
Colleges and other educational institutions post-high school	Documentation of receipt of two doses after the first birthday or other evidence of measles immunity*
Medical personnel beginning employment	Documentation of receipt of two doses after the first birthday or other evidence of measles immunity*

*Prior physician-diagnosed measles disease, laboratory evidence of measles immunity, or birth before 1957.
Source: Centers for Disease Control: MMWR 1989;38(S-9).

ble to rubella provides an opportunity to offer measles vaccine if indicated. Patients can receive either measles–rubella or measles–mumps–rubella vaccine. Susceptibility to measles need not be based on serologic testing, since immunization of persons already immune is not associated with an increased risk of adverse events. As is the case with any woman of childbearing age, counseling to avoid conception for 3 months following vaccination is necessary. Breast-feeding is not a contraindication to vaccination with measles, mumps, and rubella vaccines. Although rubella vaccine virus may be excreted in breast milk and may infect breast-fed infants, it has not been shown to produce significant adverse effects. While there are no direct data for measles and mumps vaccine viruses, the experience with rubella vaccine indicates that administration of measles or mumps vaccine is also not contraindicated in this situation.

Management during pregnancy
Widespread immunity in adults as a result of vaccination or early infection accounts for the naturally low incidence of gestational measles. Measles infection during pregnancy progresses along the same course as that in the nonpregnant woman and lasts about

8 days. However, when measles reached the previously unexposed population of Greenland in 1951, mortality among pregnant women was nearly threefold greater than among nonpregnant women. This difference may have reflected the combined effects of the lack of "herd immunity" coupled with the well-known modulation of cellular immunity that occurs as an accommodation of the female to pregnancy.

Although the fetus can become infected from the maternal virus through transplacental transmission, such infection is infrequent. No specific pattern of congenital malformations has been associated with transplacentally acquired measles virus. However, measles infection, like other acute febrile illnesses, may interfere with carriage of the pregnancy to term. Thus, increments in the incidence of spontaneous abortion and premature delivery have been recorded during measles epidemics.

When measles infection occurs near the time of delivery, the fetus may be infected at birth or within 12 days after delivery. Severe respiratory disease in the infant is a serious complication that may be attenuated by administering immunoglobulin to the affected newborn.

Although there is no specific treatment for pregnant women with measles, immune globulin can be given to prevent or modify measles in a susceptible patient. Therefore, immune globulin, at 0.25 mL/kg IM, should be given to susceptible exposed pregnant women. To be effective, this dose must be given within 6 days of exposure.

Children born to women who have measles in the last week of pregnancy or the first week postpartum should receive immune globulin as soon as possible.

SUGGESTED READING

Amstey MS: Measles in pregnancy, in Gleicher N (ed): *Principles of Medical Therapy.* New York, Plenum, 1985, pp 561-562

Atmar RL, Englund JA, Hammill H: Complications of measles during pregnancy. Clin Infec Dis 1992;14:217

Centers for Disease Control: Measles prevention: recommendations of the Immunization Practices Advisory Committee (ACIP). MMWR 1989;38(S-9):1-18

Korones SB: Infectious complications of pregnancy: influenza, mumps and measles. Clin Perinatol 1988;15:267

Modlin JF: Measles virus, in Belshe RB (ed): *Human Virology.* Littleton, Mass, PSG Publishing, 1984, pp 333-360

South MR, Sever JL: Viral and protozoan diseases, in Danforth DN, Scott JR (eds): *Obstetrics and Gynecology,* ed 5. Philadelphia, JP Lippincott, 1986, pp 551-561

23
Mumps
in pregnancy

By R. David Miller, MD, and W. David Hager, MD

Background and incidence

Mumps virus is a member of the paramyxovirus family, which also includes rubeola virus. Mumps is primarily a disease of children aged 5 to 15 and has a world-wide distribution. In the United States, incidence increases in the winter, peaking in March and April. Epidemics tend to occur in confined populations such as boarding schools and military encampments.

Since the introduction of mumps vaccine in 1967, when 152,209 cases were reported in the US, the incidence of clinical mumps has declined dramatically to 2,900 to 5,800 cases annually. Incidence in pregnancy has been estimated to be from 0.8 to 10 cases per 10,000 pregnancies. Death from mumps in adults with intact immune systems is rare.

Pathophysiology

Mumps is transmitted by droplet nuclei, saliva, and fomites. Since there is no good animal model, the precise pathogenesis of infection has not been established. The virus initially replicates in the epithelium of the upper respiratory tract. A viremia follows, after which the agent localizes in glandular or central nervous system tissues. Parotitis is believed to occur as a result of the viremia.

Studies of the pathology of mumps are few because it is rarely a fatal disease. The histologic changes in the parotid gland and the testis are similar. There is necrosis of acinar and ductal epithelial cells in the salivary glands and of the germinal epithelium of the seminiferous tubules. The significance of this disease in obstetrics, however, rests with its effects on the fetus.

Diagnosis

History plays an important role in making a diagnosis of mumps, since the patient presenting with a suspicion of the disease will have been in close contact with a person who has acquired mumps. Mumps patients have a typical viral prodrome of fever, anorexia, malaise, and myalgia. These symptoms are followed within the next 24 hours by infection and swelling of the glands, which will resolve in 1 week or less.

Parotitis is a bilateral infection, although the onset of disease may be asynchronous. The submaxillary and sublingual glands are only rarely involved. Mumps may involve the gonads of the male and rarely will cause aseptic meningitis, mastitis, thyroiditis, myocarditis, nephritis, or arthritis in both sexes.

Maternal effects. Mumps in pregnancy is generally a benign illness and not appreciably more severe than it is in other adult women. Mastitis and thyroiditis can occur in postpartum women, but not more frequently than in nonpregnant women.

Fetal effects. Studies comparing women who have mumps during the first trimester with uninfected pregnant women show a significant increase in spontaneous abortion rates. Most of these pregnancy losses occur within 2 weeks of the infection.

There is no increased risk of prematurity among women who acquire mumps in the second or third trimester. Although there is evidence of an increased risk of congenital anomalies such as endocardial fibroelastosis associated with mumps in animal models, data are lacking to support such a relationship in humans. Presence of maternal mumps infection is not an indication for therapeutic abortion.

Congenital mumps or postnatally acquired perinatal mumps has rarely if ever been documented virologically or serologically. Among the possible explanations for this are:

- protection of the neonate by passive maternal antibodies;
- exclusion of mumps virus from the fetus by a hypothetical placental barrier;
- relative insusceptibility of fetal and neonatal tissues to infection by the virus; and
- occurrence of infections that are predominantly subclinical.

Treatment

Treatment of mumps parotitis is symptomatic. The use of analgesics and antipyretics is indicated, plus application of cold packs to the parotid gland and breasts. There is no evidence that mumps immune globulin has a beneficial effect in treating established disease. Some severe cases of orchitis have been reported to respond to systemic corticosteroids.

Immunization. The use of live attenuated mumps virus vaccine induces the production of protective antibodies in 95% of recipients. The vaccine is usually administered along with measles and rubella vaccines at 15 months of age. It should never be administered to infants less than 1 year old, to pregnant women, or to immunocompromised patients.

SUGGESTED READING

Chretien JH, McGinniss CG, Thompson J, et al: Group B beta-hemolytic streptococci causing pharyngitis. J Clin Microbiol 1979;10:263

Garcia A, Pereira J, Vidigal N, et al: Intrauterine infection with mumps virus. Obstet Gynecol 1980;56:756

Gershon AA: Chickenpox, measles, and mumps, in Remington JS, Klein JO (eds): *Infectious Diseases of the Fetus and Newborn Infant*, ed 3. Philadelphia, WB Saunders, 1990, pp 432-445

Lim DV, Morales WJ, Walsh AF: Lim group B strep broth and coagglutination for rapid identification of group B streptococci in preterm pregnant women. J Clin Microbiol 1987;25:452

Nahmias AJ, Armstrong G: Mumps virus and endocardial fibroelastosis. N Engl J Med 1966;275:1449

Monif GR: Maternal mumps infection during gestation: observations on the progeny. Am J Obstet Gynecol 1974;119:549

Stagno S, Whitley RJ: Herpesvirus infections of pregnancy. N Engl J Med 1985;313:1272

Swan C: Congenital malformations associated with rubella and other virus infections, in Banks HS (ed): *Modern Practice in Infectious Fevers*. New York, PB Hoeber, 1951, vol 2, pp 528-552

24
Rubella
in pregnancy

By John H. Grossman III, MD, PhD

Background and incidence

In 1988 the Centers for Disease Control reported an all-time annual low of 225 cases of rubella in the United States. However, the number of reported cases increased twofold in 1989 and an additional three-fold in 1990, reaching 1,093, the highest total since 1982.

In 1990 ten confirmed cases of congenital rubella syndrome (CRS) in US-born infants were reported to the CDC's National Congenital Rubella Syndrome Registry. In contrast, during 1988 only two infants were born with CRS, and in 1989 only one.

These reports indicate a moderate resurgence of rubella and a major increase in CRS in the United States. This resurgence follows the substantial reduction in reported rubella cases seen during the mid-1980s, associated with an increased emphasis on vaccinating adolescents and adults, particularly women of childbearing age. Because a substantial proportion (6% to 25%) of women in this age group remain susceptible, the potential risk for CRS persists.

Pathophysiology

Rubella is a single-stranded RNA virus belonging to the togavirus family. It is acquired as a respiratory disease 2 to 3 weeks after exposure. Infectious virus is usually present in the nasopharynx and upper respiratory tract 1 week before symptoms develop. When clinical illness becomes apparent, a discrete pink–red maculopapular rash appears on the face and then spreads to the trunk and extremities. The rash lasts 3 days. Postauricular and suboccipital lymphadenopathy, fever, and arthralgias may also be present. From 25% to 50% of all rubella infections are subclinical. Conversely, skin rashes resembling rubella may occur as a result of adenovirus, enterovirus, or other respiratory virus infections. Thus, laboratory testing is necessary to confirm the diagnosis of infection.

In 1941, Gregg, an Australian ophthalmologist, associated the development of cataracts in children with an epidemic of maternal rubella infection. Long-term follow-up of children born during US epidemics has established the clinical features of congenital rubella syndrome. The eyes, heart, and CNS are most frequently affected at birth. Cataracts, glaucoma, microphthalmia, and chorioretinitis are common ophthalmologic problems. Peripheral pulmonic stenosis, patent ductus arteriosus, and septal defects are frequent manifestations of congenital heart disease. Mental retardation, microcephaly, and, rarely, encephalitis are neurologic manifestations of illness. Sensorineural deafness is the most common consequence.

A direct effect of rubella virus infection is decreased cell replication. This may result in growth retardation and failure of normal cellular differentiation during embryogenesis. The inflammatory response to infection or autoimmune reactions that may be triggered by infection may also produce tissue damage. Myocarditis, pneumonitis, hepatosplenomegaly, and vascular stenosis may be manifestations of these processes. In approximately 20% of individuals, late manifestations of infection develop at 10 to 20 years of age. These include endocrinopathies (insulin-dependent diabetes, thyroid abnormalities, hypoadrenalism), hearing loss or additional ocular damage, and, rarely, progressive rubella panencephalitis.

Several large studies have conclusively demonstrated that first-trimester maternal infection is associated with a high (70% to 90%) incidence of developmental malformation. Deafness and mental retardation may result when infection occurs as late as the sixth gestational month. Structural defects, however, do not appear to occur as a consequence of third-trimester gestational infection. The absence of clinical manifestations of disease at birth does not exclude the possibility of subclinical damage or subsequent impairment. Consequently, offspring of women who have sustained rubella infections during pregnancy should undergo careful long-term follow-up.

Diagnosis

The presence of subclinical rubella among adults and newborns underscores the importance of laboratory confirmation in clinically suspicious cases. Although virus can be isolated from nasopharyngeal secretions, this approach is largely of historic and research interest. Few laboratory facilities provide this service, and rubella isolation usually takes 4 to 6 weeks to complete.

Serologic testing is the cornerstone of laboratory confirmation of recent rubella infection or immunity. With very few exceptions, demonstration of detectable rubella antibody constitutes proof of immunity from subsequent systemic infection. Conversely, demonstration of serologic conversion using paired acute and convalescent specimens implies recent infection even among asymptomatic individuals.

The "gold standard" for serologic testing has historically been the hemagglutination inhibition test. The presence of antirubella antibody in test serum blocks agglutination of chick red blood cells by rubella virus. Technical difficulties with this reference method have led to the development of less expensive and less labor-intensive alternative approaches. Reliable serologic methods based upon latex agglutination, fluorescence immunoassay, passive hemagglutination, and enzyme immunoassay are all examples of available alternatives.

Rubella-specific IgG, whether the consequence of natural infection or immunization, persists for life and can be detected by enzyme immunoassay at least 16 years after seroconversion. Recent rubella infection can be confirmed by demonstrating the presence of rubella-specific IgM antibody. This becomes detectable about 1 week after the onset of illness and persists for about 1 month.

Recently, new scientific technologies have been applied to the diagnosis of congenital rubella infection. Demonstration of rubella-specific IgM in fetal blood obtained by cordocentesis has been used to establish diagnosis in utero. Seroreactivity has been shown as early as the 19th gestational week.

At least one false-negative serology associated with subsequent congenital infection has been reported when testing was performed at the 20th gestational week. Although experience with this approach is still limited, serologic testing of fetal blood appears reliable once fetal immunoresponsiveness has developed (gestational weeks 20 to 24). Chorionic villus sampling with recovery of virus by culture has also been used to diagnose such first-trimester infections.

Immunoblotting with rubella-specific monoclonal antibodies and hybridization with cloned radioactively labeled rubella-complementary DNA probes appear to be more sensitive methods for detecting first-trimester infection than virus isolation from chorionic villus tissue samples. Although experience with these approaches is currently limited, they are clearly feasible and represent promising approaches for directing management of certain cases.

Treatment
Since 1969, vaccines for rubella have been available in the US. Vaccination produces seroconversion with long-term immunity from infection in 95% of all cases. Rashes, arthropathy, and lymphadenopathy are occasional self-limited complications of vaccination.

Transient peripheral neurologic complaints also very rarely occur.

It is currently recommended that all children be immunized against rubella infection when they reach 15 months of age. Additionally, women of childbearing age who do not have detectable rubella IgG antibody should also be immunized, provided that they are not pregnant when they receive the vaccine and will not become pregnant for at least 3 months after immunization.

Since 1971, the CDC has maintained a registry for women who have been inadvertently vaccinated against rubella during their pregnancy. There have been no observed cases of congenital rubella syndrome among more than 500 individuals in the registry who have been exposed. Although rubella vaccination is still not recommended during pregnancy, the risks of congenital rubella syndrome following vaccination within 3 months of conception are now considered to be negligible. Consequently, inadvertent rubella vaccination is no longer considered by itself to be an indication for the termination of pregnancy. The Centers for Disease Control still states, however, that the patient and her physician should make the final decision regarding continuation of pregnancy in individual cases.

Based upon this experience, the CDC currently recommends that routine laboratory screening for both pregnancy and the rubella antibody is unnecessary before administering vaccine and that health-care workers should routinely offer the rubella vaccine whenever they encounter a potentially susceptible woman lacking contraindications for vaccination. As of April 30, 1989, the Centers for Disease Control discontinued accepting new enrollees into the Rubella Vaccine in Pregnancy Registry.

Prevention
Despite the increased incidence of rubella in 1990, the rate still represented a decline of 98% from that for 1966–1968, the period immediately before vaccine licensure. Limited data from outbreaks reported in 1990 suggest that failure to vaccinate, rather than vaccine failure, has been responsible for the recent increase in rubella. This conclusion is supported by studies showing the long-term persistence of vaccine-induced immunity to rubella.

Many of the rubella outbreaks in 1990 occurred in crowded or closely contained settings which facilitated transmission to susceptible persons. In California, for example, at least 14 pregnant women were exposed to rubella as a result of prison exposure.

The CDC has suggested the following strategies for improving rubella prevention and control:

(1) Encourage health-care providers to implement recommended immunization guidelines to improve rubella vaccine coverage levels

among children and adults, particularly women of childbearing age.

(2) Establish prevention and control programs in all correctional facilities.

(3) Identify missed or underused opportunities for vaccinating susceptible adults and adolescents (such as immediate postpartum vaccination of susceptibles).

SUGGESTED READING

Centers for Disease Control: Rubella vaccination during pregnancy—United States, 1971-1988. MMWR 1989;38:289

Centers for Disease Control: Increase in rubella and congenital rubella syndrome—United States, 1988-1990. MMWR 1991;40:93

Cradock-Watson JE, Miller E, Ridehalgh MK, et al: Detection of rubella virus in fetal and placental tissues and in the throats of neonates after serologically confirmed rubella in pregnancy. Prenat Diagn 1989;9:91

Daffos F, Forestier F, Grangeot-Keros L, et al: Prenatal diagnosis of congenital rubella. Lancet 1984;2:1

Mann JM, Preblud SR, Hoffman RE, et al: Assessing risks of rubella infection during pregnancy. JAMA 1981;245:1647

South MA, Sever JL: The congenital rubella syndrome, in Sever JL, Brent RL (eds): *Teratogen Update: Environmentally Induced Birth Defect Risks.* New York, Alan R Liss, 1986, p 81

Terry GM, Ho-Terry L, Warren RC, et al: First trimester prenatal diagnosis of congenital rubella: a laboratory investigation. Br Med J 1986;292:930

25
Viral influenza in pregnancy

By Joseph J. Apuzzio, MD

Background and incidence

Viral influenza is still a common and potentially serious problem for pregnant women. In the pandemic of 1918, the mortality rate was higher in pregnant than in nonpregnant women. Many fatalities probably resulted from secondary infection with bacterial pneumonia, frequently caused by coagulase-positive staphylococci. No antibiotics were available to treat this complication.

Today, fatalities related to viral influenza infections are still primarily from complications of pneumonia, but they are not common, as in the preantibiotic era. Researchers have estimated that 0.01% to 0.1% of the population at large is at risk for death from influenza. One death, reported in the fall of 1988, was that of a 32-year-old woman at 36 weeks' gestation who died of swine flu pneumonia despite intensive medical support. Other less common complications of influenza include myocarditis, pericarditis, aseptic meningitis, and postinfection neuritis.

Etiology

Influenza is caused by an orthomyxovirus that has three distinct types—A, B, and C. Type A is the epidemic type, type B is less common, and type C is least likely to cause epidemics.

The virus contains RNA and has an enveloped helical nucleocapsid enclosing two types of glycoprotein antigens, hemagglutinin (HA) and neuroaminidase (NA). NA is concentrated in that region of the viral envelope where newly formed virus particles are released from the host cell. Thirteen different subtypes of HA and nine subtypes of NA exist, allowing antigenic shifts in the virus to cause new epidemics. Alterations in the amino acid sequence of these proteins change their antigenic ability and thus recognition by a host cell.

During the 1987–1988 influenza season, influenza A (H_3N_2) dominated, with few cases of influenza B. However, during the 1988–1989 season, influenza B dominated, with most cases reported in children. Influenza B epidemics have often resulted in excess mortality compared with influenza A epidemics. During the 1989–1990 season, influenza A caused the most influenza activity in the US and worldwide.

Aerosol droplets spread the influenza viruses when an infected person coughs or sneezes. People in the immediate area may inhale these virus-laden droplets. If the virus is not neutralized by a specific antibody from previous exposure, replication begins. Because of the aerosol spread, there is a very high attack rate of the influenza virus, especially in closed environments, such as classrooms, vehicles, and workplaces.

Diagnosis

Illness may range from occasional asymptomatic infection to more serious and occasionally fatal primary influenza pneumonia. The usual clinical course begins within 1 to 4 days after exposure with a sudden rise in temperature—often up to 39.2°C (102.5°F)—accompanied by myalgias, lassitude, sore throat, nasal congestion, cough, and headache. Because of the severe physical lassitude and malaise, the patient may spend several days in bed. Symptoms usually subside within several days, and patients usually can resume their customary activities.

Pneumonias, the most serious complication of influenza, are of two types. The more frequent is a secondary bacterial infection, with the most common infecting organisms being *Staphylococcus aureus*, *Streptococcus pneumoniae*, and *Haemophilus influenzae*.

The second type, caused solely by the influenza virus, is uncommon but potentially more lethal. A patient may have paroxysms of coughing, shortness of breath, and scant sputum. Hypoxia may occur and chest x-ray may reveal an infiltrate. These patients may need aggressive medical therapy with respiratory support, as well as a trial of antiviral agents.

Diagnostic aids. The diagnosis of influenza is made primarily by the history and clinical evaluation. The virus may be grown in the laboratory, but this is usually not practical in most clinical situations. Serologic confirmation of the infection is usually not required, although complement fixation and hemagglutination tests are available.

When you suspect superimposed pneumonia, a chest x-ray, as well as examination of the sputum with a Gram stain and culture, is important. Appropriate antibiotic therapy, as determined by Gram staining and culture, is needed for patients suspected of having bacterial pneumonia.

Treatment

The treatment of uncomplicated viral influenza infection is supportive. Antipyretics, such as acetaminophen for myalgias and fever, as well as bed rest, will comfort the patient. Aspirin may increase the risk of Reye's syndrome in children and teenagers, especially when type B influenza predominates.

In nonpregnant patients, early treatment with amantadine hydrochloride often diminishes the severity of symptoms and may hasten clinical recovery from infections with influenza A. Amantadine also reduces the titer and duration of viral excretion, as well as the altered pulmonary function that may last for several weeks after the infection.

The use of amantadine is relatively contraindicated in pregnancy, however. Although there are no large-scale studies of its use in pregnancy, the drug is embryotoxic and teratogenic when used in high doses in animals. In an isolated case report, its use in the first trimester was associated with the development of a complex cardiovascular defect in the infant. It was hypothesized that agents that inhibit lymphocyte stimulation, such as amantadine and thalidomide, share teratogenic potential. The absence of other case reports may reflect the probable infrequency of use of the drug in pregnant patients. In view of these concerns, symptomatic treatment for influenza in most pregnant women would seem to be a safer course than the use of amantadine, unless it is needed as a lifesaving measure.

Pregnant patients experiencing respiratory failure from influenza pneumonia may benefit from therapy with amantadine and other agents. Kirshon and co-workers reported a favorable outcome for a pregnant patient with influenza pneumonia and respiratory failure who was treated with oral amantadine and ribavirin inhalation therapy. Ribavirin has antiviral activity against influenza virus, respiratory syncytial virus, and herpes simplex virus, but it is teratogenic and embryotoxic in animals. There are no human studies. Therefore, its use during pregnancy must be limited to clearly lifesaving indications.

Prevention

Because there is no specific treatment for influenza, an attempt at prevention is appropriate in pregnant women at increased risk for influenza-related complications (Table 1). Vaccinate these patients in November before the flu season begins. In the US, high levels of influenza activity are usually not seen before late December.

TABLE 1
Pregnant women at increased risk for influenza-related complications

Those with chronic disorders of the pulmonary or cardiovascular systems

Those who have required regular medical followup or hospitalization during the preceding year because of chronic metabolic diseases (including diabetes mellitus), renal dysfunction, hemoglobinopathies, or immunosuppression (including immunosuppression caused by medications)

Teenagers up to 18 years of age who are receiving long-term aspirin therapy and therefore may be at risk of developing Reye's syndrome after influenza

Those infected with HIV

Influenza vaccine is considered safe for pregnant women and should be offered to patients who have medical conditions that increase their risks of complications from influenza.

If possible, wait until the second trimester before vaccinating such a pregnant patient to preclude the theoretic risk of teratogenesis. However, it may be unwise to wait for the second trimester if influenza activity in the community is imminent or has already begun. The inactivated vaccine is modified each year in anticipation of the new viral antigens. Since influenza-associated excess mortality among pregnant women has not been documented except in the pandemics of 1918–1919 and 1957–1958, it is probably unnecessary to routinely vaccinate low-risk pregnant women. Amantadine should not be given to pregnant women for influenza prophylaxis except as a lifesaving measure.

Sequelae
The influenza virus crosses the placenta and has been considered a cause of fetal malformation. However, the literature is not clear on this issue. Several studies have indicated a 1% increase in congenital malformation over the control group. But other, larger series, including the Collaborative Perinatal Research Study, have not been able to show an increased risk of congenital malformation from first-trimester influenza infection.

Therefore, it is unlikely that there is an increased risk of congenital malformation. If it exists, this risk is very small, especially considering the background rate of 3% to 5% for congenital malformations during any pregnancy.

SUGGESTED READING

Centers for Disease Control: Human infection with swine influenza virus. MMWR 1988;37:61

Centers for Disease Control: Prevention and control of influenza. MMWR 1990;39(RR-7):1-15

Coulson AA: Amantadine and teratogenesis. Letter. Lancet 1975;2:1044

Elizan T, Ajero-Froehich L, Fabiyi A, et al: Viral infection in pregnancy and congenital CNS malformations in vivo. Arch Neurol 1969;20:115

Kirshon B, Faro S, Zurawin R, et al: Favorable outcome after treatment with amantadine and ribavirin in a pregnancy complicated by influenza pneumonia. J Reprod Med 1988;33:399

McGregor J, Burns J, Levin M, et al: Transplacental passage of influenza A/Bangkok mimicking amniotic fluid infection syndrome. Am J Obstet Gynecol 1984;149:856

Nora JJ, Nora AH, Way GL: Cardiovascular maldevelopment associated with maternal exposure to amantadine. Letter. Lancet 1975;2:607

Sever J, Larsen J, Grossman J: *Handbook of Perinatal Infection*. Boston, Little, Brown & Co, 1989

26

Hepatitis B infection in pregnancy

By David A. Baker, MD

Background and incidence

Each year in the United States, an estimated 300,000 persons, primarily young adults, are infected with hepatitis B virus (HBV). One quarter become ill with jaundice, more than 10,000 require hospitalization, and an average of 250 die of fulminant disease. The pool of infectious carriers in the US is currently estimated at 750,000 to 1,000,000.

Transmission of HBV from mother to infant during the prenatal period represents one of the most efficient modes of HBV spread and often leads to severe long-term sequelae. However, the availability of a safe and effective vaccine offers the opportunity to prevent fetal infection and its serious consequences.

Etiology

This infection is caused by a small, double-stranded DNA virus. Several well-defined antigen–antibody systems are associated with HBV infection. Hepatitis B surface antigen (HBsAg) is produced in excess amounts, circulating in blood as 22-nm spherical and tubular particles. HBsAg can be identified in serum 30 to 60 days after exposure to HBV and persists for variable periods. Anti-HBs develops after a resolved infection and is responsible for long-term immunity.

Antibody to core antigen (anti-HBc) develops in all HBV infections and persists indefinitely. IgM anti-HBc appears early in infection and persists for 6 months or longer. It is a reliable marker of acute or recent HBV infection. A third antigen, hepatitis B e antigen (HBeAg), may be detected in samples from persons with acute or chronic HBV infection. The presence of HBeAg correlates with viral replication and high infectivity. Antibody to HBeAg (anti-HBe) develops in most

TABLE 1

Commonly encountered serologic patterns of hepatitis B infection

HBsAg	Anti-HBs	Anti-HBc	HBeAg	Anti-HBe
+	−	IgM	+	−
+	−	IgG	+	−
+	−	IgG	−	+
+	+	+	+/−	+/−
−	−	IgM	+/−	+/−
−	−	IgG	−	+/−
−	+	IgG	−	+/−
−	+	−	−	−

HBV infections and correlates with the loss of replicating virus and with lower infectivity.

Epidemiology

The major modes of HBV transmission are contact with blood, sexual activity, and vertical transmission from mothers to newborns.

The newborn will be infected if the mother has acute HBV infection during the third trimester or is a chronic carrier. Perinatal transmission is very high (70% to 90%) if the mother is not only HBsAg-positive but also HBeAg-positive. If the mother is positive only for HBsAg, the chances of transmission in the newborn period are approximately 15%.

The role of the HBV carrier is central in the epidemiology of HBV transmission. A carrier is defined as a person who is HBsAg-positive

Interpretation

Acute HBV infection, high infectivity

Chronic HBV infection, high infectivity

Late-acute or chronic HBV infection, low infectivity

1. HBsAg of one subtype and heterotypic anti-HBs (common)
2. Process of seroconversion from HBsAg to anti-HBs (rare)

1. Acute HBV infection
2. Anti-HBc window

1. Low-level HBsAg carrier
2. Remote past infection

Recovery from HBV infection

1. Immunization with HBsAg (after vaccination)
2. Possible remote past infection
3. False-positive

on at least two occasions at least 6 months apart. Although the degree of infectivity is best correlated with HBeAg-positivity, any person positive for HBsAg is also potentially infectious. The likelihood of developing the carrier state varies inversely with the age at which infection occurs. During the perinatal period, HBV transmitted from HBeAg-positive mothers results in HBV carriage in up to 90% of infected infants, whereas only 6% to 10% of acutely infected adults become carriers.

Diagnosis

Precise diagnosis is carried out by use of serologic tests for the HBV antigens (HBsAg and HBeAg), and for antibodies to HBsAg, HBcAg, and HBeAg. Table 1 lists the common serologic patterns of HBV infection. Sensitive and specific techniques have been developed to

TABLE 2

Current recommendations for prenatal HBV screening and prevention of perinatal transmission

1. All pregnant women should be tested routinely for HBsAg during an early prenatal visit. When acute hepatitis is suspected, when a history of exposure to hepatitis has been reported, or when the mother has a particularly high-risk behavior such as IV drug abuse, an additional HBsAg test can be ordered later in pregnancy. No other HBV marker tests are necessary for the purpose of maternal screening, although HBsAg-positive mothers identified during screening may have HBV-related acute or chronic liver disease and should be evaluated by their physicians.

2. For patients not tested prior to delivery, HBsAg testing should be done on admission.

3. Infants born to HBsAg-positive mothers
   (a) should receive HBIG, 0.5 mL IM within 12 hours of birth;
   (b) should be given HB vaccine concurrently with the HBIG, but at a different site; completion of the HB vaccine series should be carried out as recommended for specific vaccine preparations

4. Infants should be tested for HBsAg and its antibody (anti-HBs) at 12 to 15 months of age.

5. The mother's sexual partners and household members should be tested and vaccinated appropriately

6. Obstetric and pediatric staff should be notified directly about HBsAg positivity in mothers, so that neonates can receive therapy after birth without delay and be given follow-up doses of vaccine.

identify markers in serum of suspected cases. Knowing both the clinical presentation and the serologic pattern, one can identify the specific stage of hepatitis B infection.

Usually there is a prodrome of symptoms that are gradual in onset. The disease may present as a flu-like syndrome, with fatigue, anorexia, nausea, and vomiting. Myalgia, malaise, headache, and pharyngitis may also occur. Approximately 2 weeks after these symptoms appear, jaundice may be clinically evident along with a low-grade fever.

Clinical manifestations parallel the severity of the disease. In 10%

to 20% of patients, signs of hepatomegaly, splenomegaly, and lymphadenopathy may appear. Jaundice may persist for 4 to 6 weeks while symptoms slowly resolve. There is a slow healing phase that may take up to 3 months, but the overwhelming majority of patients recover completely from hepatitis B infection. Approximately 5%, however, will become chronic carriers.

It appears that the chronic carrier state is much more common among those who acquired the infection vertically and among patients infected while immunosuppressed.

Treatment
There is currently no specific therapy for HBV infection aside from supportive care.

Prevention
Because they are frequently exposed to body fluids, health-care workers should be considered at high risk and should receive hepatitis B vaccine. In the US, approximately 15% of health-care workers contract HBV infection. The principal source of these infections is the asymptomatic hospital patient who gives no history of HBV exposure and has not been screened for it.

Current recommendations include screening all health-care workers for serologic evidence of hepatitis B and immunizing those who are seronegative with hepatitis B vaccine. Both passive prophylaxis with hepatitis B immunoglobulin and active prophylaxis with hepatitis B vaccine are currently available. The vaccine is based on HBsAg, the surface antigen, and has been demonstrated to be safe and highly effective.

In the US, an estimated 18,000 births occur to HBsAg-positive women each year, producing approximately 4,000 infants who become chronic HBV carriers. In many populations, including the indigent, selective screening has failed to identify one half to two thirds of infected mothers. Accordingly, the Centers for Disease Control has recommended prenatal HBsAg screening of all pregnant women. This practice makes it possible to treat newborns of infected women, which is 85% to 95% effective in preventing development of the HBV chronic carrier state. The CDC recommendations are outlined in Table 2.

Sequelae
Between 6% and 10% of young adults with HBV become carriers. Chronic active hepatitis develops in over 25% of carriers and often progresses to cirrhosis. Furthermore, HBV carriers' risk of developing primary liver cancer is 12 to 300 times higher than that of other

persons. It is estimated that 4,000 persons die from hepatitis B–related cirrhosis each year in the US and that more than 800 die from hepatitis B–related liver cancer.

As noted previously, infants born to HBsAg-positive and HBeAg-positive mothers have a 70% to 90% chance of acquiring perinatal HBV infection, and 85% to 90% of infected infants will become chronic HBV carriers (as opposed to 6% to 10% of infected adults). Estimates are that more than 25% of these carriers will die from primary hepatocellular carcinoma or cirrhosis. Infants born to HBsAg-positive and HBeAg-negative mothers have a lower risk of acquiring perinatal infection. However, such infants have had acute disease, and fatal fulminant hepatitis has also been reported in this group.

SUGGESTED READING

American Academy of Pediatrics Committee on Infectious Diseases: Prevention of hepatitis B virus infection. Pediatrics 1985;75:362

Arevalo JA, Washington E: Course effectiveness of prenatal screening and immunization for hepatitis B virus. JAMA 1988; 259:365.

Beasley RP, Hwang LY, Lee GC, et al: Prevention of perinatally transmitted hepatitis B virus infections with hepatitis B immunoglobulin and hepatitis B vaccine. Lancet 1983;2:1099

Centers for Disease Control: Prevention of perinatal transmission of hepatitis B virus: prenatal screening of all pregnant women for hepatitis B surface antigen. MMWR 1988; 37:341

Centers for Disease Control: Protection against viral hepatitis: recommendations of the Immunization Practices Advisory Committee. MMWR 1990;39(RR-2):1-26

Cruz AC, Frentzen BH, Behnke M: Hepatitis B: a case for prenatal screening of all patients. Am J Obstet Gynecol 1987;156:1180

Dinstag JL, Wants JR, Koff RS: Acute hepatitis, in Braunwald E, Isselbacher KJ, Petersdorf RG, et al (eds): *Harrison's Principles of Internal Medicine.* New York, McGraw-Hill, 1987, pp 1325-1335

Jonas MM, Schiff ER, O'Sullivan MJ, et al: Failure of Centers for Disease Control criteria to identify hepatitis B infection in a large municipal obstetrical population. Ann Intern Med 1987;107:335

Jonas MM, Reddy RK, DeMedina M, et al: Hepatitis B infection in a large municipal obstetrical population: characterization and prevention of perinatal transmission. Am J Gastroenterol 1990;85:277

Koretz R: Universal perinatal hepatitis B testing: is it cost-effective? Obstet Gynecol 1989;74:808

Summers PR, Viswas MJ, Pastorek JG, et al: The pregnant hepatitis B carrier: evidence favoring comprehensive antepartum screening. Obstet Gynecol 1987;69:701

27
Toxoplasmosis in pregnancy

By John L. Sever, MD, PhD

Background and incidence

Studies of pregnant women in the US have shown that about 15% to 40% have antibody to *Toxoplasma gondii* and thus have experienced infection with this organism. Prospective investigations indicate that the rate of primary infection during pregnancy is approximately one in 1,000. Almost all of these infections are asymptomatic.

Among the children of mothers who have had a primary infection during pregnancy, about 10% have later evidence of damage, including lower than normal IQ and deafness. In addition, severe congenital toxoplasmosis is apparent at birth in about one of every 10,000 births.

Chemotherapy is available for *T gondii*, as are tests for both immunoglobulin G and M antibody. However, the laboratory data frequently do not enable the physician to distinguish a primary infection during pregnancy from a prior infection. This distinction is extremely important since a primary infection, particularly early in pregnancy, can result in fetal infection and damage, whereas a prior infection is of importance only if the mother is severely immunocompromised.

Diagnosis

Mother. The great majority of women infected with *T gondii* are asymptomatic. In one prospective study, we had the opportunity to examine five women who had documented infection. Only one had any signs or symptoms possibly related to the infection, and these were mild bilateral occipital lympadenopathy. Occasionally, women with primary infection have a "monolike" illness or, rarely, *Toxoplasma* infection of the eye with visual impairment.

Tests of IgG and IgM antibody are readily available from many laboratories. However, the fact that 15% to 40% of women have IgG antibody limits the use of this test to documenting past infection. In the US, one in 1,000 women seroconvert during pregnancy. To document the time of these seroconversions, it would be necessary to perform serial antibody tests on antibody-negative women. Unfortunately, in addition to the low rate of seroconversion, standard laboratory tests are often quite unreliable, making IgG data difficult to use.

IgM antibody appears at the time of infection but may persist at a high titer for several years. Thus, its presence does not necessarily indicate recent or current primary infection. Although its absence may help exclude the diagnosis, it must be remembered that IgM antibody may disappear in 6 months in some patients.

Problems with reliability and interpretation of IgG and IgM results make these tests difficult to apply clinically. We have recommended that until improved methods are available, tests should be limited to patients who have clinical symptoms suggesting the diagnosis. Presence of IgG and IgM antibody would then be consistent with a diagnosis of toxoplasmosis.

For special "high-risk" patients, such as an individual with many cats, serial IgG determinations can be performed every 1 to 2 months on antibody-negative patients. If a seroconversion occurs, the patient can be treated or counseled. This approach requires having a reliable laboratory to send the specimens to. With many laboratories, reliability is a problem.

Child. Children infected in utero with *T gondii* may have severe brain damage, hydrocephaly, microcephaly, chorioretinitis, deafness, and other abnormalities. Studies from France have shown that transmission of infection to the fetus is lower in the first trimester (15%) than in the third (60%) but that infection of the fetus early in pregnancy is more likely to cause fetal death or damage.

French laboratory studies of fetal blood and amniotic fluid indicate that toxoplasmal organisms can be isolated by mouse inoculation from blood samples of most infected fetuses. In addition, a panel of enzymatic and hematologic laboratory tests, such as a platelet count, run on fetal blood reveals some abnormalities in most infected children. Ultrasound, too, can detect evidence of some in utero infections. IgM tests of fetal blood are positive only after 22 weeks' gestation and, even then, only 10% to 20% of infected fetuses have specific IgM antibody.

A recent study by Grover and co-workers used polymerase chain reaction tests to detect gene sequences of *T gondii* in amniotic fluid from proven cases of congenital infection. This approach has the advantages of speed, sensitivity, and ease of transport of specimens.

Treatment

If a pregnant patient is diagnosed as having acute toxoplasmosis because of symptoms plus IgM-specific antibody or a seroconversion, treat her with 25 mg of oral pyrimethamine daily plus 1 g of oral sulfadiazine four times daily for 28 days, followed by one half the dose of each drug for an additional 28 days. In addition, give 6 mg of folinic acid IM or orally three times weekly. If the mother has severe, symptomatic toxoplasmosis, you may have to continue therapy for several months.

In general, we recommend omitting pyrimethamine in the first trimester because of possible teratogenic effects associated with the drug. In addition, we discontinue sulfadiazine in the last weeks of pregnancy.

There have been a few reports of pregnant patients who had malignancies, immunosuppressive diseases, or immunosuppressive chemotherapy and who had had prior *T gondii* infection that was reactivated during pregnancy and transmitted to the infant. Fortunately, these were rare occurrences. However, it will be important to determine whether IgM tests can be used to detect reactivation of *Toxoplasma* infection in immunosuppressed pregnant patients.

Prevention

Toxoplasmosis is acquired by eating infected raw meat or unpasteurized goat's milk or by exposure to a *T gondii* oocyst excreted in the feces of infected cats. Instruct pregnant women not to eat raw meat or drink unpasteurized milk. If cats are in the environment, the pregnant woman should avoid exposure to the feces, litter, or soil where feces may be present. Another family member should daily discard litter and clean the box by wiping it with household bleach diluted with ten parts of water.

SUGGESTED READING

Daffos F, Forestier F, Capella-Pavlovsky M, et al: Prenatal management of 746 pregnancies at risk for congenital toxoplasmosis. N Engl J Med 1988;318:271

Grover CM, Thulliez P, Remington JS, et al: Rapid prenatal diagnosis of congenital *Toxoplasma* infection by using polymerase chain reaction and amniotic fluid. J Clin Microbiol 1990;28:2297

Sever JL, Ellenberg JH, Ley AC, et al: Toxoplasmosis: maternal and pediatric findings in 23,000 pregnancies. Pediatrics 1988;82:181

Sever JL, Larsen JW, Grossman JH: *Handbook of Perinatal Infections.* Boston, Little, Brown & Co, 1989, pp 160-167

28
Parasitic infections in pregnancy

By Marvin S. Amstey, MD

Background

Little information is available about the effects of various human parasites on pregnancy, nor is any more known about the reverse: the effect of pregnancy on parasitic infections. Parasites about which a body of data exists—*Toxoplasma gondii, Trichomonas vaginalis, Sarcoptes scabiei,* and *Phthirus pubis*—are discussed in detail in Chapters 27, 31, 40, and 41 of this text. That leaves all the other parasitic infections to be dealt with here. Needless to say, this is not a complete exposition and will be limited only to the more common infections. We will emphasize those parasitic infections seen in North America in the order of their frequency and the use of various antiparasitic drugs in pregnancy.

Giardiasis

Several surveys have demonstrated a prevalence of 3% to 9% of all stool specimens positive for this parasite. While such surveys have not been done in pregnant women, there is no *a priori* reason why the same prevalence would not occur in pregnant women. This is an endemic infection of the gastrointestinal tract associated with contaminated water and food. The vast majority of those affected have no symptoms or only minor diarrhea and require no therapy. However, those with severe nausea, vomiting, diarrhea, and weight loss should be treated. Those left untreated are at risk for significant hypokalemia and ketosis.

There are no reports of transmission of *Giardia lamblia* to the placenta or to the fetus.

The therapy of choice is paromomycin, 30 mg/kg/day in three or four divided doses. Because this aminoglycoside is very poorly absorbed from the GI tract, fecal concentration is very high and there is very little or no effect on mother or fetus. We believe this drug is a better choice in pregnancy than the *Medical Letter's* drug of choice, quinacrine, 100 mg three times daily for 5 days. Quinacrine is an FDA class C drug in pregnancy, which means that risk cannot be ruled out. The alternative choice is metronidazole, a class B drug, whose use should be limited to the latter two trimesters of pregnancy; dosage is 250 mg three times daily for 5 days.

Enterobiasis (pinworm infection)

This agent, like *G lamblia*, rarely causes symptoms leading to illness. However, it can cause intense anal and perineal itching that can be disabling, and ridding the body, family members, and clothing of eggs, larvae, and adult worms can be difficult. Other than the rare anecdotal case of pinworm salpingitis (with worms actually seen protruding from the fimbriated end of the tube), no other gynecologic or obstetric complication is known. Pinworm should not be treated during pregnancy unless the woman is incapacitated by itching or very concerned about having worms.

MacLeod recommends pyrantel pamoate in a single dose of 10 mg (base)/kg (maximum dose of 1 g of pyrantel base) after the first trimester if treatment is elected. The entire family should be treated, and clothing and bedding washed in hot water or chlorine bleach to avoid reinfection by viable eggs. MacLeod cautions against the use of mebendazole and thiabendazole. All three of these drugs are FDA class C drugs in pregnancy.

Hookworm

This infection used to be seen most commonly in the Southern US, where it is still endemic. In addition, a series of prevalence studies have shown that various hookworms are the most common parasites in the stools of Southeast Asian refugees. The most common result of infestation with *Ancylostoma duodenale* or *Necator americanus* is anemia due to bloodsucking in the GI tract by the adult worms. A single worm consumes 0.2 mL of blood per day. After it detaches, the old wound continues to bleed, adding to the blood loss.

Ancylostoma braziliense and *Ancylostoma caninum* are not true parasites of man. As in scabies, cutaneous larva migrans (creeping eruption) results from penetration of the skin by filariform larvae. This infestation causes intense itching and usually secondary infection. There does not appear to be any effect, other than the results of anemia, of these parasites on the placenta or fetus.

The mainstay of therapy for the intestinal hookworm is iron. Oral iron supplements are usually all an infected pregnant woman will need. Heavy infestations that do not respond well to iron should be treated with pyrantel, 11 mg/kg (up to 1.0 g/day) for 3 days. For cutaneous larval migrans, topical therapy with thiabendazole suspension or a 0.5-g tablet triturated with 5 g of petroleum jelly has been suggested as effective and free of toxic side effects. Teratogenicity of this regimen is unknown.

Amebiasis

Infection with *Entamoeba histolytica* is less common in the US than in new immigrants to this country. Approximately 10% of immigrants have stool specimens positive for this parasite. While the infection is commonly symptomatic as diarrhea, intestinal ulceration and severe diarrhea may occur. A later stage of infestation is amebic liver abscess. In one report, administration of corticosteroids as treatment for "chronic colitis" (due to amebiasis) hastened the development of liver abscess.

The effect of this parasitic infection on pregnancy is an indirect one—secondary to the chronic diarrhea, anemia, and weight loss. Even liver abscess does not seem to have an adverse effect on pregnancy.

First choice for therapy of asymptomatic to moderately severe amebiasis is paromomycin, 30 mg/kg/day in three doses for 7 days; metronidazole, 750 mg three times daily for 10 days, is an alternative. For severe intestinal disease and for hepatic abscess, metronidazole is the drug of choice. The alternative for severe disease is dehydroemetine, 1.5 mg/kg/day (maximum, 90 mg/day) IM for 5 days. This drug is obtainable only from the Centers for Disease Control Drug Service [404-639-3670]. There is no information about its use in pregnancy. Several other alternative drugs are recommended, including chloroquine, iodoquinol, and emetine.

Malaria

There is very little malaria in the United States, and it is a rare medical problem in pregnancy. It is seen more commonly as relapses in immigrants or in citizens who have travelled to endemic areas. It is not the purpose of this chapter to detail the effects of malaria on pregnancy or vice versa because it is so uncommon. The reader is referred to the Suggested Reading list. One should remember that the effects on the fetus are usually secondary to the severity of the anemia and nutritional status of the mother. Severe illness leads to excess pregnancy wastage and intrauterine growth retardation. It has been suggested that malarial illnesses are worse in pregnancy. It is also known that pregnant women living in endemic areas are more susceptible to *Plasmodium falciparum* infection than are nonpregnant women. In one study of malaria in West Africa, 40% of mothers and 16% of placentas were parasitized. No parasites were found in cord blood. However, congenital malaria is documented in 1% to 4% of nonimmune, infected mothers.

Therapy for non–chloroquine-resistant malaria of all types is chloroquine, 1.0 g of the salt, then 500 mg at 6, 24, and 48 hours. This dosage should then be continued on a once-a-week basis for *P vivax* and *P ovale* disease until after delivery. Radical cure of the tissue forms of these organisms is accomplished with primaquine, one tablet (15-mg base) daily for 14 days. Primaquine should not be used during pregnancy, however, and is best reserved for the postpartum period. Treatment of resistant *P falciparum* malaria is accomplished with quinine, 650 mg three times daily for 3 to 7 days, plus pyrimethamine/sulfadoxine, three tablets at once. One needs to be careful in using sulfadoxine close to delivery. Quinine can stimulate uterine contractions and may provoke abortion if given in high doses. However, quinine has been used successfully to treat seriously ill women in the third trimester of pregnancy.

The CDC has recently reviewed data on the management of severe life-threatening infectious *P falciparum* malaria and has concluded that the drug of choice in the US for treatment of complicated *P falciparum* infections is parenteral quinidine gluconate. Because of this decision, parenteral quinine dihydrochloride is no longer available from the CDC Drug Service.

Prophylaxis during pregnancy. The most common question about malaria that arises in this country is whether to use prophylaxis for pregnant women traveling to endemic areas. Up-to-date information on the occurrence of malaria in specific countries and on antimalarial chemoprophylaxis can be obtained from the Malaria Branch, Division of Parasitic Diseases, Center for Infectious Diseases, CDC [404-488-4046]. The CDC Voice Information Service [404-332-4555] has added facsimile capability to the malaria hotline. By following the recorded instructions, callers can receive fax information on the risk for malaria and on malaria prevention measures in Africa, Southeast Asia, South America, Central America, Mexico, the Caribbean, the Indian subcontinent, and Oceania, as well as information on children and pregnancy and a world map showing areas with malaria transmission. This service is available 24 hours a day.

Malaria infection may be more severe in pregnant than in nonpregnant women. There may also be increased risk of prematurity, abortion, and stillbirth. For these reasons, and because chloroquine has not been found harmful to the fetus when used in doses recommended for malaria prophylaxis, pregnancy is not a contraindication for prophylaxis with chloroquine or hydroxychloro-

TABLE 1
Therapy for parasite infection in pregnancy

Infection	Parasite	Pregnancy effects
Giardiasis	*Giardia lamblia*	Secondary to maternal disease
Pinworms	*Enterobius vermicularis*	None known
Hookworm	*Ancylostoma duodenale* *Necator americanus*	Secondary to maternal anemia
Cutaneous larva migrans	*Ancylostoma braziliense* *A caninum*	None known
Amebiasis	*Entamoeba histolytica*	Secondary to maternal illness
Malaria	*Plasmodium ovale* *P vivax* Nonresistant *P falciparum*	Secondary to maternal disease
	Chloroquine-resistant *P falciparum*	Secondary to maternal disease

quine. In areas free of chloroquine-resistant malaria, weekly therapy with 500 mg of chloroquine salt (300-mg base), beginning 1 week before and continuing until 4 weeks after returning, is satisfactory.

Women pregnant or likely to become so should avoid travel to areas with chloroquine-resistant *P falciparum* because alternative drugs such as mefloquine, doxycycline, and primaquine should not be used during pregnancy. Women with childbearing potential who are taking mefloquine for malaria prophylaxis should use reliable contraception until 2 months after the last dose of mefloquine. Adverse fetal effects of doxycycline and other tetracyclines include discoloration and dysplasia of the teeth and inhibition of bone

Drug of choice (FDA class)	Alternative drug
Paromomycin, 30 mg/kg/day in 3 doses × 7 days (B)	Metronidazole, 250 mg tid × 5 days (B)
Pyrantel, 10 mg/kg once (C)	
Iron; for severe infections—pyrantel 11 mg/kg × 3 days (C)	
Thiabendazole topically (C)	
Paromomycin, 30 mg/kg/day in 3 doses × 7 days for moderate infections; metronidazole, 750 mg tid × 7 days for severe infections (B)	For severe infection dehydroemetine, 1.5 mg/kg/day IM × 5 days (?)
Chloroquine, 1 g, then 500 mg at 6, 24, and 48 hours; then weekly until after delivery; reserve primaquine until postpartum	
Quinine, 650 mg tid × 3 days plus sulfadoxine/pyrimethamine, 3 tabs once	

growth. Use of tetracyclines would be indicated in pregnancy only to treat life-threatening infections due to multidrug-resistant *P falciparum*. Primaquine may be passed transplacentally to a G6PD-deficient fetus and cause hemolytic anemia in utero. Whenever radical cure or terminal prophylaxis with primaquine is indicated during pregnancy, chloroquine should be given once a week until delivery, when the decision to give primaquine may be made.

To summarize, in areas where chloroquine-sensitive *P falciparum* is present, prophylactic regimens that are safe in pregnancy have been developed. No prophylactic regimen, however, can assure complete protection against malaria; most severe complications of malaria are more common in pregnant women, and prophylactic regimens occasionally produce unwanted side effects. In areas where chloroquine-resistant *P falciparum* is present, there is no completely safe regimen for pregnant women, and travel should be avoided unless the need is imperative.

Other agents

There are a host of other parasitic infections that are less common but important on an endemic basis in some countries. Congenital infection with *Trypanosoma cruzi* occurs in infants born to mothers with the chronic form of Chagas' disease (American trypanosomiasis). These infants have a characteristic edema of the face and eyelids—Romaña's sign. Transplacental infection by the blood-borne organism is thought to be the mechanism of infection, but adequate studies are lacking. In endemic areas, up to 2% of infants under 2 kg are thought to have this infection, but it is rare in the US, even among immigrants from Central America.

Placental infection, but probably not congenital infection, is known to occur from *Schistosoma haematobium*.

Other parasitic infections of humans with potential for harm to mother or fetus include ascariasis, trichuriasis, visceral larva migrans (toxocariasis), and tapeworms in this country; filariasis, leishmaniasis, trypanosomiasis, and fluke infections also have this potential but are not seen in the US. It is not possible in this short review—limited to the more common US infections—to present details about them. The reader is referred to the bibliography for more information. Table 1 summarizes the parasitic infections described in this chapter.

SUGGESTED READING

Brabin, BJ: Epidemiology of infection in pregnancy. Rev Infect Dis 1985;7:579

Centers for Disease Control: Recommendations for the prevention of malaria among travelers. MMWR 1990;39(RR-3):1-18

Centers for Disease Control: Treatment of severe *Plasmodium falciparum* malaria with quinidine gluconate: discontinuation of parenteral quinine from CDC drug service. MMWR 1991;40(14):240

Drugs for parasitic infections. Med Lett 1990;34:23

Kreutner AK, DelBene VE, Amstey MS: Giardiasis in pregnancy. Am J Obstet Gynecol 1981;140:895

Lee RV: Protozoan infections in pregnancy, in Gleicher N (ed): *Principles of Medical Therapy in Pregnancy*. New York, Plenum, 1985.

MacLeod CL (ed): *Parasitic Infections in Pregnancy and the Newborn*. Oxford, England, Oxford University Press, 1988

Roberts NS, Copel JA, Bhutani V, et al: Intestinal parasites and other infections during pregnancy in Southeast Asian refugees. J Reprod Med 1985;30:720

Villar J, Klebanoff M, Kestter E: The effect on fetal growth of protozoan and helminthic infection during pregnancy. Obstet Gynecol 1989;74:915

Infection Protocols in the Gynecologic Patient

29
Candidal vaginal infections

By Hans A. Hirsch, MD

Background and incidence

Lower genital tract infections are a common cause of symptoms that lead women to seek medical care, and vaginitis in its various forms may be the most frequent of these infections. Candidiasis accounts for 20% to 30% of vaginitis complaints. Few women escape having at least one candidal infection in their lifetime.

Candidal infections are a major cause of vulvar and vaginal morbidity. But accurate incidence and prevalence data for candidal vaginitis are difficult to obtain since many women may harbor the organism and remain asymptomatic, and many others self-treat with home remedies and over-the-counter preparations. Candidal organisms commonly exist in the vagina as part of an elaborate ecosystem without causing symptoms; culture data may therefore not be representative of true infection.

Among women with candidal vaginal infections, 20% to 30% will have dual or multiple infections involving other pathogens. These mixed infections cause significant diagnostic and therapeutic problems for the practicing physician.

Etiology

Vulvovaginal candidiasis is caused by *Candida albicans* in 80% to 90% of patients. The remaining cases are due primarily to infection by *C glabrata*, *C tropicalis*, and other candidal species.

In 15% to 25% of asymptomatic women, candidal organisms can be isolated from the vagina. These agents usually become pathogenic only when present in large numbers. Candidal species also occur as commensals at various sites, principally in the gastrointestinal tract. Asymptomatic colonization has been found in 30% to 40%

of pregnant women.

The circumstances leading to symptomatic infection are not fully understood. Several host factors have been associated with elevated incidence of vaginal yeast colonization and symptomatic infection. Predisposing factors for candidal overgrowth are administration of antimicrobials, primarily broad-spectrum antibiotics; high blood glucose levels, as in diabetics; and depressed cell-mediated immunity, as in AIDS patients or patients given immunosuppressive drugs. Promotion of candidal infection by oral contraceptives has not been unequivocally proven.

Diagnosis

Typical symptoms of genital candidiasis are vulvar and vaginal pruritus, burning, and dysuria. Some patients complain about discharge and dyspareunia. Examination often reveals erythema and edema of the vulva, sometimes extended perianally and to the groin. The mostly scant discharge is nonodorous, white or gray, and liquid or thick. Only about 20% of patients display the characteristic white, cottage-cheese-like plaques adherent to the vaginal wall. The pH of the vaginal discharge is usually less than 4.5, and addition of potassium hydroxide (KOH) does not produce amine odor.

For clinical purposes, the diagnosis is usually made by microscopic examination of a wet mount at 100× magnification. Samples are taken from pooled vaginal discharge, or are scraped from plaques or the edges of vulvar erythematous lesions. On microscopic examination, characteristic branching hyphae and spores can best be seen when a vulvar or vaginal sample is mixed with a drop of 10% KOH. Spores in large numbers without associated filaments are suggestive of *C glabrata*. Occasionally, the entire slide must be thoroughly scanned because the yeasts may be present only in small numbers or clumped in only one area of the slide. On saline preparation, leukocytes usually are absent and lactobacilli morphotypes present.

Reports of the sensitivity of the KOH preparation have ranged from 22% to 80%, whereas that of Gram stain approaches 100%; that of a Papanicolaou stain is only about 50%. The most sensitive means of detecting candidal infection or asymptomatic candidal carriers is culture on Sabouraud's or other fungal media. For clinical purposes, however, cultures are indicated only when candidal infection is suspected on the basis of symptoms and signs and the diagnosis cannot be confirmed by microscopic examination.

Treatment

In general, local therapy should be administered to patients with symptoms. Under certain circumstances, asymptomatic carriers should also be treated (for example, when immune suppression is a factor). During pregnancy, elimination of candidal colonization of the vagina is indicated to avoid infecting the baby during vaginal passage. Male partners should be treated only when they have symptoms. Routine treatment of asymptomatic male partners has not been shown to reduce subsequent female infection.

Among the large number of antifungal agents currently available, only nystatin, a polyene antibiotic introduced in the 1950s, and the more recent azole derivatives are widely used. Azole agents for topical application include imidazole derivatives such as clotrimazole, miconazole, butoconazole, and econazole. These agents are available as vaginal creams, vaginal tablets, capsules, or suppositories; like nystatin, they are not absorbed orally. Terconazole, one of the newer triazoles, is also for local use only.

Ketoconazole and the more recently developed azole derivatives fluconazole and itraconazole can be administered orally for systemic therapy. For acute infection, however, systemic treatment is not superior to topical therapy. Furthermore, hepatotoxic reaction has occurred in some patients after systemic treatment with ketoconazole.

As an alternative, boric acid may be used effectively when applied as 600-mg vaginal capsules once daily for 2 weeks. Local treatment of pregnant women with nystatin and azole derivatives has not been shown to be harmful to the fetus, but boric acid should definitely be avoided in pregnancy.

The application of a 1% aqueous solution of gentian violet to the vagina and the vulva twice weekly for about 2 weeks is also effective but less practical. This approach has been recommended mainly for treatment of recurrent infection. In general, candidal lesions of the vulva should be treated with cream preparations from azole derivatives or nystatin.

Local treatment of acute candidiasis with azole derivatives or boric acid for 7 to 14 days offers clinical and mycologic cure rates of 80% to 90%. Cure rates are similar among this group of agents and somewhat higher than with nystatin. Patient preference and better compliance have produced a trend toward 3-day, 1-day, or single-dose therapy. For single-dose therapy, vaginal preparations are used at higher dosages. In patients with infrequent episodes of acute infection, the shorter regimens achieve cure rates similar to conventional 7- to 14-day therapy.

There is a subset of women, however, who have frequent recurrence or chronic intractable symptoms. These patients improve after intravaginal therapy, but develop recurrent symptoms a month or two later [see Chapter 30: Chronic recurrent vaginal candidiasis]. Characteristic risk factors should be investigated and eliminated whenever possible. But these are often lacking. Defects in the cell-mediated immunologic system have been demonstrated in some of these patients. Oral treatment with 400 mg of ketoconazole daily for 10 to 14 days may be effective.

SUGGESTED READING

Eschenbach DA: Lower genital tract infections, in Galask RP, Larsen B (eds): *Infectious Diseases in the Female Patient*. New York, Springer-Verlag, 1986, pp 163-186

Odds FC: *Candida and Candidiasis*. Baltimore, University Park Press, 1979

Oriel JD, Partridge BM, Denny MY, et al: Genital yeast infections. Br Med J 1972;4:761

Sobel JD: Epidemiology and pathogenesis of recurrent vulvovaginal candidiasis. Am J Obstet Gynecol 1985;152:924

30
Chronic recurrent vaginal candidiasis

By Steven S. Witkin, PhD

Background

The lay press has popularized the unproven idea that *Candida* infections are the underlying cause of a multitude of symptoms in every body part. Consequently, most women who seek help for recurrent symptoms of vaginitis will claim to have a "yeast infection." Unfortunately, most of these self-attempted diagnoses are incorrect, with evidence of *Candida* being detected on subsequent examination only 30% of the time. It's not surprising, therefore, that antifungal medications have no effect on most of these conditions.

Of private patients at our institution, about 5% with an initial episode of candidal vaginitis will have recurrent infection after apparently successful treatment with antifungal medications. To prevent frequent episodes, we must identify underlying factors predisposing to *Candida* growth and take measures to reduce these risks.

Pathophysiology

More than 95% of candidal vaginal infections are caused by *C albicans*, and the remainder primarily by *C glabrata* and *C tropicalis*. Although all women have antibodies to *Candida*, these antibodies are nonprotective and do not prevent its growth. Moreover, women with defective B-cell immunity don't have an increased rate of vaginal candidiasis.

Cell-mediated immunity appears to be the major, if not the only, immune mechanism limiting vaginal proliferation of *C albicans*. Polymorphonuclear leukocytes aren't noticeably present in the vagina. Rather, mononuclear lymphoid cells, macrophages and T lymphocytes, appear to be the major regulators of vaginal *Candida* growth. Women with genetic defects that affect T lymphocyte or macrophage functions have an increased rate of candidal mucous membrane infections.

In healthy women with normally functioning immune systems, infection of mucosal surfaces by *Candida* is readily treated and rarely recurs. Conversely, a defective in vitro cellular immune response to *Candida* is readily demonstrable in many women with recurrent candidal vaginitis. It is sometimes not appreciated that recurrent *C albicans* vaginal infections are often opportunistic and secondary to a transient deficiency in cell-mediated immunity.

In about 20% of cases, a vaginal allergic response can be implicated as a predisposing factor for recurrent candidal vaginitis. Semen components, contraceptive spermicides, vaginal douches, other chemicals or medicines that may come into contact with the vagina, and *C albicans* itself can serve as allergens in sensitized women. The vagina's immediate hypersensitivity response causes release of histamine, which stimulates macrophages to produce prostaglandin E_2. The PGE_2 inhibits production of interleukin-2 by T lymphocytes, thereby transiently paralyzing the cell-mediated immune response. Under these conditions, the low levels of *Candida* normally present in many women's vaginas are able to proliferate and trigger a clinical infection.

Allergy-related candidal vaginitis can also be induced in nonallergic women if the male partner has a genital tract allergic response. In these cases, immunoglobulin E antibodies are transferred to the woman by coitus and bind to her basophils and mast cells. The allergen, also present in the ejaculate, then reacts with the bound IgE, initiating an allergic response.

Candidal vaginitis most often reappears during the late luteal phase of the menstrual cycle, when the elevated level of progesterone down-regulates cellular immune response and lessens inhibition of *Candida* growth. Similarly, women with endocrinopathies may also be especially susceptible to recurrent candidal vaginitis.

Infectivity of *C albicans* is associated with ability of the yeast forms to germinate. Recent evidence indicates that germination, too, may be regulated by cellular immune system components. Compounds such as PGE_2, which increase the intracellular level of cyclic adenosine monophosphate (cAMP), promote *Candida* germination. Thus, medications that increase cAMP levels may also increase susceptibility to candidal vaginitis. Conversely, gamma interferon, a product of activated T lymphocytes, inhibits it.

Candida albicans can also sometimes be present in the male genital tract. Recurrent infection in the woman, therefore, may sometimes result from failure to eliminate the reservoir of infection in the man.

Diagnosis

Recurrent candidal vaginitis may show the classical symptoms of pruritus, inflammation, and curdlike, cheesy discharge. Sometimes, intense pruritus may be the only symptom. Unfortunately, many patients have been treated by numerous physicians, nutritionists, and other health-care providers and have tried various home remedies that often complicate and mask presenting symptoms. Therefore, the gross appearance of vaginal secretions is not diagnostic.

You can confirm diagnosis in some cases by finding branched budding pseudohyphae on wet mounts of vaginal secretions in 10% potassium hydroxide. In many symptomatic patients in whom *Candida* infection is suspected but wet mounts are negative, a more sensitive and specific test is to inoculate Sabouraud agar slants with a vaginal swab. Identify the yeast as *C albicans* by inoculating a small colony into serum or glucose beef extract and examining for germ tube formation after 90 to 120 minutes.

Question patients about such classic risk factors as frequent antibiotic or steroid usage, pregnancy, diabetes or other endocrinopathies, poor perianal hygiene, or wearing of tight clothing or nylon or silk undergarments. Typically, most patients will be negative for all these risk factors.

Ascertain the relationship between sexual activity and vaginal symptoms. Are the symptoms temporally related to coitus with just the present partner or with all partners? Does the sexual partner have symptoms of genital, oral, or digital *Candida* infection? Was he taking any medication or drug to which the woman might be sensitized? What is the means of contraception?

At our institution, women with recurrent vaginitis are tested for evidence of a vaginal allergic response. We obtain a vaginal wash sample by instilling 5 to 10 mL of sterile saline into the vagina with a needle and syringe, directing the injection flow against the vaginal sidewalls, withdrawing the solution, and separating it into pellet and supernatant fractions by centrifugation. ELISA is used to test the supernatant for IgE antibodies to *Candida* and semen, and the pellet for bound IgE. In coitus-related vaginitis, we obtain cultures for *Candida* from semen samples and test for total IgE and specific IgE antibodies to the vaginal wash pellet.

Although not performed routinely, a lymphocyte proliferation assay on a sample of peripheral-blood mononuclear cells isolated from heparinized blood may be useful when immunosuppression might be suspected, such as in women with concomitant oral thrush or condyloma. In such instances, a defective proliferative response to *Candida* and plant mitogens might indicate a more serious underlying disease.

Treatment

To treat recurrent *Candida* infection, use a local antifungal medication to reduce the high level of organisms, and initiate a protocol to lessen risk factors associated with reappearance. Short courses of treatment with imidazole drugs are usually successful. More recalcitrant infections respond to 400 mg of oral ketoconazole given daily for 7 to 14 days, although this drug is currently not approved in the US for treatment of candidal vaginitis. Should it become available, you will need to periodically monitor patients receiving it by liver function tests and advise them to contact you if they become nauseated. Most patients tolerate it without symptoms.

Sobel has reported that an effective regimen for limiting vaginal candidiasis recurrence is a daily prophylactic low dose of ketoconazole for 6 months. Unfortunately, when the drug is stopped, recurrences are experienced at the prior frequency. Another new oral antifungal, fluconazole, is currently being evaluated for its ability to prevent recurrences of candidal infection of mucous membranes.

One should eliminate or limit risk factors for recurrence, such as use of hormones or immunosuppressive medications, whenever possible. Whether or not oral contraceptives should also be discontinued remains unclear. The increased risk associated with their use is probably small.

If candidal vaginitis is associated with coitus with one particular partner, it's important to find out if he is ingesting any medications or drugs that may enter his semen and elicit a vaginal response. Reports exist of vaginal allergic reactions to semen that contained products of ingested penicillin or thioridazine. Change or eliminate the offending medication, if possible. Similarly, evaluate the effect on vaginitis recurrence of changing the contraception method or spermicide brand.

If the woman has vaginal fluid IgE antibodies to her partner's semen, or the man has IgE antibodies in his ejaculate, using a condom will eliminate vaginal contact with the allergen. An untested alternative is the use of an oral antihistamine before intercourse.

Vaginal allergic responses to *Candida* appear to be relatively common in women with recurrent candidal vaginitis. In one study, we reported that 18% of 64 patients tested had anticandidal IgE in their vaginal washes. In women who are hypersensitive to *Candida* or to an unidentified component of a vaginal wash sample, the best treatment at present is to prevent growth of *Candida* by aggressive use of antifungal agents plus use of oral antihistamines to obtain symptomatic relief of vaginal symptoms and reduce the incidence of histamine-mediated immunosuppression.

Hyposensitizing the patient to *Candida*, semen, or any other allergen associated with a vaginal allergic response may ultimately provide the best therapy. However, improved methodology and standization along with controlled clinical trials are needed to evaluate the effectiveness of these experimental immunizations.

SUGGESTED READING

Hobbs JR, Brigden D, Davidson F: Immunological aspects of candidal vaginitis. Proc R Soc Lond (Med) 1977;70(suppl 4):11

Green RL, Green MA: Postcoital urticaria in a penicillin-sensitive patient: possible seminal transfer of penicillin. JAMA 1985;245:531

Kalo-Klein A, Witkin SS: *Candida albicans*: cellular immune system interactions during different stages of the menstrual cycle. Am J Obstet Gynecol 1989;161:1132

Kalo-Klein A, Witkin SS: Prostaglandin E_2 enhances and gamma interferon inhibits germ tube formation in *Candida albicans*. Infect Immun 1990;58:260

Odds FC: *Candida and Candidosis*, ed 2. Philadelphia, Bailliere Tindall, 1988, p 273

Sell MB: Sensitization to thioridazine through sexual intercourse. Am J Psychiatry 1985;142:271

Sobel JD: Recurrent vulvovaginal candidiasis: a prospective study of the efficacy of maintenance ketoconazole therapy. N Engl J Med 1986;315:1455

Sobel JD, Muller G, Buckley HR: Critical role of germ tube formation in the pathogenesis of candidal vaginitis. Infect Immun 1984;44:576

Witkin SS: Immunology of recurrent vaginitis. Am J Reprod Immunol Microbiol 1987;15:34

Witkin SS, Hirsch J, Ledger WJ: A macrophage defect in women with recurrent *Candida* vaginitis and its reversal in vitro by prostaglandin inhibitors. Am J Obstet Gynecol 1986;155:790

Witkin SS, Jeremias J, Ledger WJ: A localized vaginal allergic response in women with recurrent vaginitis. J Allergy Clin Immunol 1988;81:412

Witkin SS, Jeremias J, Ledger WJ: Recurrent vaginitis as a result of sexual transmission of IgE antibodies. Am J Obstet Gynecol 1988;159:32

Witkin SS, Yu IR, Ledger WJ: Inhibition of *Candida albicans*-induced lymphocyte proliferation by lymphocytes and sera from women with recurrent vaginitis. Am J Obstet Gynecol 1983;147:809

31
Trichomoniasis

By Michael R. Spence, MD, MPH

Background and incidence

Trichomonas vaginalis, the protozoan parasite that causes trichomoniasis, was first described in 1836. The organism is unicellular, flagellated, and motile. It forms pseudopods and is slightly larger than a polymorphonuclear neutrophilic leukocyte. It prefers an environment of high pH and has its maximum growth and metabolic functions at pH 6.0. Most commonly found in vaginal secretions of pH greater than 4.5, it proliferates at the time of menstruation and is frequently associated with a large number of leukocytes.

Since long-term longitudinal studies of at-risk populations have not been conducted, incidence has not been defined. Prevalence varies significantly, depending on the population evaluated and the method employed. The organism has been found in as few as 3% of college students attending a student health clinic and as many as 37% of women working in the sex industry.

Since the primary and only significant mode of transmission is sexual intercourse, increased risk of infection is associated with increased numbers of new, different, or casual sex partners. Therefore, whenever trichomoniasis is diagnosed, the patient should be evaluated for other sexually transmitted diseases, such as gonorrhea, syphilis, chlamydial infection, and HIV infection. It is also possible for trichomoniasis to be associated with bacterial vaginosis or monilial infection, or both, in a combined vaginitis.

Diagnosis

The clinical presentation of persons infected with *T vaginalis* is varied, with many women harboring the organism asymptomatically. Vaginal discharge may vary from minimal to copious, purulent, frothy, and irritating. Dysuria, frequency of urination, vaginal pruritus, dyspareunia, offensive genital odor, and low back pain can also be present. The "classic" frothy, yellow, copious discharge with vaginal wall erythema and "strawberry" cervix are seen in fewer than 10% of infected women. Disagreeable odor associated with a slight increase in homogeneous, nonsticky, yellow–white discharge that pools in the posterior vaginal fornix is the most common presentation.

Since the organism is so often harbored asymptomatically and the clinical signs of infection can be subtle, it is advisable to do normal saline wet preparation evaluations of the vaginal secretions of all sexually active women undergoing speculum examination. The sensitivity of this method varies from 22% to 76% and is highly dependent on the reagents employed, the handling of the specimen, and the compulsiveness of the observer. Fresh saline intended for IV use and not containing preservative should be employed. If dropper bottles are used, they should be washed and refilled at least monthly; leaving them open to air promotes evaporation and hypertonicity, which inhibits motility. If test tubes are used for the saline, they should be firmly capped and should not contain additives.

Specimens should be kept warm in one's breast or vest pocket from the time obtained to the time visualized. They should be evaluated by first scanning the entire slide at low power and then examining any suspicious areas at high power. The organisms are frequently found on the periphery of clumps of white blood cells or epithelial cells. One should never diagnose "dead trich" on wet mount. If motile organisms are not found, the diagnosis cannot be made with this technique.

The diagnosis of trichomonal infection is occasionally made on a Papanicolaou smear. In a research setting, the sensitivity of this method varies from 52% to 67%, too low to permit its use as a screening method. Moreover, unless vital stains are used, its specificity can vary and false positives will be reported.

Another option for diagnosis is culture, and many preparations, both liquid and semi-solid, have been formulated for this purpose. Culture diagnosis, however, is labor intensive and costly and, to date, employed only in research settings.

Treatment

Before 1959, when Durel and colleagues introduced the 5-nitroimidazole metronidazole, therapy provided only symptomatic relief. Intermittently, patients would have spontaneous cures, but specific therapy was not available. When metronidazole was first introduced, therapeutic regimens were determined empirically and varied from three to four 250-mg doses per day for 7 to 14 days. In 1971, Csonka demonstrated that a single 2-g dose of metronidazole was as effective as the prolonged multidose regimens. The 2-g regimen is now the standard, administered as a single dose or in two divided doses of 1 g each over 8 to 12 hours. The cure rate with this regimen exceeds 90%.

Occasionally, a treatment failure will occur. The most common cause of treatment failure is reexposure to an untreated partner. When this problem is encountered, one should re-treat with the standard dose and try to determine whether the woman's sexual partner or partners have been treated. In those rare instances when the organism persists even after adequate therapy has been provided for the patient and her partner or partners, antibiotic resistance should be considered.

Since absolute resistance has never been described, the first approach should be to treat with a prolonged regimen at increased dosage. A reasonable starting point is 500 mg to 1 g orally twice daily for 7 days. Failure with this level of therapy may result from malabsorption of the drug or inability to get adequate amounts to the infection site. In past years, these problems were overcome by using prolonged high-dose intravenous therapy. Now, before resorting to high-dose IV therapy, we try intravaginal therapy with two uncoated 500-mg tablets twice daily in addition to high-dose oral therapy. If failure persists, even with combined oral and intravaginal therapy, intravenous therapy may be required.

Trichomoniasis in pregnant women presents a dilemma. There is no question that metronidazole should not be given at any dosage during the first trimester. However, it is acceptable to use it for symptomatic infections after the first trimester. An alternative that has been described is intravaginal clotrimazole cream. However, in a randomized prospective trial employing clotrimazole to treat culture-proven trichomonal infections, it was found to be no more useful than placebo. Currently, experienced clinicians do not treat these infections in pregnant women unless symptoms are severe.

Irrespective of route of administration or level of dosage, toxic side effects of metronidazole can occur. It occasionally causes nausea with vomiting, through a central mechanism, as seen with parenteral therapy. In addition, the drug is a neurotoxin. Peripheral neuropathy, seizures, and Bell's palsy have all been reported. This antimicrobial also significantly impacts bowel flora. Therefore, although rare, pseudomembranous colitis can occur.

Prevention

The sexual partner or partners of any woman with trichomonal infection must be treated concurrently. Controls aimed at the prevention of sexually transmitted diseases, especially the use of condoms, are indicated.

SUGGESTED READING

Csonka GW: Trichomonal vaginitis treated with one dose of metronidazole. Br J Vener Dis 1972;47:456

Hager WD, Brown ST, Kraus SJ, et al: Metronidazole for vaginal trichomoniasis: seven-day vs single-dose regimens. JAMA 1980;244:1219

McCormack WM, Evrard JR, Laughlin CF, et al: Sexually transmitted conditions among women college students. Am J Obstet Gynecol 1981;139:130

Minkoff H, Grunebaum AN, Schwarz RH, et al: Risk factors for prematurity and premature rupture of membranes: a prospective study of the vaginal flora in pregnancy. Am J Obstet Gynecol 1984;150:965

Spence MA, Hollander DH, Smith J, et al: The clinical and laboratory diagnosis of *Trichomonas vaginalis* infection. Sex Transm Dis 1980;7:168

Wölner-Hanssen P, Krieger JN, Stevens CE, et al: Clinical manifestations of vaginal trichomoniasis. JAMA 1989;261:571

32
Bacterial vaginosis

By Jessica L. Thomason, MD, Sheldon M. Gelbart, PhD, and N.J. Scaglione, NP

Background and incidence

Bacterial vaginosis (formerly known as nonspecific vaginitis; *Haemophilus, Corynebacterium,* or *Gardnerella* vaginitis; nonspecific vaginosis; anaerobic vaginitis; or anaerobic vaginosis) is the most common form of vaginitis in reproductive-aged women. Prevalence rates vary from 5% in college populations to more than 60% in sexually transmitted disease clinics. Risk factors associated with increasing incidence include lower socioeconomic status, IUD usage, multiple or uncircumcised sexual partners, smoking, and increasing parity.

Pathophysiology

The exact etiology of bacterial vaginosis (BV) is unknown. The theory that a single organism was responsible for the disease has given way to the knowledge that BV is polymicrobial. Massive overgrowth of the vaginal bacterial flora occurs, with anaerobic bacteria predominating. Both *Gardnerella* and mycoplasmas are generally present in high numbers.

An initiating factor upsetting the normal vaginal bacterial ecosystem is the virtual disappearance of hydrogen peroxide–producing lactobacilli that normally are the predominant flora of the vagina. With the loss of this natural host defense, bacteria like *Gardnerella*, mycoplasmas, and anaerobes proliferate to attain excessively large numbers.

The anaerobes produce catabolic enzymes, such as aminopeptidases and decarboxylases. These enzymes degrade proteins and amino acids to amines. In turn, the amines contribute to the signs and symptoms of BV by elevating the vaginal pH and producing the characteristic odor associated with the syndrome. The decarboxyla-tion of betaine, derived from choline, produces trimethylamine, which may be responsible for the rotting fish odor that is a strong diagnostic clue for this syndrome.

Large numbers of the various types of bacteria harbored by BV patients attach to vaginal epithelial cell surfaces to form "clue" cells. These clue cells are also a principal diagnostic marker for the syndrome.

Diagnosis

Just as a woman may be asymptomatic with chlamydial or gonococ-cal infections, patients may be asymptomatic with BV. In fact, more than half the women with BV will present with no symptoms. Therefore, physicians must rely on objective diagnostic data ob-tained during the pelvic speculum examination rather than simply accept that the patient's vaginal discharge must be "normal" if she does not complain of symptoms.

If symptoms occur, the patient will complain of a profuse, mal-odorous, nonirritating discharge, which classically has the appear-ance of a cup of milk (homogeneous) poured into the vagina. This discharge may adhere to, but can easily be wiped from, the vaginal walls. In addition, the woman may complain of an offensive odor, most noticeable after intercourse.

Certain indicators of the disease are both sensitive and specific (Table 1):

- **Clue cells.** The disease is best diagnosed by microscopic exami-nation (wet prep) of freshly collected vaginal secretions for clue cells, which are vaginal epithelial cells so covered with attached bacteria that the cell borders are no longer clearly discernible. These cells are virtually pathognomonic for the syndrome and can be observed at 400× magnification.

- **Fishy amine odor.** The odor can best be elicited by adding 10% to 20% potassium hydroxide to freshly collected vaginal secre-tions. This odor is also considered virtually pathognomonic for the syndrome. The same volatile amines are released when vaginal secretions are alkalinized by seminal fluid during intercourse in patients with bacterial vaginosis.

- **Mobiluncus bacteria.** The highly characteristic motility of the crescent-shaped Mobiluncus bacterium also is pathognomonic for BV. Motility is wavelike, with rapid movements of short duration in a straight line or slightly arched direction, rarely out of the view field. Characteristic corkscrew or spinning activity is seen as one end of the bacterium appears to attach to epithelial cells or to the

TABLE 1

Diagnosis of bacterial vaginosis

Highly specific signs

Clue cells present

Fishy amine odor

Mobiluncus bacteria motility

Less specific signs

Vaginal pH >4.5

Lactobacilli fewer than background bacteria

For highly specific signs, best sensitivity and specificity is when clue cells and amine odor are detected.

glass slide. The bacterium then breaks away and moves in its characteristic wavelike pattern before stopping again.

Seeing these bacteria in the vaginal secretions of a patient assures the diagnosis of BV. Unfortunately, only about 50% of patients with BV have *Mobiluncus* bacteria visually present at wet prep examination, making this objective sign highly specific but not very sensitive.

Other objective signs that indicate BV are less sensitive:

■ ***pH greater than 4.5.*** Normally, vaginal (not endocervical) pH is about 4.0 except during menses. In bacterial vaginosis, the pH is elevated by the amines to above 4.5. However, many conditions, such as recent intercourse or douching, can falsely elevate pH. A finding of a vaginal pH of less than 4.5 virtually excludes the diagnosis of BV. The finding of a vaginal pH greater than 4.5 by itself does not establish the diagnosis. Use of other objective criteria is necessary.

■ ***Absence of lactobacilli.*** On Gram stain, patients with BV have a large number of small rods and coccobacillary bacteria rather than the lactobacilli that predominate in normal healthy vaginal flora. This valuable indicator that the vaginal flora is not normal appears to be only an early change in the BV disease process. Many women do not go on to develop BV, and their lactobacilli return to normal predominance.

■ ***Homogeneous discharge.*** The weakest and most subjective of the original classical signs of bacterial vaginosis is homogeneous discharge. Variation in quantity adds to difficulty of evaluation, making this sign basically unreliable.

■ ***Laboratory test results revealing bacterial enzymes and products.*** An enzymatic test to detect proline aminopeptidase from bacteria present in high quantity in the secretions of patients with BV is currently available. Although reliable, it is presently found in few clinical laboratories. Other laboratory tests found to have limited usefulness include gas–liquid chromatography and

DNA probes for various bacteria.

■ *Vaginal culture for Gardnerella or anaerobes.* Since up to 40% of healthy women may have high numbers of these organisms present as normal flora, detection is not a reliable predictor of the syndrome and culture is not advised. Furthermore, although anaerobic bacteria diminish with cure, *Gardnerella* levels can persist.

Treatment

While symptomatic cases must be treated to alleviate patient discomfort, treatment of asymptomatic patients is controversial. Because of the large number of bacteria present in vaginal secretions from patients with BV and recent data linking it to serious infectious sequelae, the following guidelines are suggested:

■ *Gynecologic.* In asymptomatic women about to undergo elective vaginal or abdominal surgical procedures, treat to decrease the risk of postsurgical infections. Treat asymptomatic women about to undergo outpatient ambulatory invasive procedures, such as endometrial biopsy or hysterosalpingography. Consider treating asymptomatic woman at risk for PID.

■ *Obstetric.* Consider treating the asymptomatic patient with a history of preterm labor or previous infant of low birthweight.

■ *Sexual partners.* Although sexual intercourse is believed to be a primary method of transmitting BV, unequivocal proof is lacking and the syndrome has been identified in young virgins. Currently, treatment of sexual partners is advised in cases where recurrent BV is identified.

The only medications considered effective for treating BV are metronidazole and clindamycin. You may give 500 mg of metronidazole orally twice daily for 7 days. Metronidazole in a gel preparation is effective, but currently is available only through research protocol. You may give clindamycin either orally, in 300-mg doses two or three times daily for 7 days, or as a 2% vaginal cream, one application at bedtime daily for 7 days. The cream, although effective, is currently available only through research centers.

Douching and vaginal medications designed to lower vaginal pH may relieve symptoms but do not cure BV. Although once thought to be effective, antibiotics such as amoxicillin and sulfa are now considered less useful alternatives.

Treatment of pregnant women with metronidazole is complicated by the fact that the drug readily crosses the placenta. Metronidazole has not been shown to be carcinogenic or teratogenic in humans, but because of the theoretical risk, you should weigh whether benefit justifies use. Defer treatment of pregnant women at least until the second trimester, and consider using clindamycin as an alternative to metronidazole.

Sequelae

Although vaginitis generally is considered benign, serious sequelae have been associated with BV. Obstetric patients are at significant risk for development of preterm labor and delivery of low-birthweight infants. More recently, postpartum endometritis following vaginal or operative delivery and chorioamnionitis also have been identified as serious sequelae.

Gynecologic infectious sequelae include an increased frequency of laparoscopically proven pelvic inflammatory disease and posthysterectomy cuff cellulitis. In addition, patients with BV are at significant risk for recurrent urinary tract infections and nonpuerperal endometritis. Moreover, patients with BV have a higher incidence of cervical dysplasia.

SUGGESTED READING

Gardner HL, Dukes CD: *Haemophilus vaginalis* vaginitis. Am J Obstet Gynecol 1955;69:962

Hillier SL: In vitro inhibition of vaginal microorganisms by lactobacilli. Abstract No. 14. Annual Meeting, Infectious Disease Society for Obstetrics and Gynecology, Snowmass Village, Colo, Aug 6, 1988

Livingood CH, Thomason JL, Hill GB: Bacterial vaginosis: treatment with topical intravaginal clindamycin phosphate. Obstet Gynecol 1990;76:118

Spiegel CA, Amsel R, Holmes KK: Diagnosis of bacterial vaginosis by direct Gram stain of vaginal fluid. J Clin Microbiol 1983;18:170

Thomason JL, Gelbart SM, Anderson RJ, et al: Statistical evaluation of diagnostic criteria for bacterial vaginosis. Am J Obstet Gynecol 1990;162:155

Thomason JL, Gelbart SM, Broekhuizen FF: Advances in the understanding of bacterial vaginosis. J Reprod Med 1989;34(S8):580

Thomason JL, Gelbart SM, Wilcoski LM, et al: Proline aminopeptidase activity as a rapid diagnostic test to confirm bacterial vaginosis. Obstet Gynecol 1988;71:607

Totten PA, Amsel R, Hale J, et al: Selective differential human blood bilayer media for isolation of *Gardnerella (Haemophilus) vaginalis*. J Clin Microbiol 1982;15:141

33
Mucopurulent cervicitis

By Newton G. Osborne, MD, PhD

Background and incidence

Mucopurulent cervicitis (MPC) is a distinct clinical entity characterized by yellow mucopus and polymorphonuclear leukocytes (PMNs) in the endocervical exudate of reproductive-aged women who are not in the bleeding phase of their menstrual cycle. Since this type of discharge may also be seen in women with endometritis or salpingitis, it is important to differentiate these disorders by other diagnostic criteria.

The true incidence of MPC is not known since it is not a reportable disease; however, estimates have been made based on the incidence of *Chlamydia trachomatis* infection in given populations. In a 1984 study, Brunham and co-workers found that among women selected randomly for testing in a sexually transmitted disease clinic, 40% were diagnosed according to strict criteria as having MPC. Up to 75% of women identified as the sexual partners of men with chlamydial urethritis had positive cultures for *C trachomatis*, and many of these women had MPC.

Etiology

At least three organisms are recognized as causing cervicitis in women: *C trachomatis*, *Neisseria gonorrhoeae*, and herpes simplex virus (HSV). From 50% to 70% of MPC is caused by *N gonorrhoeae* or *C trachomatis*, or both. Nongonococcal urethritis (NGU), the male counterpart of MPC, is caused by *C trachomatis* in 40% to 50% of cases. It is possible that gram-negative facultative bacilli or anaerobes such as *Bacteroides* sp are involved as secondary invaders in the disease process, but this relationship is not well documented.

Diagnosis

Criteria for presumptive diagnosis include:

- mucopurulent endocervical secretion, usually yellow or green when viewed on a white cotton-tipped swab (positive swab test);
- 10 or more polymorphonuclear leukocytes per microscopic oil immersion field in a gram-stained smear of endocervical secretions; and
- cervicitis, determined by cervical friability (bleeding when the first swab culture is taken) and/or presence of erythema or edema within a zone of cervical ectopy.

The clinical diagnosis of MPC can be confirmed by laboratory tests documenting the presence of *N gonorrhoeae, C trachomatis*, or HSV. Specimens for gonococcal isolation should be inoculated on modified Thayer–Martin media or other appropriate selective media. Endocervical Gram stains for *N gonorrhoeae* in women are quite specific but only about 50% sensitive.

The gold standard for *C trachomatis* detection is culture on pretreated McCoy cell cultures. When culture is not available, direct immunofluorescence techniques using fluorescein-labeled monoclonal antibodies applied to endocervical specimens can be used, and are 97% sensitive and 99.8% specific. Recently marketed DNA probes are approximately as sensitive and specific as fluorescent antibody tests and are much less labor intensive for the laboratory. Culture for *C trachomatis* is mandatory, however, in cases involving rape or child abuse.

Cell culture is still the most sensitive and specific technique for establishing the diagnosis of herpes simplex virus infection. The presence of intranuclear inclusions and multinucleated giant cells on Papanicolaou smears suggests HSV infection but is only about 50% sensitive. Recently developed ELISA and other rapid antigen detection methods hold promise for providing immediate confirmation of HSV involvement in suspicious cervical lesions, but current tests are less sensitive than cell culture.

Clinical findings. Women with MPC may be completely asymptomatic. If symptoms are present, they may include abnormal discharge, postcoital spotting, and dyspareunia. Although some cases of asymptomatic disease may resolve spontaneously, most persist or ascend progressively to culminate in acute salpingitis.

At the time of clinical examination, certain signs may assist in making the diagnosis. The columnar epithelium of the endocervix is often friable and bleeds on contact with a swab or Ayre's spatula used to obtain a cytologic specimen. The classic mucopus should be seen after the cervical portio has been cleaned of debris. There may be tenderness with palpation and movement of the cervix.

In prepubertal females who are infected as a result of abuse or rape, vaginitis may be the presenting finding if chlamydial infection is involved. Lack of estrogenization of the vaginal epithelium allows for infection if *C trachomatis* is inoculated. Thickening of the epithelium after estrogen begins to be produced prevents vaginal invasion in reproductive-aged women.

Treatment

Once the diagnosis of MPC is made and appropriate cultures are obtained, antibiotic therapy must be instituted. If *N gonorrhoeae* is found on Gram stain or culture of endocervical or urethral discharge, a treatment regimen effective against both gonococcal and chlamydial infection should be used. The treatment of choice is ceftriaxone, 250 mg IM once, plus doxycycline, 100 mg orally twice daily for 7 to 10 days, or tetracycline, 500 mg orally four times daily for 7 to 10 days. [For alternative gonococcal regimens, see Chapters 34 and 35.]

When only chlamydial infection is proven or suspected, therapy should consist of either tetracycline or erythromycin. Erythromycin base, 500 mg orally four times daily for 7 days, is the recommended treatment for women who are tetracycline allergic or are pregnant. Recently, Crombleholme and co-workers have reported success in treating chlamydial infection with amoxicillin, and since nausea may be a significant side effect of erythromycin therapy, this drug may be an acceptable second choice.

The sexual partner or partners of all patients with MPC must be encouraged to seek medical care and be treated with an antibiotic regimen appropriate for coverage of *N gonorrhoeae* and *C trachomatis*.

Sequelae

Women with MPC who are undiagnosed and therefore untreated are at risk for a wide variety of diseases caused by *C trachomatis* or *N gonorrhoeae*. Chlamydial infection has been associated with the presence of atypical cells on cervical cytologic exams. Treatment of the infection will usually resolve the atypia.

Failure to treat MPC promptly may allow *C trachomatis* or *N gonorrhoeae* to invade the urethra and cause acute urethritis with purulent discharge and dysuria. Chlamydial infection has been associated with acute urethral syndrome, characterized by symptoms of cystitis in the absence of abnormal microscopic findings in the urinary specimen.

If *C trachomatis* or *N gonorrhoeae* remain untreated in the endocervix, they may ascend into the uterus and fallopian tubes and cause endometritis or salpingitis, or both. Chlamydial infection causes a very insidious type of salpingitis with minimal to moderate symptoms and yet severe damage to the tubal mucosa. Further consequences of salpingitis may be tubo-ovarian abscess, which occurs in 3% to 10% of cases, and ectopic pregnancy, which is increasing in incidence in the US.

Perihepatitis was once felt to be almost always caused by *N gonorrhoeae*; we now recognize that *C trachomatis* causes 75% of these cases. This disorder may often be confused with gallbladder disease and be improperly treated.

Mucopurulent cervicitis must be considered in any woman who presents with a history of dyspareunia and postcoital spotting or who is found to have mucopurulent cervical discharge and easily induced cervical bleeding on exam. Early appropriate therapy should diminish the number of women who can transmit their infection as well as prevent the consequences of ascending infection.

SUGGESTED READING

Brunham RC, Paavonen J, Stevens CE, et al: Mucopurulent cervicitis—the ignored counterpart in women of urethritis in men. N Engl J Med 1984;311:1

Crombleholme WR, Schachter J, Grossman MA, et al: Amoxicillin therapy for *Chlamydia trachomatis* in pregnancy. Obstet Gynecol 1990;75:752

Katz BP, Caine VA, Jones RB: Diagnosis of mucopurulent cervicitis among women at risk for *Chlamydia trachomatis* infection. Sex Transm Dis 1989;16:103

Osborne NG, Hecht Y, Gorsline J, et al: A comparison of culture, direct fluorescent antibody test, and a quantitative indirect immunoperoxidase assay for detection of *Chlamydia trachomatis* in pregnant women. Obstet Gynecol 1988;71:412

Shafer MA, Chew KL, Kromhout LK, et al: Chlamydial endocervical infections and cytologic findings in sexually active female adolescents. Am J Obstet Gynecol 1985:151:765

34
Uncomplicated anogenital gonorrhea

By Daniel V. Landers, MD

Background and incidence

Despite a recent overall decline, gonococcal infections continue to be among the most commonly reported sexually transmitted diseases in the United States, with an estimated 2 million cases occurring annually. The vast majority of uncomplicated anogenital gonorrhea cases occur in the 15- to 29-year-old age group. Sexually active 15- to 19-year-olds have twice the incidence seen in 20- to 24-year-olds. However, the highest incidence overall is found among 20- to 24-year-olds, since this group has a higher proportion of sexually active individuals than the teenaged group. Interestingly, there are also seasonal variations of about 20% in the incidence of gonorrhea in the US, with the peak in late summer.

Numerous risk factors have been associated with gonococcal infections, including low socioeconomic status, urban residence, non-Asian and nonwhite race and ethnicity, early onset of sexual activity, unmarried marital status, illicit drug use, prostitution, and past history of gonococcal infections. Contraceptive choices may affect risk. Spermicides, diaphragms, and condoms have been found to reduce the risk.

Etiology

Transmission of gonorrhea is almost entirely by sexual contact. It has been estimated that the risk of transmission from male to female is 80% to 90%, compared with only 20% to 25% for female to male after a single sexual encounter.

Although uncomplicated anogenital gonorrhea can frequently be asymptomatic, myriad clinical manifestations are associated with it. The primary site of urogenital gonococcal infection in women is the endocervix. Isolated colonization of the urethra is uncommon, but such infection may often be seen in association with endocervical infection. Occasionally, Bartholin's, Skene's, and the periurethral glands may be involved in gonococcal infections.

Most women either develop symptoms within 10 days of infection or remain asymptomatic. Symptoms that do occur are most commonly vaginal discharge, dysuria, intermenstrual bleeding, and menorrhagia. Mucopurulent endocervical discharge may be seen along with erythema and edema around the squamocolumnar junction.

In up to 50% of women with gonococcal cervicitis, there is a concurrent gonococcal rectal infection with or without a history of acknowledged rectal sexual contact. Anal examination may frequently be normal or may reveal erythema, discharge, or both. Anoscopy may reveal mucoid or purulent exudate, edema, and mucosal friability.

Diagnosis
Definitive diagnosis of gonococcal infection depends on identifying the causative agent, *Neisseria gonorrhoeae*, a gram-negative intracellular diplococcus. Isolation in culture is the standard means of diagnosis. The Centers for Disease Control's 1989 guidelines for sexually transmitted diseases advocate diagnosing or confirming all gonorrhea cases by culture to aid antimicrobial susceptibility testing.

Culturing is best accomplished by using selective media containing antibiotics. Modified Thayer–Martin medium has a diagnostic sensitivity of 96% in cultures from the endocervix. Sensitivity can be increased by duplicate endocervical swabbings or consecutive endocervical and anal swabbings. One should collect specimens by first cleansing the cervix to remove external exudate and then inserting a swab 1 to 2 cm up to the internal os and rotating it gently for 5 to 10 seconds.

Gram staining can be useful when culture is unavailable or as an adjunct to culture. Gram-negative diplococci with typical morphology identified or closely associated with polymorphonuclear leukocytes are considered diagnostic. The Gram stain is primarily used when there is a high index of suspicion of infection.

Treatment
Antimicrobial therapy for gonococcal infections derives from in vivo resistance patterns. The rising incidence of infection due to penicillinase-producing or tetracycline-resistant *N gonorrhoeae* (PPNG and TRNG, respectively) and strains of chromosomally mediated resistance to multiple antibiotics has led the CDC to alter treatment

TABLE 1

Treatment guidelines for uncomplicated urethral endocervical or rectal infections

Recommended regimen	Ceftriaxone, 250 mg IM once
Alternative regimen for patients who cannot tolerate ceftriaxone	Spectinomycin, 2 g IM once
Other alternatives for which there is less experience	Ciprofloxacin, 500 mg orally once
	Norfloxacin, 800 mg orally once
	Ofloxacin, 400 mg orally once
	Cefuroxime axetil, 1 g orally once with 1 g probenecid
	Cefotaxime, 1 g IM once
	Ceftizoxime, 500 mg IM once
	Amoxicillin, 3 g orally with 1 g probenecid (may be used only when infection is from a source proven not to have penicillin-resistant gonorrhea)
All regimens to be followed by	Doxycycline, 100 mg orally twice daily for 7 days

Source: Centers for Disease Control: MMWR 1989;38(S-8):21.

recommendations over the years. Guidelines were also influenced by the high frequency of chlamydial infections in individuals with gonorrhea and the absence of a rapid, inexpensive, and accurate test for these infections.

Thus, the current recommendation for treatment of uncomplicated anogenital gonorrhea is a single IM dose of ceftriaxone, followed by a 7-day course of oral doxycycline (Table 1). Ceftriaxone is highly effective against PPNG. While the recommended ceftriaxone dose for treatment of gonorrhea is 250 mg IM, the CDC points out that some experts prefer a dose of 125 mg IM because it is less expensive and can be given in a smaller volume, making deltoid administration easier. However, the 250-mg dose may delay emergence of ceftriaxone-resistant strains. Presently, both doses are considered highly effective for mucosal gonorrhea at all sites. A single 2-g dose of spectinomycin can be given in place of ceftriaxone. This agent has long been an alternative treatment for gonorrhea in the penicillin-allergic patient.

For the several additional options listed in the guidelines, there is considerably less experience. These include the quinolones ciprofloxacin, given as a single oral 500-mg dose, and norfloxacin, given as a single oral 800-mg dose. Ofloxacin, in a single oral dose of 400 mg, is another option. However, these agents are contraindicated for pregnant women and children up to the age of 16.

Three advanced-spectrum cephalosporins are listed as well, including cefuroxime axetil given as a single 1-g oral dose along with 1 g of probenecid. The other two cephalosporins, cefotaxime (1 g) and ceftizoxime (500 mg), do not require probenecid. Treating uncomplicated gonorrhea with a penicillin such as oral amoxicillin (3 g) together with oral probenecid (1 g) is appropriate only if the infection was acquired from a source proven not to have penicillin-resistant gonorrhea.

All alternatives to ceftriaxone are also followed with a 7-day course of oral doxycycline. Although tetracycline is a possible substitute for doxycycline, compliance may be worse with this drug since it must be administered four times a day instead of twice. Also, at current prices, tetracycline costs slightly more than generic doxycycline. Neither doxycycline nor tetracycline alone is considered adequate therapy for gonococcal infections but only for coexisting chlamydial infection.

Follow-up
Since treatment failure after the ceftriaxone/doxycycline regimen is rare, the CDC considers follow-up cultures ("test-of-cure") nonessential. A more cost-effective strategy may be reexamination with culture 1 to 2 months after treatment ("rescreening"). This approach detects both treatment failure and reinfections. Patients treated with regimens other than ceftriaxone/doxycycline should have follow-up cultures taken 4 to 7 days after completion of therapy.

Persons exposed to gonorrhea within the preceding 30 days should be examined, cultured, and treated presumptively. All patients with gonorrhea should have a serologic test for syphilis and should be offered confidential counseling and testing for HIV infection. Most patients with incubating syphilis will be cured by a regimen containing ceftriaxone, another ß-lactam, or tetracyclines. Patients treated with other regimens (for example, spectinomycin, ciprofloxacin, or norfloxacin) should have a serologic test for syphilis in 1 month.

Treatment failure

Persistent symptoms after treatment should be evaluated by culture for *N gonorrhoeae*, and any gonococcal isolate should be tested for antibiotic sensitivity. Because of reinfection rather than treatment failure, infections occurring after treatment with one of the recommended regimens are common.

Prevention

As with all sexually transmitted diseases, reducing the incidence of gonorrhea depends on education of patients and public awareness of modes of transmission and means of prevention. Among contraceptives, condoms are the most capable of preventing transmission and acquisition of *N gonorrhoeae*. The diaphragm, cervical cap, and to a lesser degree topical bacteriocidal agents may reduce risk of acquisition in women. Other practices, such as douching, washing, or urinating after intercourse, have not been shown to significantly reduce risk of acquiring *N gonorrhoeae*. In fact, douching may be associated with other potentially harmful effects.

Most important to any prevention effort is the tracing and treating of sexual contacts. This task is easier in areas where reporting gonococcal infections is mandatory, as in the US. The private physician, as well as public health departments, should make every attempt to refer or treat the partners of infected individuals.

Efforts are continuing toward developing a vaccine for the prevention of gonorrhea and gonococcal pelvic inflammatory disease. Thus far, however, there is no effective vaccine on the immediate horizon.

SUGGESTED READING

Barlow D, Phillips I: Gonorrhea in women: diagnostic, clinical and laboratory aspects. Lancet 1978;1:761

Centers for Disease Control: 1989 Sexually transmitted diseases treatment guidelines. MMWR 1989;38(S-8):21

Dans PE: Gonococcal anogenital infection. Clin Obstet Gynecol 1975;18:103

Hook EW III, Handsfield HH: Gonococcal infections in the adult, in Holmes KK, Mårdh PA, Sparling PF, et al (eds): *Sexually Transmitted Diseases.* New York, McGraw-Hill, 1990, pp 149-165

Klein EJ, Fisher LS, Chow AW, et al: Anorectal gonococcal infection. Ann Intern Med 1977;86:340

Louv WC, Austin H, Perlman J, et al: Oral contraceptive use and the risk of chlamydial and gonococcal infections. Am J Obstet Gynecol 1989;160:396

35

Disseminated gonococcal infection

By David E. Soper, MD

Background and incidence

Disseminated gonococcal infection (DGI) is a rare but important complication of *Neisseria gonorrhoeae* mucosal infection. Although the exact incidence is not known, it is estimated that approximately 1% of women with an uncomplicated gonococcal infection will develop DGI. The disseminated form is the most common cause of septic arthritis or tenosynovitis in adults.

Pathophysiology

Dissemination occurs when the *N gonorrhoeae* infecting the genital tract, pharynx, or rectum invade the bloodstream. This bacteremia leads to infection of the skin, synovia, and joints and accounts for clinical manifestations of the disease. Associated strains of *N gonorrhoeae* are usually of transparent-colony phenotype, have growth requirements for arginine, hypoxanthine, and uracil, and have a low-molecular-weight protein I. These factors may be associated with an increase in the invasiveness of the microorganism.

Host factors also play an important role. Patients with deficiencies in one of the late-acting complement components (C5, C6, C7, or C8) responsible for the bactericidal action of serum are predisposed to disseminated infection. Hormonal influences may also be important, because most cases in women occur close to menstruation or during pregnancy.

Diagnosis

The infection may be considered a two-stage process: an initial bacteremia associated with skin lesions, followed by a secondary phase associated with septic arthritis. Patients may present with

TABLE 1
Positive cultures from various sites

Site	Culture	Gram stain
Skin lesions	10%	10%
Joint fluid	20%–30%	10%–30%
Blood	10%–30%	—
Mucosal*	80%–90%	—

*Pharynx, urethra, cervix, or rectum
Source: Mills J, Brooks GF: Disseminated gonococcal infection, in Holmes KK, et al: *Sexually Transmitted Diseases.* 1984

different degrees of severity ranging from uncomplicated cases with skin lesions alone to such metastatic infections as endocarditis.

The primary manifestations are fever, usually with temperatures between 38°C (100.4°F) and 39°C (102.2°F), and skin lesions. The skin lesions begin as erythematous macules, 1 to 5 mm in diameter, and rapidly become pustular. They are located on the extremities, commonly near the small joints of the hands or the feet. It is important to look for these lesions between the fingers and toes.

Tenosynovitis, involving the extensor and flexor tendons and sheaths of the hands and feet, is also a common finding. Erythema, swelling, and tenderness are found along the tendon sheath. Marked pain is associated with tendon motion.

Arthritis is the third most common clinical manifestation. The knee is the most commonly affected joint, followed by the elbow, ankle, and small joints of the hand. Erythema, edema, pain, and effusion are the most frequent manifestations of a septic joint. Endocarditis and meningitis, the most serious complications, rarely occur.

Consider the diagnosis in any patient with tenosynovitis, polyarthritis, or peripheral pustular skin lesions. The differential diagnosis includes other bacteremias and noninfectious causes of tenosynovitis and arthritis. Meningococcemia may mimic gonococcal infection. However, when this occurs, the skin lesions are more likely to be petechial or purpuric, and tenosynovitis is rarely associated with meningococcal infection.

The laboratory diagnosis relies upon the Gram stain and culture. The local mucosal site is the most common source of a positive culture (Table 1). Blood cultures are positive in only about 10% to 30% of patients.

Treatment

Antimicrobial therapy is the mainstay of treatment (Table 2). Selected patients may be treated as outpatients. However, women who cannot reliably comply with treatment, pregnant patients, patients with septic arthritis, and those in whom the diagnosis is unclear should be hospitalized for observation and therapy. Although most strains of *N gonorrhoeae* causing disseminated disease are very susceptible to penicillin, a few cases caused by penicillinase-producing strains of *N gonorrhoeae* have been reported.

If an outpatient regimen is used, the patient should return for follow-up examinations in 24 hours and 1 week after the initiation of therapy. Symptoms rapidly resolve once therapy is started. Skin lesions should disappear within a few days. Tenosynovitis markedly improves within 24 hours and septic arthritis is much improved within 48 hours. Failure of symptoms to respond rapidly to appropriate antibiotic therapy should alert you to the possibility of an incorrect diagnosis such as Reiter's syndrome. Adjunctive anti-inflammatory drug therapy is not recommended. It may cloud the patient's symptomatic response to antibiotic therapy and obscure the final diagnosis.

Recovery of *N gonorrhoeae* from any site is strong evidence. The therapeutic response of patients to antibiotic therapy alone, even in the face of negative cultures, is good evidence that the diagnosis is correct.

TABLE 2
Treatment regimens

Initial therapy

Ceftriaxone, 1 g IM or IV every 24 hours

or

Ceftizoxime, 1 g IV every 8 hours

or

Cefotaxime, 1 g IV every 8 hours

If organism proves to be penicillin sensitive: ampicillin, 1 g every 6 hours

Penicillin-allergic patients

Spectinomycin, 2 g IM every 12 hours

Completion therapy

Complete therapy for a total of 1 week with an oral regimen once symptoms have resolved

Cefuroxime axetil, 500 mg bid

or

Amoxicillin, 500 mg with clavulanate tid

or

Ciprofloxacin, 500 mg bid (if not pregnant)

Source: Centers for Disease Control: MMWR 1989;38(S-8).

Contact tracing is an important element of both diagnosis and therapy. The sexual contact may have a positive culture when the index case does not, and epidemiologic treatment is important to prevent reinfection of the patient or infection of others with a strain of *N gonorrhoeae* likely to cause disseminated infection.

SUGGESTED READING

Centers for Disease Control: 1989 sexually transmitted diseases treatment guidelines. MMWR 1989;38(S-8):24

Hook EW, Holmes KK: Gonococcal infections. Ann Intern Med 1985;102:229

Mills J, Brooks GF: Disseminated gonococcal infection, in Holmes KK, Mårdh PA, Sparling PF, et al (eds): *Sexually Transmitted Diseases*. New York, McGraw-Hill, 1984

36
Syphilis in the nonpregnant patient

By George D. Wendel, Jr., MD, and Larry C. Gilstrap III, MD

Background and incidence

Syphilis is a complex, chronic systemic infection caused by the spirochete *Treponema pallidum*, which is usually transmitted through intimate or sexual contact. The incidence of syphilis has increased markedly in the past few years in the United States, primarily because of increases in large urban areas plagued by drug abuse and prostitution.

In 1988, the incidence of primary and secondary syphilis was 16.7 per 100,000 persons in the US, and 40,117 cases were reported to the Centers for Disease Control. Not surprisingly, a marked increase in the incidence of congenital syphilis has followed (766 cases in 1988), since most of the infections occur in reproductive-aged men and women. Currently, the marked increases in infectious syphilis are occurring in heterosexual men and women, with marked declines noted in gay males, presumably because of safe sex practices to prevent HIV infection. The ratio of the total cases of primary and secondary syphilis in men to women is now less than 2:1.

Etiology

T pallidum has a characteristic spiral motion and flexing about its midportion that allows easy identification by dark-field microscopy. The organism enters the body through minute abrasions in skin or a mucosal surface and begins to replicate locally. Thus, the common sites of the initial lesions of syphilis are those most likely to sustain microscopic frictional trauma during intimate contact—the fourchette, the cervix, the anus, the lips, and the nipples.

Diagnosis

The most accurate method for confirming the clinical diagnosis of syphilis is visualization of *T pallidum* by dark-field microscopy in material from a moist genital lesion or a regional lymph node aspirate. Serologic tests are the most common means of confirming infection, especially latent syphilis. Nonspecific antibody can be measured by the rapid plasma reagin (RPR) test or the Venereal Disease Research Laboratory (VDRL) test, which can be used both for screening and to follow response to therapy.

These tests are reported as nonreactive or reactive and also given a titer, which generally reflects the degree of current infection and allows for comparison with post-treatment titers. Specific antitreponemal antibody testing is used to confirm infection after a reactive RPR or VDRL test.

Two methods are used: one measures specific treponemal antibody by the microhemagglutination assay for antibodies to *T pallidum* (MHA-TP); the other approach is the fluorescent treponemal antibody-absorption (FTA-ABS) technique. Results, which are reported as nonreactive or reactive, without titers, remain positive even after therapy and are not used as an index of response to treatment or for primary diagnosis. False-positive results (reactive nontreponemal tests and nonreactive treponemal tests) occur transiently in 1% of patients, and are generally of low titer. They are often attributed to laboratory error, subclinical autoimmune disease, or IV drug abuse.

The initial clinical manifestation of syphilis is the chancre, usually accompanied by regional adenopathy. The lesion develops at the site of inoculation about 3 weeks after exposure, but can take up to 10 to 90 days to appear. It is a painless, red, round, firm ulcer with a granular base with well-formed, raised edges. A "press prep" of material squeezed from a chancre will usually show motile spirochetes under dark-field microscopy, confirming the diagnosis. Serologic testing is reactive in 80% to 90% of patients with primary infection because of a several-day delay in the production of antibody after primary infection. Chancres spontaneously heal in 3 to 8 weeks without treatment.

After several weeks, the local manifestations of primary syphilis progress to dissemination, characteristic of the secondary stage of infection. Chancres may be present as the infection progresses. Nearly all patients will progress to this stage about 6 weeks after primary syphilis develops. It is characterized by diffuse, symmetric skin lesions and systemic abnormalities. The dermatologic manifestations of secondary syphilis are numerous, leading to the prior designation as the "great imitator." Generalized lymphadenopathy, hepatitis, nephrosis, and alopecia also may occur.

TABLE 1
Regimens for treatment of syphilis

Early syphilis*
Benzathine penicillin G, 2.4 million U IM, as a single injection

Syphilis of more than 1 year's duration†
Benzathine penicillin G, 2.4 million U IM, weekly for three doses

Neurosyphilis
Aqueous crystalline penicillin G, 2 to 4 million U IV every 4 hours, for 10 to 14 days; followed by benzathine penicillin G, 2.4 million U IM weekly, for three doses

Aqueous procaine penicillin G, 2.4 million U IM daily, plus probenecid, 500 mg orally four times daily, both for 10 to 14 days; followed by benzathine penicillin G, 2.4 million U IM weekly, for three doses.

*Primary, secondary, and latent syphilis of less than 1 year's duration.
†Latent syphilis of unknown or more than 1 year's duration, cardiovascular, or late benign syphilis.
Source: Centers for Disease Control: MMWR 1989;38(S-8).

The genital manifestations of secondary syphilis are moist cutaneous external lesions called condylomas and mucous patches, the latter often resembling genital herpes simplex virus infection. Both of these lesions are moist, highly infectious, and easily diagnosable by dark-field examination. The serologic testing for syphilis is reactive in almost all cases at this stage.

After 3 to 12 weeks, the untreated lesions of secondary syphilis resolve and a latent stage develops. The diagnosis at this stage is made by a reactive serologic test for syphilis without the signs or symptoms of primary or secondary disease. This stage is often divided into early-latent syphilis and late-latent syphilis according to the length of the illness, using 1 year's duration as the reference point. This timing is used because the infectivity for sexual or fetal transmission is important during the early period when about 25% of patients will have a clinical recurrence similar to the secondary stage. In late latency, patients run a greater risk of having tertiary syphilis or neurosyphilis.

Treatment
Penicillin is the preferred drug for treating all patients with syphilis, regardless of the stage of infection (Table 1). Penicillin is the only clinically tested agent that has been widely used for patients with all

TABLE 2
Alternative regimens for penicillin-allergic patients

Early syphilis
Tetracycline, 500 mg orally four times daily for 2 weeks
Doxycycline, 100 mg orally two times daily for 2 weeks
Erythromycin, 500 mg orally four times daily for 2 weeks
Ceftriaxone, 250 mg IM daily for 10 days*

Syphilis of more than 1 year's duration
Tetracycline, 500 mg orally four times daily for 4 weeks
Doxycycline, 100 mg orally two times daily for 4 weeks

Neurosyphilis
Nonpenicillin treatment not recommended

*Probably effective; limited clinical experience.
Source: Centers for Disease Control: MMWR 1989;38(S-8).

stages of infection, including those during pregnancy. In general, barring reinfection, therapy with long-acting benzathine penicillin G is effective in eradicating early syphilis in 98% of immunocompetent adults. Penicillin desensitization is the optimal mode of therapy for patients allergic to penicillin (documented by skin testing). Oral or IV penicillin desensitization is available, and the oral regimen has been widely used clinically.

Alternative regimens of doxycycline and tetracycline are less effective but should cure over 90% of cases (Table 2). Close follow-up and compliance are necessary when using alternative regimens.

After treatment of early disease, the Jarisch-Herxheimer reaction occurs in over 60% of patients. This is manifested as an acute febrile reaction, occurring within 24 hours of therapy, with systemic symptoms such as headache, myalgia, and flushed lesions. Antipyretics may be recommended, but no proven methods exist to prevent this reaction.

Early syphilis treatment failures can occur with any regimen but are infrequent with penicillin. Patients should be reexamined clinically and serologically 3 and 6 months after treatment. Nontreponemal antibody titers should decline fourfold by 3 months with primary or secondary syphilis and by 6 months with early latent syphilis. HIV-infected patients should have more frequent follow-up with serologic testing at 1, 2, 3, 6, 9, and 12 months. Any patient with signs and symptoms of persistent infection or reinfection or a four-fold increase in nontreponemal titer should have a cerebrospinal fluid (CSF) exam by lumbar puncture and be retreated appropriately.

Ideally, patients with late-latent syphilis of more than a year's duration, gummas, or cardiovascular syphilis should have a CSF examination before treatment. However, the decision can be individualized. In the older asymptomatic patient, the lumbar puncture is likely to be normal. The CSF examination is indicated in specific cases. The recommended regimen for the treatment of this stage of infection consists of benzathine penicillin G given weekly for three doses on consecutive weeks. The alternative regimen of doxycycline or tetra-cycline given daily for 4 weeks for penicillin-allergic patients can be used for patients in whom penicillin skin testing and desensitization are unavailable (Table 2). Quantitative serologic tests should be repeated at 6 and 12 months.

Clinical evidence of neurologic involvement, such as optic and auditory symptoms or cranial nerve palsy, warrants CSF examination. The treatment of neurosyphilis is not well established, but requires prolonged parenteral penicillin. If initial CSF pleocytosis was present, spinal fluid should be examined every 6 months until the cell count is normal. If it has not decreased in 6 months or is not normal by 2 years, retreatment should be considered.

HIV-infected patients. All sexually active patients with syphilis should be encouraged to have counseling and testing for HIV anti-body because of frequent coinfection and implications for clinical management. Neurosyphilis should always be considered in a differ-ential diagnosis of neurologic abnormalities in HIV-infected persons. Bizarre high nontreponemal antibody titers have been noted as well as seronegative secondary syphilis in HIV-infected patients. Penicillin regimens should be used whenever possible for all stages of syphilis in HIV-coinfected patients, but no change in the dosage for early syphilis is recommended by the CDC. Careful follow-up is necessary to ensure the adequacy of treatment, as treatment failures have been reported in HIV-coinfected adults.

Epidemiologic treatment. Sexual partners of individuals with early syphilis should be evaluated clinically and serologically. If the contact occurred within 3 months, the partner may be infected but seronegative and should be presumptively treated. The current recommended treatment for gonorrhea (ceftriaxone and doxycy-cline) probably is effective for incubating syphilis. If a nonpenicillin antimicrobial is used to treat gonorrhea, the patient should undergo serologic testing for syphilis in 3 months.

Sequelae

After prolonged latency of many years, 20% to 30% of untreated patients will develop late complications of syphilis. Today, these entities are quite rare, as fewer patients escape early diagnosis and treatment. Additionally, because of the long latency period, most of the signs of late syphilis are rare in young, reproductive-aged women. Benign late syphilis, characterized by gummas, develops in 15% of patients. Cardiovascular syphilis, with aortitis, develops in a least 10% of patients. Late neurosyphilis, causing meningovascular disease, paresis, and tabes dorsalis, develops in 7% of untreated adults.

Unfortunately, neurosyphilis cannot be diagnosed accurately by any single testing technique. Moreover, the decision on when to perform a lumbar puncture for CSF analysis in patients with latent syphilis is controversial. The CDC recommends that a lumbar puncture be considered for all patients with latent syphilis of unknown or greater than a year's duration, especially in specific situations such as the following:

■ treatment failure;

■ nonpenicillin treatment planned;

■ neurologic signs or symptoms (optic, auditory, cranial nerve, or meningeal);

■ serum RPR or VDRL titer ≥ 1:32;

■ other evidence of active late syphilis (aortitis, gumma, iritis);

■ positive HIV test.

As CSF abnormalities are common in adults with early (primary, secondary, or early latent) syphilis, a lumbar puncture is not recommended unless signs and symptoms of neurologic involvement exist in immunocompromised and HIV-infected patients.

As most of the patients with early syphilis and abnormal CSF findings do not develop neurosyphilis, there are no clear data to indicate that these patients need additional therapy. CSF tests should include a cell count, a quantitative protein determination, and a VDRL test. The CSF white blood cell count is usually elevated to greater than 5 WBC/mm^3 when neurosyphilis is present. The VDRL should be considered diagnostic of neurosyphilis when positive. However, it may be negative when neurosyphilis is present and, thus, cannot be used to rule out neurosyphilis.

SUGGESTED READING

Centers for Disease Control: 1989 sexually transmitted diseases treatment guidelines. MMWR 1989;38(S-8):5-13

Centers for Disease Control: Recommendations for diagnosing and treating syphilis and HIV-infected partners. MMWR 1988;37:600,607

Hart G: Syphilis tests in diagnostic and therapeutic decision making. Ann Intern Med 1986;104:368

Holmes KK, Mårdh PA, Sparling PF, et al (eds): *Sexually Transmitted Diseases*, ed 2. New York, McGraw-Hill, 1989

Wendel G: Early and congenital syphilis. Obstet Gynecol Clin North Am 1989;16:479

Zenker PN, Rolfs RT: Treatment of syphilis, 1989. Rev Infec Dis 1990; 12(suppl 6):S590

37
Chancroid

By H. Hugh Allen, MD

Background and incidence

Chancroid is a common sexually transmitted disease in many parts of the developing world, especially in Africa. The global incidence far exceeds that of syphilis. The disease is less common in North America, although the incidence appears to be rising.

Between 1971 and 1980, a mean of 878 cases was reported annually in the United States, with most cases in the southern part of the country. Since 1981, a steady increase in cases has been reported, to a maximum of 5,047 in 1987. However, there may be many more unreported cases at present. Recent outbreaks in Greenland, Canada, and the United Kingdom (Sheffield, England) emphasize the disease potential in temperate climates.

Etiology and Epidemiology

Because *Haemophilus ducreyi*, the causative organism, is a difficult organism to grow in culture, suspected cases are not often confirmed in clinics. Since certain physicians, especially those in sexually transmitted disease clinics, are more aware of the disease, geographic clustering is a prominent feature of reports. The actual incidence and overall rate in North America, therefore, is difficult to assess.

The male:female ratio for chancroid ranges from 3:1 to 25:1. Since prostitutes are important transmitters of the disease, a few women can infect a large number of men. Case findings and culture efforts in some areas where outbreaks have occurred have not been helpful in pinpointing the source of infection. Attempting to find women who harbored *H ducreyi* without symptoms or signs has not proven useful. A few women without symptoms were found with cervical ulcers. Efforts to eliminate the disease have not been successful in any reported areas over the past decade. The role of asymptomatic carriers is unclear. Outside of the United States, chancroid has been associated with increased HIV infection rates.

Diagnosis

Chancroid must be considered in the differential diagnosis of any patient with a painful genital ulcer. Painful inguinal lymphadenopathy is present in about half of all chancroid cases. Chancroid lesions typically present as painful, sharply demarcated, nonindurated ulcers. These ulcerations are often ragged and undermined in appearance, with an erythematous halo. The base of the ulcer is composed of granulation tissue that bleeds easily on manipulation and may be covered by a necrotic exudate. A single ulcer is usual, but multiple ulcers and even extragenital lesions are occasionally reported.

Clinical diagnosis of chancroid based on the appearance of the ulcer is often inaccurate. In comparing bacteriologic with clinical diagnosis, accuracy of diagnosing lesions caused by *H ducreyi* has varied from 33% to 53%. However, in areas where chancroid was prevalent and clinicians more experienced, the diagnostic accuracy rose to 75%. These reports emphasize the necessity of definitive laboratory testing, because a wide variety of aerobic and anaerobic bacteria can be isolated from ulcers that clinically resemble chancroid. Agents such as herpes simplex virus and *Treponema pallidum* are sometimes isolated together with *H ducreyi*. Aids in making the diagnosis include:

- clinical suspicion when a genital ulcer is seen;
- cultures from the genital ulcer material (aspirates from inguinal nodes are less reliable);
- transporting the swab in Amies or Stuart transport media (a sterile swab transported on chocolate agar has also been shown to be successful).

Direct examination of Gram staining has not been consistent. The Ito-Reenstierna skin test and the complement fixation test formerly used have shown both false-negative and false-positive reactions. Poor sensitivity and specificity preclude their clinical use. There are qualitative and quantitative differences in the immune response to *H ducreyi* and the factors controlling this response are not clearly understood.

Circulating immune globulins (IgM and IgG) have been detected in patients with a clinical diagnosis of chancroid. Immunobinding and enzyme immunoassays have been used to investigate culture-confirmed and clinically suspected cases of chancroid. However, the geographic differences in the protein on the outer membrane add to the difficulty in selecting a cross-reacting antigen. There are both qualitative and quantitative differences in the immune response to chancroid, but the underlying factors are not clearly understood.

Treatment

Antibiotic resistance has been observed to trimethoprim, gentamicin, tetracycline, chloramphenicol, streptomycin, kanamycin, penicillin, ampicillin, and sulfonamides. The genetics and mechanisms of the antibiotic resistance by various strains of *H ducreyi* have been fairly well investigated. *H ducreyi* appears to have remained susceptible to erythromycin and ceftriaxone and most strains are susceptible to the quinolones.

The recommended treatment regimens for chancroid infection are erythromycin, 500 mg orally four times a day for 7 days, and ceftriaxone, 250 mg in one IM dose. Alternative regimens include ciprofloxacin, 500 mg orally every 12 hours for a total of 3 days; amoxicillin, 500 mg, plus clavulanic acid, 125 mg, orally every 8 hours for 7 days; and sulfamethoxazole, 800 mg, with trimethoprim, 160 mg (one double-strength tablet), orally twice daily for 7 days (in areas where trimethoprim resistance is not prevalent).

Because of the resistance spectrum, susceptibility testing of isolates from patients who fail therapy should always be performed. With effective treatment, ulcers should improve symptomatically within 3 days and objectively within 7 days after institution of therapy. Clinical resolution of lymphadenopathy is slower than that of ulcers. If no clinical improvement is evident in 7 days, consider the following: (1) Is the *H ducreyi* a resistant strain? (2) Is the diagnosis incorrect? (3) Is there coinfection with another sexually transmitted disease? (4) Is the patient also infected with HIV?

Sex partners within the 10 days preceding onset of symptoms in an infected patient, whether symptomatic or not, should be examined and treated with a recommended regimen.

SUGGESTED READING

Chouinard A: Winnipeg suffered second chancroid outbreak: team reports. Can Med Assoc J 1989;140:18

Johnson AP, Abeck D, Davies HA: The structure, pathogenicity, and genetics of *Haemophilus ducreyi*. J Infec 1988;17:99

Morse B, Stephen A: Chancroid and *Haemophilus ducreyi*. Clin Microbiol Rev 1989;4:137

Schmid GP: The treatment of chancroid. JAMA 1986;255:1757

Schmid GP, Sanders LL, Blount JH, et al: Chancroid in the United States. JAMA 1987;258:3265

38

Lymphogranuloma venereum

By Gael P. Wager, MD, MPH

Background and incidence

Lymphogranuloma venereum (LGV) is a systemic disease caused by the L-serotypes of *Chlamydia trachomatis* (L1, L2, L3). These serovars are often referred to as *C trachomatis biovar lymphogranuloma* and are identified by means of microimmunofluorescence techniques.

LGV has the potential for systemic dissemination and often persists as a chronic disorder. It is endemic in Africa, India, parts of Southeast Asia, South America, and the Caribbean. However, it can appear sporadically anywhere in the world. Data on prevalence rates are unreliable even in endemic areas.

The lymphadenitis of LGV was recognized by Greek, Roman, and Arab physicians. Durand, Nicolas, and Favre established the infection as a clinical and pathologic entity in 1913. Frei, in 1924, developed a specific skin test that permitted more accurate diagnosis.

Pathophysiology

The organism is generally transmitted by sexual contact. Once it has gained entry into the host, it incubates at the infection site and induces a primary lesion. It then invades the lymphatic system to cause a thrombolymphangitis and perilymphangitis. The inflammatory process spreads from infected lymph nodes into the surrounding tissue. The infected nodes become enlarged and develop areas of necrosis, which then form "stellate abscesses." As the inflammation progresses, the abscesses coalesce and rupture the node, forming loculated abscesses, fistulas, or sinus tracts.

The acute inflammatory process lasts several weeks to months before subsiding. Healing takes place by fibrosis, which destroys the normal structure and function of the lymph nodes and vessels. The resulting chronic edema and fibrotic changes cause induration and enlargement of the affected areas. Fibrosis also compromises the blood supply to the overlying skin and mucous membrane, leading to ulceration.

Diagnosis

LGV is predominantly an infection of lymphatic tissue. It has a variety of acute and late manifestations. Three stages usually characterize the clinical course of the disease: a primary stage extending from the incubation period through formation of the initial lesion; a secondary stage with inflammation and swelling of the regional lymph nodes (the inguinal syndrome); and a tertiary stage that includes the late sequelae of the infection (anogenital syndrome).

Primary stage. The infection is believed to occur primarily during sexual contact. Since chlamydial organisms cannot penetrate intact skin or mucous membranes, they probably enter through minute lacerations or abrasions. The incubation period after exposure is uncertain but appears to range from 3 to 21 days. After this period, a primary lesion may develop. It may appear as a papule, a small or shallow ulcer or erosion, a small herpetiform ulcer (the most common presentation), or even as nonspecific urethritis. This lesion is generally small, transient, and painless. It often goes unnoticed by the patient.

Healing is spontaneous and without scarring. The most common sites in men are the coronal sulcus, glans, penile shaft, urethra, and scrotum. In women, the lesion is most commonly located on the posterior vaginal wall, the fourchette, the posterior lip of the cervix, or the vulva.

Secondary stage (inguinal syndrome). The secondary stage is characterized by painful inflammation and enlargement of the inguinal nodes. This presentation is seen primarily in men, probably because the penis and scrotum are the most common sites of primary infection and because the lymphatic drainage from this area is to the inguinal nodes. In women, the vagina and cervix are the primary sites and the principal lymphatic drainage is to the deep iliac, perirectal, and lumbrosacral nodes. Involvement of the deep iliac and retroperitoneal lymph nodes may be signified by a pelvic mass. Abdominal, pelvic, and lower back pain are also frequently seen.

When the femoral nodes are concomitantly involved, a characteristic cleft is found between the inguinal and femoral nodes because of the presence of Poupart's ligament. This finding is referred to as the "groove sign" and is considered pathognomonic for LGV. At this stage, many patients will also manifest systemic symptoms such as fever, headache, malaise, and anorexia in addition to the enlarging femoral nodes.

The lymph nodes may suppurate as a result of inflammatory enlargement. Rupture through the overlying skin may occur, with immediate relief of pain and fever. Numerous sinus tracts are then formed that continue to drain thick, yellowish pus for long periods.

The organism may also gain access to the bloodstream and cause systemic disease. Manifestations of such a dissemination may include arthritis, pericarditis, pneumonia, hepatitis, erythema nodosum, and erythema multiforme.

Tertiary stage (anogenital syndrome). This stage is characterized by proctocolitis, rectal stricture, rectovaginal fistulae, esthiomene, and elephantiasis. The vast majority of patients with these late complications are women or homosexual men.

The early symptoms of rectal infection include anal pruritus and a mucous rectal discharge resulting from edema and hyperemia of the anorectal mucosa. The mucosa becomes friable, easily traumatized, and prone to ulceration. Ulcers are replaced by granulation tissue and the granulomatous process progressively involves all layers of the bowel wall. The muscle layers are replaced by fibrous tissue that contracts over time.

The region 2 to 10 cm above the rectal sphincter is the area most commonly affected. Patients may complain of colicky pain, abdominal distension, constipation, and narrow-caliber stools ("pencil stools"). The rectal mucosa distal to the stricture and the skin around the anus are frequent sites of perirectal abscesses and anal fissures.

The combination of chronic inflammation and lymphatic stasis will induce marked changes in the genital structures. Perianal outgrowths of lymphatic tissue that grossly resemble hemorrhoids (lymphorrhoids) may be seen. In women, there may be severe edema and enlargement of the vulvar structures. Subsequent compromise of the blood supply to the superficial tissues will lead to development of painful ulcers. This presentation is referred to as esthiomene (Greek: "eating away"). In men, penile, scrotal, or perineal sinuses may develop. Penoscrotal elephantiasis may also be seen.

Other manifestations. Autoinoculation of infectious discharge to the conjunctiva may occur. In this situation, the maxillary and posterior auricular lymph nodes may become involved.

LGV lesions of the mouth and pharynx may appear when infection is acquired by fellatio or cunnilingus. Cases of supraclavicular lymphadenitis with mediastinal lymphadenopathy and pericarditis have been reported with the presentation of LGV.

The literature also records the recovery of *C trachomatis* from the gallbladder wall in cases of chronic cholecystitis as well as from fibrous perihepatic abdominal and pelvic adhesions (in cases of Fitz-Hugh–Curtis syndrome).

Laboratory confirmation. For decades, the Frei antigen skin test was the definitive method for confirming the diagnosis of LGV. The Frei antigen is no longer available in the US and the Frei test is mentioned only for its historical significance. The diagnosis is now based on (1) a positive serologic test, either complement-fixation (CF) or microimmunofluorescence (MIF); (2) isolation of chlamydial organisms; or (3) histologic identification of chlamydial elementary and/or inclusion bodies in infected tissue.

The CF test was introduced in the 1930s. This test will detect antibodies to either *C trachomatis* or *C psittaci*. The CF antigen is common to all members of the *Chlamydia* genus. In LGV, the CF test usually becomes positive within the first 2 weeks of infection. Titers may remain positive for life. Titers of 1:64 or greater are generally associated with LGV infection. Titers in individuals with other *C trachomatis* infections are generally 1:16 or less.

The MIF test was developed by Wang and Grayson to serotype strains of *C trachomatis*. The test detects type-specific antibodies produced against each chlamydial serotype. The specimen is run against a panel of antigens and the diagnosis is based on the pattern of reactivity. The disadvantage of the MIF test is that it is available only in a few specialized laboratories.

Chlamydial organisms can be isolated from infected tissue by inoculation into HeLa-229 or McCoy cells. Specimens of pus obtained from a fluctuant lymph node yield the highest rates. However, most laboratories do not maintain active cell lines for chlamydial isolation. Reported recovery rates range from 24% to 30%.

Histologic identification of chlamydial elementary and inclusion bodies can be made both outside and inside cells in secretion and infected tissues. Fluorescent antibody staining and Giemsa's iodine are used. Overall, the diagnosis of LGV by histologic and cytologic methods has not been very successful.

Differential diagnosis. Conditions to exclude when findings suggest LGV are genital herpes, donovanosis (granuloma inguinale), chancroid, cat-scratch fever, bacterial lymphadenitis, Hodgkin's disease, and non-Hodgkin's lymphoma. Because other sexually transmitted infections may occur at the same time, it is also important to exclude common infections such as syphilis and gonorrhea when entertaining a diagnosis of LGV.

Treatment

A number of antibiotics have been shown to be effective in treating

LGV. However, no single drug has demonstrated superior effectiveness. Antibiotics that have been used in the treatment of LGV have included the tetracyclines, chloramphenicol, erythromycin, sulfadiazine, sulfamethoxazole, and rifampin. Treatment administered in the early stages of the infection achieves a better clinical response than therapy begun at the later, more chronic stages.

The most recent CDC recommendations for LGV suggest that patients be treated for 3 weeks. The drug of choice is doxycycline, 100 mg orally two times per day. Alternative regimens include tetracycline, 500 mg orally four times per day; erythromycin, 500 mg orally four times per day; or sulfisoxazole, 500 mg orally four times per day (or equivalent sulfonamide course).

SUGGESTED READING

Centers for Disease Control: 1989 sexually transmitted diseases treatment guidelines. MMWR 1989;38(S-8):15

Faro S: Lymphogranuloma venereum, chancroid, and granuloma inguinale. Obstet Gynecol Clin North Am 1989;16:517

Hammerschlag MR: Lymphogranuloma venereum, in Felman YM (ed): *Sexually Transmitted Diseases*. New York, Churchill Livingstone, 1986, chap 7

Perine PL, Osoba AO: Lymphogranuloma venereum, in Holmes KK, Mårdh PA, Sparling PF, et al (eds): *Sexually Transmitted Diseases*. New York, McGraw-Hill, 1984, chap 26

Sweet RL, Gibbs RS: *Infectious Diseases of the Female Genital Tract*. Baltimore, Williams & Wilkins, 1985, pp 34-36

39
Donovanosis

By Rudolph P. Galask, MD, and Noelle Bowdler, MD

Background and incidence

Donovanosis is an ulcerative bacterial infection of the genitalia that is found most commonly in tropical and subtropical areas. First described by McLeod in 1882, the disease has carried several names, including granuloma inguinale and granuloma venereum. The causative agent, identified by Donovan in 1905, is currently known as *Calymmatobacterium granulomatis*. Infection can lead to significant scarring and may be associated with the subsequent development of carcinoma. Recently, concern has arisen that genital ulcers due to this and other infectious agents may be sites for transmission of the human immunodeficiency virus.

The disease occurs primarily in India, the west coast of Africa, the West Indies, Brazil, southern China, and New Guinea and is endemic in the aboriginal population of central Australia. Although uncommon in the United States, it has been found in the Southeast, particularly among the black population.

Donovanosis is believed to be transmitted sexually, although it is not thought to be highly contagious. In various studies, between 12% and 52% of the sexual partners of affected patients were found to have the disease after repeated unprotected sexual contact. The fact that lesions almost always occur on the genitalia or uterine cervixes of sexually active women supports the concept that the disease is transmitted sexually. The occasional appearance of oral lesions is believed to be due to orogenital contact. Because the organism requires living tissue in order to grow in vitro, it has been suggested that a break in the host's skin or mucous membranes is needed to allow infection.

Pathophysiology

After an incubation period, which varies from 8 to 80 days, single or multiple subcutaneous nodules appear and erode through the skin to produce ulcers. Ulcerated areas are sharply defined but irregular in contour, and the base is often described as "beefy red." The lesions are granulomatous, and may become secondarily infected. Fibrosis occurs as the primary lesion extends, and lymphedema distal to the lesions is common.

In women, the lesions of donovanosis are found most often on the inner labia, particularly near the clitoris. The uterine cervix is also a primary site. In men, the lesions are generally on the glans or prepuce. The inguinal regions are involved in approximately 10% of cases, with formation of pseudobuboes. The perianal tissues are affected in 5% to 10% of cases.

Local extension from the cervix to the endometrium, fallopian tubes, and ovaries occurs occasionally. Distant sites are involved in up to 6% of cases. Primary infections of the head, in particular the mouth and throat, have been reported. Infections of the liver, spleen, thorax, and bone have also been described. Distant disease of this type is usually, but not always, associated with genital involvement. It is assumed that the organism spreads hematogenously to these sites.

Diagnosis

A diagnosis of donovanosis may be suggested by the patient's history and physical findings. Confirmation depends on the identification of Donovan bodies in a smear or biopsy specimen taken from the margin of an ulcer. Donovan bodies are calymmatobacteria located within the cytoplasmic vacuoles of macrophages. The bacteria are pleomorphic rods that turn blue with Giemsa staining. Wright's stain and various silver stains can also be used to identify the organism. A recent report suggests that the Rapidiff stain is another satisfactory alternative.

Although complement fixation and skin testing have been studied experimentally in patients with donovanosis, no immunologic test is yet available for use clinically in the diagnosis of this disease.

The differential diagnosis includes infectious diseases such as chancroid that cause genital ulcers. Early lesions may resemble the syphilitic chancre. Perianal lesions are often verrucous, and can be confused with the condylomata lata of secondary syphilis. Differentiation of donovanosis from other disorders is hampered by the fact that it often coexists with other sexually transmitted diseases.

When lesions are chronic, they must be differentiated from those of carcinoma of the vulva. Evaluation for carcinoma is particularly important in this setting because it may occur as a complication of donovanosis.

Treatment

The drug of choice is tetracycline, 500 mg orally every 6 hours. There is disagreement about whether this dosage should be continued until all visible lesions have healed, or whether a 10- to 14-day course is sufficient. Resistance of the organism to tetracycline has been reported. An alternative oral regimen is trimethoprim/sulfamethoxazole, two tablets twice a day for 14 days. This regimen can be used during pregnancy, except in the late third trimester.

Gentamicin, 1 mg/kg parenterally three times a day, was found to be an effective treatment in a small study. Chloramphenicol, 2 g per day orally in divided doses for 10 to 14 days, is also effective but is not recommended because of its rare potential for causing profound bone marrow depression. Recently, norfloxacin, 400 mg orally twice a day for 7 to 10 days, was shown to be useful for treating donovanosis in a study of ten patients.

Erythromycin, 500 mg orally every 6 hours, is another option for use in pregnancy. It is most effective, however, when combined with agents such as ampicillin or lincomycin. Ampicillin may be effective as a single agent, but penicillin is not.

With appropriate antibiotic treatment, lesions usually begin to decrease in size within days after the initiation of therapy. Generally, they are completely healed within 2 to 3 weeks.

Vulvectomy is undertaken in cases resistant to antibiotic treatment. Surgery may also be necessary if there is significant residual lymphedema of the vulva after antibiotic treatment, or if there has been extensive destruction of vulvar tissues.

Patients with donovanosis should be screened for other sexually transmitted diseases. Their sexual partners should also be treated. Abstinence from sexual activity is recommended until the lesions have healed.

Sequelae

Long-standing infection with *C granulomatis* may lead to destruction of the affected tissues and scarring at the site of involvement. Stenosis of the vagina or anus can result. An increased incidence of vulvar carcinoma has been reported in patients with a history of donovanosis, although the strength and nature of this association is unclear.

In one study, an increased incidence of HIV infection was noted in patients with genital ulcers. Because the lesions of donovanosis bleed easily, there is concern that these may be sites for the transmission of HIV.

SUGGESTED READING

Faro S: Lymphogranuloma venereum, chancroid, and granuloma inguinale. Obstet Gynecol Clin North Am 1989;16(3):517

Hart G: Donovanosis, in Mandell GL, Douglas RG Jr, Bennet JE (eds): *Principles and Practice of Infectious Diseases*, ed 3. Edinburgh, Churchill Livingstone, 1990, p 393

Latif AS, Mason PR, Paraiwa E: The treatment of donovanosis (granuloma inguinale). Sex Transm Dis 1988;15(1):27

O'Farrell N, Hoosen AA, Coetzee K, et al: A rapid stain for the diagnosis of granuloma inguinale. Genitourin Med 1990;66:200

Schwartz RH: Chancroid and granuloma inguinale. Clin Obstet Gynecol 1983;26(1):138

Sehgal VN, Shyamprasad AL, Beohar PC: The histopathological diagnosis of donovanosis. Br J Vener Dis 1984;60:45

40
Pediculosis pubis

By Mahmoud A. Ismail, MD

Background and incidence

Lice infestations have been recognized for centuries both as endemic and as epidemic disorders. Conditions of poor personal hygiene and overcrowding have been associated with such epidemics. Recently, a resurgence of skin disease caused by the pubic or crab louse has been recognized, paralleling the current increased incidence of other sexually transmitted diseases.

Lice infestations have been observed in virtually every inhabited area of the world. Sexual permissiveness has aided spread to all strata of society. Pediculosis pubis is usually spread through sexual contact. It is more contagious than any other sexually transmitted disease; the chance of contracting the disease during a single sexual encounter is 95%.

After infection, pubic lice can be found on any terminal hair of the body. The organism's transfer from the pubic hair is probably mechanical, assisted by animated scratching, fingernails, towels, and other similar means rather than self-propulsion. The perineal and axillary hair is often infected, and the hair of trunk, beard, scalp, and eyelashes is occasionally contaminated. Pediculosis pubis is most commonly encountered during adolescence and young adulthood.

Etiology

Phthirus pubis, the crab louse, is the organism that causes pediculosis pubis. The organism is 1 to 2 mm long, gray, tough skinned, and square, resembling a crab—whence it derives its nickname. It tends to remain in a restricted area in the genital region, where it attaches to the base of pubic hairs and feeds through mouth parts adapted to piercing skin. The sites of feeding nits are sometimes marked by small bluish hemorrhages into the skin.

The life cycle is 25 to 30 days from egg to egg. The female begins to lay eggs within 24 hours after mating, attaching them to a hair near the root. After an incubation time of 7 days, a nymph hatches and proceeds through three molts over the next 13 to 17 days. Once the louse reaches sexual maturity, the adult's life expectancy is 3 to 4 weeks.

Diagnosis

Pediculosis pubis infestations usually cause pruritus and itching. The intense itching is believed to be due to allergic reactions to foreign material injected by the organism during feeding. Bites often exhibit a hemorrhagic component thought to be the result of injections of anticoagulant material at the time of feeding. Pubic lice infestations of eyelashes may produce a pruritic and occasionally secondary infected marginal blepharitis.

Visualization of adult lice and their eggs (nits) with a magnifying glass is diagnostic for pediculosis pubis. Diagnosis should be confirmed by microscopic examination of a crab or its nit, or both. On occasion, the patient may see the crab louse moving over the skin.

Treatment

The recommended regimen is permethrin (1%) cream rinse applied to the affected area and washed off after 10 minutes. Alternatives are pyrethrins and piperonyl butoxide applied to the affected area and washed off after 10 minutes, or lindane (1%) shampoo applied for 4 minutes and then thoroughly washed off. Lindane treatment is not recommended for pregnant or lactating women.

Patients should be reevaluated after 1 week if symptoms persist. Retreatment may be necessary if lice are found or eggs are observed at the hair–skin junction. Sex partners should also be treated.

Pediculosis of the eyelashes should be treated by applying occlusive ophthalmic ointment to the eyelid margins two times a day for 10 days to smother lice and nits. Lindane or other drugs should not be applied to the eyes. Clothing or bed linen that may have been contaminated by the patient within the past 2 days should be washed and dried by machine (hot cycles) or dry-cleaned.

SUGGESTED READING

Centers for Disease Control: 1989 sexually transmitted diseases treatment guidelines. MMWR 38(S-8):39

Couch JM, Green WR, Hirst LW, et al: Diagnosing and treating *Phthirus pubis palpebarum*. Surv Ophthalmol 1982;26:219

Felman YM, Nikitas JA: Pediculosis pubis. Cutis 1980;25:482,487-489,559

Orkin M: Pediculosis today. Minn Med 1974;57:848

41
Scabies

By Mahmoud A. Ismail, MD

Background and incidence

Scabies is a disease of great antiquity and possibly the cause for the "Seven Year Itch" known to medicine for centuries. Napoleon's troops during the Russian campaign were thought to have had rampant scabies. It is common throughout the world and appears to increase in prevalence in 30-year cycles. Scabies has been on the rise in the US since 1973.

The disease is world-wide in distribution, but the actual prevalence is unknown. Epidemics have been associated with world wars. Overcrowding, poor hygiene, malnutrition, and sexual promiscuity probably are contributing factors.

Scabies is now considered a sexually transmitted disease, but prolonged contact with an infected person is required for transmission. Nonsexual transmission has been reported in hospitals during nursing activities such as sponge bathing patients and applying body lotions. Transfer of mites through infested bedding, clothes, or other fomites has also been implicated as a major mode of transmission.

Etiology

Human scabies is caused by the itch mite *Sarcoptes scabiei var hominis*. The full-grown adult female is only about 0.35 mm long and is rounded, with three pairs of short stubby legs. *S scabiei* moves briskly across the skin and can travel from neck to waist in a few hours.

Eggs are laid by the fertilized female in burrows several millimeters to several centimeters long, created at the base of the stratum corneum of the epidermis. Approximately 72 to 84 hours later nymphs emerge and undergo several molts to become adult mites. The adult mites mate 17 days later; shortly afterward the male dies, but the grown female proceeds to burrow and complete the life cycle.

Diagnosis

Scabies manifests itself by causing intense itching in the host, usually worse at night. The rash has an insidious onset and a characteristic pattern of involvement that includes the interdigital web spaces, wrists, elbows, anterior axillary folds, periumbilical skin, genitals, buttocks, and sides of the feet. In infants and small children, the palms, soles, face, and scalp may be affected.

The physical findings in scabies include classic linear burrows, particularly in the interdigital spaces and on the penis. The burrows are 5 to 10 mm long and the organisms may be seen as tiny brown and white specks at the inner ends of them. In infants, scabies may also at times be vesicular or even bullous, and secondary pyoderma may obscure the underlying cause.

Scabies may present as eczematous or urticarial eruptions. Approximately 7% of infected persons exhibit a nodular variant with scattered, pruritic, reddish-bown nodules, particularly on the penis and in the axillae and perineum. These lesions are possibly a manifestation of strong delayed hypersensitivity to retained mite products and may take weeks or months to disappear. Immunocompromised or debilitated patients may be infested with large numbers of mites found in thickened psoriasis-like skin lesions. This condition, known as Norwegian scabies, is extremely contagious.

The burrow of *S scabiei* is pathognomonic. However, burrows may not be apparent in many cases. Application of blue or black ink to the skin overlying a suspected burrow can aid diagnosis. By capillary action, the ink will be pulled into the burrow. Removal of the excess external ink with an alcohol swab will leave a line of ink in the burrow to demonstrate its presence. It is the burrow containing the organism's egg and feces that will yield a positive scraping and confirmation of the diagnosis on microscopic examination. Fresh lesions should be used for obtaining mites.

Scabies is called the great imitator because patients may have a variety of lesions. Dermatologic conditions such as eczema, acute urticaria, impetigo, erythrasma, insect bites, neurodermatitis, and dermatitis herpetiformis must be considered in the differential diagnosis. The history of insidious onset and the presence of nocturnal pruritus, pleomorphic lesions, and the characteristic distribution of lesions are strongly suggestive of scabies.

Treatment

Treatment of scabies remains controversial. Success depends on correct application of scabicide to the patient, sexual contacts, and family members.

For adults and older children, the recommended regimen is lindane (1%), 1 oz of lotion or 30 g of cream, applied thinly to all areas of the body from the neck down and washed off thoroughly after 8 hours. Sex partners and close household contacts should also receive this treatment, but it is not recommended for pregnant or lactating women.

An alternative regimen is crotamiton (10%), applied to the entire body from the neck down nightly for 2 nights and washed off thoroughly 24 hours after the second application. This treatment should be used for infants, children up to 2 years old, and pregnant and lactating women.

Pruritus may persist for several weeks even after adequate therapy. A single retreatment after 1 week may be considered if there is no clinical improvement. Additional weekly treatments are appropriate only if live mites continue to be found.

Clothing or bed linen that may have been contaminated by the patient within the past 2 days should be washed and dried by machine (hot cycles) or dry-cleaned.

SUGGESTED READING

Cohen HKB: Scabies continues. Int J Dermatol 1982;21:134

Centers for Disease Control: 1989 sexually transmitted diseases treatment guidelines. MMWR 38(S-8):39-40

Oriel JD: Ectoparasites, in Holmes KK, Mårdh PA (eds): *International Perspectives on Neglected Sexually Transmitted Diseases*. Washington, DC, Hemisphere Publishing, 1983, pp 131-138

42
Molluscum contagiosum

By David E. Soper, MD

Background

Molluscum contagiosum is a benign dermatologic infection caused by an unclassified poxvirus. In children, the lesions appear sporadically in a generalized distribution and usually involve the face, trunk, and arms. After puberty, lesions are found typically on or near the genitalia.

Pathophysiology

Most investigators feel the molluscum contagiosum virus (MCV) is spread by direct contact. Patient histories and clinical data support the assumption that MCV may be sexually transmitted in some cases. Skin-to-skin contact associated with sexual intercourse is considered the most common method of transmitting the virus in adults. Non-sexual transmission has been reported in patients treated by a surgeon who had hand lesions and in association with wrestling, tattooing, and the use of gymnastic equipment and towels.

Initially, MCV infects the basal keratinocytes. The virus persists in the epidermis in a progressively maturing form similar to that seen in human papillomavirus infections. MCV lesions consist of focal areas of hyperplastic epidermis that surround cystic lobules filled with keratinized debris and degenerating molluscum bodies. The molluscum bodies (Henderson–Paterson bodies) are composed of large masses of maturing virions. The pathologic changes are limited to the epidermis. In some cases, dermal inflammation may occur as a reaction to viral antigen or keratin infiltration. Resolution usually follows.

The average incubation period for MCV infections is 2 to 3 months. Most patients are asymptomatic, the MCV lesions being incidental to a variety of nonvenereal and nondermatologic conditions. Occasionally, patients complain of pruritus, tenderness, and pain.

The lesions are usually flesh colored, but can appear gray–white, yellow, or pink. They begin as tiny pinpoint papules that grow over several weeks to a diameter of 3 to 5 mm. The papules are smooth, firm, and dome-shaped. They have a highly characteristic central umbilication from which caseous material can be expressed.

One to 20 lesions are commonly found on the skin of the labia majora, mons pubis, buttocks, and inner thighs. They rarely, if ever, cover mucosal surfaces. The linear orientation of some lesions suggests autoinoculation by scratching. Occasionally, multiple lesions become confluent and converge into a "giant molluscum."

Individuals with deficiencies of cell-mediated immunity (for example, AIDS patients) are at risk for extensive outbreaks.

Diagnosis

The diagnosis of molluscum contagiosum can be made reliably on clinical grounds alone. Excisional biopsy reveals typical enlarged epithelial cells with intracytoplasmic inclusion bodies. Diagnostic confirmation may also be obtained by noting sheets of ovoid, homogenous bodies up to 25 µm in diameter after crushing the contents of a lesion on a slide and staining with Giemsa, Wright, or Gram stain. Electron microscopic examination will identify the typical poxvirus particles. It is impossible to grow this organism in vitro.

Treatment

The natural history of MCV infection is characterized by spontaneous regression of mature lesions followed by continued emergence of new lesions. Molluscum contagiosum persists from 6 months to 3 years in the absence of therapy. Lesions may be eradicated by mechanical destruction or techniques that induce local epidermal inflammation. While such treatment may hasten the resolution of individual lesions and reduce the incidence of autoinoculation and transmission to other individuals, recurrence is frequent. The benign and self-limited nature of the infection must therefore be weighed against the potential harm of destructive therapies.

The most widely used method of therapy is excisional curettage. Individual lesions are curetted, and the bases are treated with light electrodesiccation. Cryotherapy and topical treatment with podophyllin or trichloroacetic acid have also been used with favorable results. No therapy has been found to be effective in immunocompromised patients, however, probably because of persistent recurrence of new lesions.

Cryotherapy with a liquid nitrogen spray apparatus is one practical approach. Such units can be purchased or are available in most dermatologist's offices. The lesions are sprayed until they turn white and are surrounded by a white ring approximately 1 mm in diameter. Large lesions can be sprayed twice with a freeze–thaw–freeze technique.

SUGGESTED READING

Brown St, Nalley JF, Kraus SJ: Molluscum contagiosum. Sex Transm Dis 1981;8:227

Douglas JM: Molluscum contagiosum, in Holmes KK, Mårdh PA, Sparling PF, et al (eds): *Sexually Transmitted Diseases*. New York, McGraw-Hill, 1990

Wilkin JK: Molluscum contagiosum venereum in a women's outpatient clinic: a venereally transmitted disease. Am J Obstet Gynecol 1977;128:531

43

Genital herpes simplex infections

By James H. Harger, MD

Background and incidence

Genital herpes simplex virus (HSV) infections appear to be common in women, although the majority are asymptomatic or produce such mild symptoms that they are overlooked. In a recent longitudinal study by Pazin and co-workers of 4,781 sexually active women attending five family planning clinics in southwestern Pennsylvania, 27.4% had antibodies to glycoprotein (gG-2) of HSV type 2 (HSV-2). However, only 4.9% of the 4,781 women gave a history of genital HSV infection. Of the history-positive women, 95.1% tested positive for antibodies to gG-1 or gG-2. In that same population, it was previously found that only 63% of the isolates from the initial case of genital HSV infections were HSV-2. The other isolates (37%) were HSV-1.

The actual prevalence of genital HSV infection in the community is difficult to determine because of this marked disparity between symptomatic and asymptomatic cases. The finding by Whitley and co-workers that more than half of all cases of neonatal HSV infection arise in babies born to women with no known history of genital HSV infections shows that such women harbor the disease and are contagious. Similarly, asymptomatic genital HSV infection has been found in men.

The subtle and highly variable course of the disease is vexing to patients and those who would counsel them. But its nature must be understood in order to plan an effective and appropriate management strategy.

Pathophysiology

Initial episodes. The first episode of genital HSV infection is as variable as the recurrences. The classic, severe "primary" episode occurs in the 30% of women who have no preexisting antibodies against either HSV-1 or HSV-2. It lasts a mean of 20 days; but evidently most initial episodes are less severe and may even produce no symptoms. These milder "initial, nonprimary" episodes of genital HSV infection may occur because anti-HSV antibodies developed during previous oral HSV infections afford partial protection.

Both true primary (seronegative) and initial nonprimary (history-negative but seropositive) genital HSV infections usually begin with a flu-like syndrome of fatigue, malaise, myalgia, nausea, and fever developing 3 to 5 days after sexual activity with the source contact. Vulvar burning and pruritus precede the multiple vesicles that occur in two or more anatomic regions of the vulva, the vagina, and (rarely) the cervix. These vesicles may remain intact for 24 to 36 hours before evolving into painful, tender, shallow ulcers. During the first several days of initial infection, crops of vesicles may appear at new sites or near old ones.

Several studies have revealed that the mean duration of pain in primary lesions is 9 to 13 days and the mean time to crusting 9 to 15 days. Complete healing of the genital lesions requires a mean of 10 to 22 days, and HSV cultures remain positive ("HSV shedding") for a mean of 8 to 14 days.

We have observed continuous HSV shedding from the cervix for 41 days after the onset of a primary episode, even when vulvar lesions were entirely healed. The correct duration of drug therapy for such initial episodes, therefore, remains difficult to establish.

Recurrent episodes. After the initial episode resolves, the pattern of recurrence varies, but there is a rough correlation between the severity of the first episode and the frequency of recurrences in the first year. After a severe primary episode of genital HSV infection, there are usually one to six recurrences in the first year. In some women, the recurrences become farther and farther apart from the beginning, but a few unfortunate patients will have monthly bouts for several years.

After a mild or equivocal initial episode, most women develop only sporadic recurrences. Often, these do not even result in lesions. Rather, the attack consists only of prodromal lancinating pain, vulvar pruritus, and vulvar tenderness and localized swelling without ulceration. Infrequently, however, women with mild primary episodes will develop frequent recurrences.

Whatever the overall pattern, many women will experience stretches of several months in which the recurrence frequency actually increases temporarily. At such times, the patient often seeks medical advice about therapy when none was deemed necessary before.

The duration and severity of recurrent genital HSV lesions is less than that of the initial episodes. Most recurrences result in the formation of one or two vesicles, and these usually ulcerate within 12 hours. Usually, only one area on the vulva is affected, and that site is often the same from one recurrence to another. The mean duration of HSV shedding varies from 3.1 to 7.4 days. The mean duration to crusting of the lesions is 2.7 to 5.0 days, and to complete healing, 9.0 to 11.3 days. Patients experience pain in the lesions for a mean of 3.1 to 8.6 days.

Just as these mean values for the recurrences vary considerably from study to study, so do the severity and duration of the recurrences vary markedly and unpredictably from one episode to another in the same patient. This pattern makes assessment of the efficacy of therapy very difficult.

Diagnosis

Although the diagnosis of genital HSV ulcers is generally made on clinical grounds, it should be confirmed at least once by laboratory methods before pharmacologic therapy is instituted. If the patient has an ulcerated or vesicular lesion or cornified squamous epithelium, a Tzanck smear can be obtained by gently scraping the base of the lesion and transferring the cells obtained to a glass slide and fixing them immediately. The cytologist will then study the slide for multinucleated giant cells that have a characteristic appearance. The Tzanck smear's sensitivity ranges from 85% to 95% and its specificity exceeds 95%. Papanicolaou smears of moist mucous membranes for HCV shedding also exceed 95% specificity, but their sensitivity is only 60% to 70% (that is, 30% to 40% are false negative).

The correct standard method for detecting HSV shedding is tissue culture on primary rabbit kidney cells or human foreskin fibroblasts. A swab moistened in Hanks balanced salt solution should be rubbed gently but persistently over the mucous membrane or the base of the lesion to dislodge and obtain viable cells infected with HSV. The swab is then placed into the transport medium and sent as soon as possible to the tissue culture laboratory. If the delay in transport is more than one hour, the transport tube should be cooled to 4°C (refrigerator temperature) or frozen at −70°C in a special virology freezer. Freezing the transport medium at −20°C, the temperature usually maintained in the freezer portion of a household refrigerator, will result in rapid reduction in the viral titer and might cause a false-negative result.

Once the specimen is inoculated into tissue culture, 95% of HSV can be detected within 3 days by observing the cell monolayer for cytopathic effect (CPE) with an inverted microscope. If typing of HSV is desired, the growing HSV can be stained with monoclonal antibodies to distinguish HSV-1 from HSV-2, though this step is rarely of any clinical use. Similarly, since 70% of the adult population is seropositive for HSV-1 because of prior oral HSV lesions, usually acquired in childhood, serologic studies for specific antibodies to HSV-1 or HSV-2 are hardly ever clinically useful.

Treatment

The goals and methods of treatment for genital HSV infections depend on the nature and severity of the episode. Although most primary episodes of genital HSV infection in the adult do not result in HSV encephalitis or disseminated HSV infection, around 10% are associated with headache, photophobia, nausea, and meningeal signs. Also, nearly all women with multiple genital HSV lesions of primary disease have severe pain when they urinate. For that reason, they usually limit their liquid intake to decrease the necessity of voiding frequently. Advise such women that the pain can be reduced by pouring warm water over the vulva while urinating (to dilute the urine) or by urinating while sitting in a tub of warm water.

A much smaller proportion of women with primary genital HSV infection, however, develop a true sensory neurogenic bladder and cannot urinate at all. These women probably require hospitalization, a suprapubic bladder catheter, and IV antiviral drug therapy. Antibiotics have no place in the treatment of primary genital HSV infections. Analgesics are of little value but may help patients sleep. Topical antiviral agents don't shorten episodes, and topical lidocaine gel provides only temporary relief (and may lead to allergic reaction).

In contrast, recurrent genital HSV infections are rarely frequent enough or painful enough to warrant pharmacologic treatment. Yet the loss of self-esteem, the loss of a sense of control over her own body, and the fear of transmitting HSV infections to others usually encourages the patient to seek help in preventing and treating recurrences. Many women have tried such unproven therapies as (1) dietary manipulation to avoid foods high in arginine, (2) megadoses of lysine and vitamins, and (3) stress management and stress reduction techniques.

While counseling and education help patients understand their disease and reduce the risks of HSV transmission, the only effective antiviral agent currently available in the US is acyclovir. This drug is a DNA-polymerase inhibitor that is activated only in the nucleus of HSV-infected cells by an HSV-encoded thymidine kinase. Acyclovir has few side effects when administered orally and is usually well-tolerated over prolonged periods. When given IV to treat adults seriously ill with HSV infections, it can be nephrotoxic. Renal function must, therefore, be monitored carefully. Long-term effects of acyclovir are not known to be harmful.

Treating primary infections. Pharmacologic therapy for the initial episode of genital HSV infection can diminish the duration of symptoms and lesions. Once the diagnosis of initial genital HSV infection has been made and a culture of the lesion obtained to confirm the diagnosis, initiate oral acyclovir at a dosage of 200 mg every 4 hours.

In prospective, randomized, placebo-controlled studies by Mertz and co-workers that demonstrated a significant improvement in the course of the disease among acyclovir recipients, 200-mg capsules were given five times a day (omitting a dose in the middle of the night) and continued for 10 days. When used in this fashion, acyclovir reduced HSV shedding from 9 days in controls to 2 days with acyclovir therapy. Mean time to crusting of lesions was reduced from 10 to 7 days in acyclovir-treated men and women. Duration of lesions was reduced from 16 days to 12 days and mean duration of local pain from 7 days to 5 days. Acyclovir also decreased the mean duration of constitutional symptoms from 6 days to 3 days.

In studies of acyclovir therapy of first episodes of genital HSV infections, the 10-day therapy was mandated by protocol. In clinical practice, it would be reasonable to continue the therapy beyond 10 days if the patient's lesions weren't healing well by that time. Continuing therapy in a prophylactic fashion is not warranted, however, because the onset of the first recurrence, if one does occur at all, cannot be predicted. Rather, it would be best to stop therapy once the initial episode has resolved and observe the severity and frequency of subsequent recurrences before deciding whether further treatment is warranted.

While hospitalization is rarely necessary for initial episodes, there are some reasonable indications for parenteral acyclovir therapy in the hospital. Patients with severe constitutional symptoms that include emesis may be unable to take oral acyclovir. Patients with meningeal signs, including nuchal rigidity, photophobia, and severe headache, should be evaluated by a neurologist and infectious disease specialist for the possibility of HSV encephalitis. Usually, they should be treated with IV acyclovir until these symptoms resolve. Patients with evidence of HSV hepatitis or other visceral dissemination should be treated parenterally. Finally, patients with urinary retention should have a suprapubic bladder catheter inserted until they recover from the overdistension. These patients may also benefit from parenteral acyclovir therapy in the hospital.

Parenteral acyclovir should be given as an infusion of 5 mg/kg of body weight, administered over 15 to 60 minutes and repeated every 8 hours. In the severely ill patient, the dosage can be pushed to 7.5 mg/kg. Serum creatinine should be determined daily to detect nephrotoxicity, a reversible condition that represents the major complication of IV acyclovir. As soon as the disease begins to resolve, the parenteral acyclovir can be changed to oral doses of 200 mg given every 4 hours.

Therapy for recurrent disease. Once a patient develops recurrent genital HSV infections, confirm by culture on one occasion to be certain that the lesions represent recurrent HSV infection. If the signs and symptoms are consistent and typical, further HSV cultures are unnecessary. Obtain a careful history to determine the frequency and duration of the episodes. There are three alternative strategies available to manage recurrent genital HSV infections.

(1) *Education.* Pharmacologic therapy may be unnecessary or contraindicated. Since the safety of oral acyclovir therapy during pregnancy is not known, the drug should not be given to women who are attempting to conceive. In fact, it is prudent to avoid acyclovir therapy in any woman at risk for pregnancy who is not using effective contraception. In most cases of recurrent genital HSV infections, frequency is so low and severity minimal enough that the patient may be satisfied if she knows she can use pharmacologic therapy at any time she chooses. Simply having this sense of control and an understanding about the disease may allow the patient to reduce the risk of HSV transmission to sexual partners and obviate acyclovir.

(2) *Intermittent oral acyclovir.* When the recurrences develop at intervals exceeding 2 months, continuous use seems wasteful and unnecessary. If the infrequent recurrences last 5 to 10 days or more, duration can be reduced by giving acyclovir at 200 mg every 4 hours during waking hours (five times each day). In a multicenter, randomized, placebo-controlled study of 250 patients by Reichman and co-workers, oral acyclovir reduced the mean duration of HSV shedding from 3.4 days to 2.1 days, mean time to crusting of lesions from 3.2 days to 2.4 days, mean duration of pruritus from 3.6 days to 2.8 days, mean duration of pain from 3.4 days to 3.0 days, and mean duration of lesions from 6.5 days in placebo patients to 5.5 days in drug recipients.

Such differences are subtle, but all were statistically significant. Because the differences are small, however, acyclovir therapy will achieve virtually no appreciable improvement in recurrences that are typically less than 5 days in length. Some patients will benefit more from the knowledge that they have some measure of control over the recurrences than from actually using the drug.

The Reichman study demonstrated a better effect from oral

acyclovir when it was begun very early in the course of the recurrence. For that reason, the patient should not wait to see a physician for confirmation of each recurrence. Rather, the patient should purchase 20 to 25 acyclovir capsules to keep on hand until prodromal symptoms are perceived. The patient should then commence therapy immediately after symptoms appear.

(3) *Suppression.* The third strategy for recurrent genital HSV infection is prophylactic therapy. In patients whose recurrences develop more than six to eight times a year, continuous administration of oral acyclovir usually produces dramatic reductions in the frequency of recurrences. Two large studies (of 950 and of 261 patients) of 1 year of oral acyclovir at a dose of 400 mg twice daily showed that 44% and 46% of patients, respectively, had no recurrences at all, whereas only 2% and 5% of placebo-treated controls remained free of recurrences. Expressed differently, acyclovir-treated patients developed a mean of 1.8 recurrences per year in the two studies compared with mean recurrence rates in controls of 11.4 and 8.7 per year, respectively.

These and other studies of smaller populations and shorter therapy demonstrate that suppressive therapy with acyclovir can be effective and safe. No hepatic or renal toxicity of oral acyclovir has been observed in any study. Determination of long-term safety, of course, must await 15 to 25 years of post-marketing evaluation. Finally, suppression therapy with acyclovir in immunocompetent patients has not yielded any clinically significant HSV isolates that are resistant to the drug.

In clinical situations where acyclovir suppression of frequent genital HSV recurrences is employed, it is reasonable to begin with the proven dose of 400 mg twice daily and then reduce the dose gradually as long as no recurrence develops. Alternatively, the potential hazards and cost of acyclovir may be minimized by beginning at a level of 200 mg twice daily and raising the dose if this lower level is insufficient. Further, suppressive doses of acyclovir have been continued beyond 1 year to 2 years or more without any adverse effects. Although many physicians refuse to extend prescriptions for acyclovir suppression beyond the 12 months "approved" by the Food and Drug Administration, FDA approval limits only the advertising claims permitted for the manufacturer, not the physician's clinical use.

Finally, although acyclovir suppression does not, in and of itself, alter the natural history of genital HSV recurrences, the frequency of recurrences may diminish spontaneously. Patients taking long courses of acyclovir should occasionally interrupt therapy to assess any changes in the frequency of recurrence that would render further suppression unnecessary.

SUGGESTED READING

Baker DA, Blythe JG, Kaufman R, et al: One-year suppression of frequent recurrences of genital herpes with oral acyclovir. Obstet Gynecol 1989;73:84

Deardourff SL, Deture FA, Drylie DM, et al: Association between herpes hominis type 2 and the male genitourinary tract. J Urol 1974;112:126

Harger JH, Pazin GJ, Breinig MC: Current understanding of the natural history of genital herpes simplex infections. J Reprod Med 1986;31:365

Kurtz TO, Boone GS, Acyclovir Study Group: Safety and efficacy of long-term suppressive Zovirax treatment of frequently recurring genital herpes: year 5 results. Abstract 1107. 30th Interscience Conference on Antimicrobial Agents and Chemotherapy, Atlanta, Ga, Oct 21-24, 1990

Mertz GJ, Critchlow CW, Benedetti J, et al: Double-blind placebo-controlled trial of oral acyclovir in first-episode genital herpes simplex virus infection. JAMA 1984;252:1147

Mertz GJ, Jones CC, Mills J, et al: Long-term acyclovir suppression of frequently recurring genital herpes simplex virus infections: a multicenter double-blind trial. JAMA 1988;260:201

Pazin GJ, Harger JH, Armstrong JA, et al: Leukocyte interferon in the treatment of initial episodes of genital herpes. J Infect Dis 1987;156:891

Reichman RC, Badger GJ, Mertz GJ, et al: Treatment of recurrent genital herpes simplex infections with oral acyclovir. JAMA 1984;251:2103

Straus SE, Croen KD, Sawyer MH, et al: Acyclovir suppression of frequently recurring genital herpes: efficacy and diminishing need during successive years of treatment. JAMA 1988;260:2227

Whitley RJ, Nahmias AJ, Visintine AM, et al: The natural history of herpes simplex virus infection in mother and newborn. Pediatrics 1980;66:489

44

Human papillomavirus infection

By Stanley A. Gall, MD

Background and incidence

Genital warts have been recognized for centuries, but their infectious nature was not described until 1894. A virus was implicated as an etiologic agent in 1907, but the human papillomavirus (HPV) particle was not seen with electron microscopy until 1949. To this day, there has been no convincing demonstration of a method for culturing human papillomavirus in tissue culture.

The spectrum of disease includes clinical (genital warts) and subclinical HPV infection of the cervix, vagina, vulva, perineal body, and anus; an association of HPV with intraepithelial neoplasia of the vulva, vagina, cervix, and penis; and juvenile laryngeal papillomatosis. More recently, it has been demonstrated that HPV DNA is present in practically every squamous malignancy of the female and male genital tracts. Because of this association with malignant disease, the diagnosis and therapy of human papillomavirus infection has taken on a greater significance.

A case load increase of more than 1,000% has been noted in sexually transmitted disease clinics and private office consultations over the past 5 years. The prevalence of HPV correlates with sexual activity. Peak occurrence is between ages 15 and 35. HPV is also associated with other STDs. Between 50% and 70% of sexual partners have or will develop genital warts.

Human papillomavirus produces an overt infection in 30% of cases and subclinical infection in 70%. The virus can also exist in a latent state. During this period it can be identified only by recombinant DNA technology.

In studies using cervical cytology to estimate the prevalence of genital HPV infection, 2% to 3% of unselected Papanicolaou smears were positive. When HPV DNA sequencing was applied to these Pap smears, an additional 20% were positive for HPV infection.

HPV can occupy multiple sites in the female genital tract. If the cervix is infected, 77% of women will have vaginal lesions. Similarly, 36% of women who have vulvar infection will also have an infected cervix. These facts suggest that HPV satisfies the criteria for an infectious etiology as a multicentric source of carcinoma of the vulva and vagina. Although most investigators do not believe HPV is the primary etiologic agent of genital squamous tract malignancies, most believe it is a strong co-carcinogen. Finding HPV in any area of the genital tract suggests the virus will be present in the remainder of the genital tract.

Pathophysiology

It has been suggested that microtrauma allows the virus to enter the skin or mucosa of the genital tract. The virus enters the cells at the basal layer and matures as it passes through the parabasal, spinous, and granular layers of the epithelium. At the granular cell level, viral DNA replication, late protein synthesis, and viral particle assembly is carried out. Integration of the viral DNA into the host genome does not occur until the CIN III/carcinoma in situ stage of development.

Findings may be clinical or subclinical in any of the genital areas. Overt condyloma acuminatum may be seen in the perianal area, perineal body, vulva, vagina, or cervix; subclinical HPV infection may also be seen in each of these areas.

Vulvar condylomas appear as pinkish, whitish, or pigmented sessile tumors with a surface of lobulated or pointed finger-like projections. These are found most commonly on the vulvar area and less commonly in the vagina and the cervix. When HPV infection manifests itself as a flat lesion with minimal elevation or as a pink papular plaque with a smooth surface, it may be missed during routine examination.

Subclinical HPV infection is more common than overt infection. The most common lesion is the elongated vaginal papilla with clustered epithelial projections in a central capillary. Aceto-white epithelium is another common manifestation. It may be detected by a colposcopic examination of the vulva after application of 5% acetic acid, which causes the individual cells to swell, giving a white color to wart or neoplastic epithelium. The lesions are usually multifocal and are more common in the upper third of the vagina.

HPV may be detected with great frequency if attention is given to the vagina. Vaginal condylomas can be detected in as many as one third of patients who have vulvar condylomas. In general, condylomas in the upper third of the vagina are considered high risk, as the

HPV DNA types found here tend to be those associated with malignant potential (types 16, 18, and 31). Condylomas in the lower third of the vagina tend to be low risk and of HPV DNA type 6 or 11. Usually condylomas in the vagina are multiple and appear as raised white elevations. Frequently, a vaginal discharge accompanies the infection. Presence of HPV should be investigated in patients with recurrent episodes of bacterial vaginosis or *Candida albicans* infection, since mild immunosuppression allows both HPV and *C albicans* to flourish.

Condyloma acuminatum of the cervix was a rare lesion in the past but is now being seen with increased frequency. Subclinical papillomavirus infection is generally accepted as the most common manifestation of HPV disease in the cervix.

Diagnosis

Techniques for detecting HPV infection include physical examination, cytology, colposcopy, histologic studies, HPV antigen detection studies, and HPV DNA molecular hybridization.

Physical examination of the genital tract is simple and noninvasive. However, this method used alone fails to detect most HPV infections and many vulvar, vaginal, anal, and penile lesions.

Cytologic studies are a relatively inexpensive method of diagnosing HPV infection. Findings include koilocytosis, dyskaryosis, atypical parabasal cells, and multinucleation. However, HPV is underdiagnosed in routine cytologic examinations. Colposcopic examination after soaking with 5% acetic acid allows detection of 70% of subclinical papillomavirus infections. The colposcope is also helpful in selecting areas to be biopsied.

The histologic findings of genital warts are basal cell hyperplasia, papillomatosis, koilocytosis, and parakeratosis. Koilocytosis is the most commonly used marker for HPV infection. However, the specific koilocytotic atypia seen in lesions is caused by high-grade HPV DNA types such as 16/18, especially in advanced grades of CIN.

HPV antigens can be detected in cytologic and histologic specimens by using immunostaining techniques with antiserum from rabbits immunized to bovine papillomavirus. The cells carrying the virus are well differentiated. As dysplasia progresses, it is increasingly difficult to detect HPV antigen; at the CIN III/carcinoma in situ stage, it is not detectable.

Cloning techniques have now given us the ability to obtain typing of HPV DNA. HPV DNA types 6 and 11 are thought to be of low malignant potential and generally are found in the vulva and lower third of the vagina. HPV DNA types 16/18, 31, and other high-number types are found in the upper third of the vagina and the cervix and are more frequently associated with malignant conditions. Since the physician will treat the clinical or histologic condition rather than the HPV DNA type, the use of routine HPV DNA typing may not be indicated. However, in questionable situations, HPV DNA typing can be useful. These include lesions that might be confused with those of HPV, as well as cases involving koilocytosis with atypia in patients who desire to know the HPV type.

Treatment

HPV infection must be regarded as having the potential for infecting the entire genital tract, since only very early disease tends to be localized. The object of therapy is to remove all overt and subclinical HPV infections detected during the diagnostic evaluation. All currently available treatment methods have been associated with a high degree of recurrence. Therapy options that attack the HPV locally will be helpful only for conditions in which the virus is present locally.

The recurrence of HPV infection after therapy is difficult to assess. Recurrences indicate a failure of therapy, failure to treat all areas involved, resistant virus, or reinfection. Most recurrences are seen within 3 to 6 months of therapy. If the disease is present for 6 months despite repeated attempts at therapy, it is called resistant and persistent HPV disease.

Treatment options include keratolytic agents, physical agents, and immunotherapy. Because of the variety of presentations, the volume of disease, the areas infected, and possibly the DNA type of the papillomavirus, no single agent has yet emerged as a standard treatment. When a patient presents with a small amount of localized disease, a simple approach is best. When disease is more extensive, more intensive therapy may be needed.

Podophyllin resin is one keratolytic agent that has been widely used. It acts by poisoning the mitotic spindle. The resin is applied directly to the surface of the wart and washed off after 6 hours; it is then reapplied on a weekly basis.

Podophyllin resin varies from lot to lot and its side effects are unpredictable. It is contraindicated during pregnancy because of the possibility of teratogenesis and even carcinogenesis. Its use should be severely limited when applied to mucosal surfaces. It may be best to reserve it for use in patients with minimal vulvar or perianal lesions.

Trichloroacetic acid (TCA), another keratolytic agent, acts by precipitation of surface proteins. It should be used at a strength of 85% and applied directly to the vulvar, anal, or vaginal lesions with a small cotton-tipped applicator. It produces a white slough that peels in several days, leaving a small ulcer. Application of 85% TCA can be repeated every 2 to 3 weeks. Again, recurrences are frequent.

5-Fluorouracil (5-FU) is a pyrimidine antimetabolite that causes sloughing of growing tissue. At 5% concentration, 5-FU is useful in the treatment of multiple, small, nonkeratinized vaginal lesions; it may also be used for lesions of the vulva. It is more effective for small HPV lesions involving the vestibule and inside labia minora. It is usually applied on a once-a-week basis into the vagina and/or the vestibule of the vulva for 12 weeks. It is important to instruct the patient in use of 5-FU and to obtain informed consent.

Cryotherapy for HPV disease may be applied either as a single cycle or as repetitive 2-minute freeze-and-thaw cycles to destroy infected wart tissue. It may be performed either by probe or by liquid nitrogen. Patients frequently require more than one application to clear the overt or subclinical papillomavirus infection. In comparative studies, cryotherapy has been more effective than podophyllin and as effective as electrical cautery or laser therapy. Treatment of the vulvar area should be preceded by a local anesthetic agent.

The use of laser therapy is widespread and has the theoretic advantage of precise control of depth, margins, and hemostasis. Laser ablation has the disadvantage of being under operator control as well as being able to treat only the visible disease. The vulva and vestibule are the most convenient areas for laser therapy. Laser therapy of the vagina is complicated by difficulty in application and by scarring. Recurrences occur in 25% to 100% of cases. A recent development has been to extend the field of laser therapy in an attempt to destroy latent virus at the margins; however, studies have shown that this approach is of little value and increases morbidity excessively. The use of 5-FU immediately following laser therapy in the vagina or vulva has been advocated, but success and morbidity rates need to be confirmed.

The laser plume, which contains carbon, water vapor, cells, and in some cases viral DNA, represents a potential hazard to the surgeon, operating room staff, and patient. Smoke evacuation units, equipped with high-efficiency filters (0.1 µm), should be used to remove as much plume as possible. Suction tubing held within 1 cm of the tissue-impact site will remove approximately 98% of plume; at a distance of 2 cm approximately 50% of the plume will escape. Although intact viral particles have been found in laser plume, viral transmission via airborne debris has not been demonstrated to date. Masks with finer filtering ability have recently been introduced, but it has not been shown that these masks significantly reduce the number of particles inhaled by the laser surgeon. Thus, careful plume evacuation should be the mainstay of inhalation safety.

The use of electrocautery to destroy small volumes of condyloma acuminatum has been found to be effective. It is particularly convenient for office use. Surgical ablation has also been widely used to treat condyloma; however, it offers less precision than laser therapy and has the disadvantage of increasing scarring in the vulvar area. Vaccine therapy has been attempted by a number of investigators and in controlled trials has been found to be no better than placebo.

Interferons, a family of proteins with antiviral, antiprolific, and immunomodulatory properties, are also being used as therapy for HPV infection. Three preparations are currently available: α-interferon II-A, α-interferon II-B, and α-interferon N-1. These may be given by an IM injection at a dosage of 2.5 to 3 million U three times a week for a minimum of 6 weeks, or 3 million U/m^2 to a maximum of 4.5 million U three times a week for at least 6 weeks. The duration of this therapy can be extended 2 to 4 weeks if a partial response is noted.

A second route of interferon therapy is intralesional injection at a dose of 250,000 to 1 million U to each wart, up to five warts at one time, three times a week for 3 weeks. In reality, this mode of injection is a regional subcutaneous injection and the duration of therapy may need to be extended longer than 3 weeks. Because the doses are somewhat lower for the α-interferon N-1 preparation, the prescribing information should be reviewed.

Side effects are dose related and usually minimal at the 3-million-U three-times-a-week level. The most frequent side effect of interferon is transient fever for 8 to 12 hours following injection. Other side effects are fatigue, myalgia, and headache; there may be a transient decrease in WBC and function tests in fewer than 10% of individuals.

Interferons may be used for either small or large volumes of HPV disease. They are effective for intravaginal as well as vulvar warts. Recent unpublished data suggest that superior results are obtained by using interferon as initial therapy followed by cryotherapy, laser therapy, or 5-FU. It has also been suggested that this approach permits use of a lower dosage (1 million U) of interferon.

Still another chemotherapeutic option is dinitrochlorobenzene (DNCB) therapy. This treatment is unique in that the patient is sensitized to the agent first. The sensitization procedure involves application of a topical solution of DNCB (1,000 µg/0.1 mL) to the volar surface of the forearm. A challenge dose of 50 µg of DNCB is applied to the same forearm 2 weeks after the sensitizing dose. Induration of greater than 0.5 cm indicates a positive reaction.

The DNCB is then placed in a cream and applied to the lesion. The patient develops a delayed hypersensitivity reaction that destroys the wart. Disadvantages of this therapy include (1) inability to sensitize patients to DNCB, (2) hesitancy of patients to have a hypersensitivity reaction occur in the perineal area, and (3) and varied sensitivity to DNCB, with potential for severe reaction.

Therapy for HPV disease in pregnancy. In general, it can be anticipated that overt condylomas will enlarge during pregnancy. This growth is probably the result of high progesterone levels in the mother. The lesions may become large enough to cause hemorrhage. Therapy with podophyllin is contraindicated because of toxicity and risk of teratogenesis. Agents such as bleomycin and 5-FU are also contraindicated because of their antimitotic and cytotoxic action. Trichloroacetic acid solution is useful, however. Cryotherapy and the CO_2 laser have also been helpful in reducing the number and volume of warts. In almost every case, HPV disease will diminish after delivery.

Extensive condylomas may develop during pregnancy. If multiple lesions are present in and on the genitalia, cesarean section may be necessary to prevent transmission of HPV infection to the infant. A strong association between clinical maternal genital condylomas and the subsequent development of laryngeal papillomatosis in infants delivered vaginally has been documented epidemiologically and corroborated by detection of HPV DNA sequences in both genital and laryngeal papilloma tissues. In one study, 78% of children with laryngeal papilloma had mothers with genital condylomas. Possible modes of transmission include contact between the fetus and the mother's infected genital tract during delivery, transplacental transmission of maternal infection, and postnatal contact. However, despite the high prevalence of genital HPV infection, juvenile laryngeal papillomatosis is a rare disease, implying that transmission of maternal infection is uncommon. Because the method of transmission is not known and the risk is ill defined, there is currently no consensus regarding a protective benefit for the neonate from cesarean delivery.

Treatment of choice
It is recommended that for localized warts, trichloroacetic acid offers the best combination of effectiveness, low morbidity, and expense. When the labia and vulva are involved, the use of TCA or 5-FU is recommended. For extensive vulvar disease, laser therapy is best used for the labia, perineal body, or perianal areas. Alternatively, intralesional and/or IM interferon either alone or in combination with laser therapy or 5-FU may offer the best hope of controlling the virus.

SUGGESTED READING
American College of Obstetrics and Gynecology: Genital human papillomavirus infections. ACOG Tech Bull 1987 (June); No. 105

Gall SA, Hughes CE, Mounts P, et al: Efficacy of human lymphoblastoid interferon on the therapy of resistant condyloma acuminatum. Obstet Gynecol 1986;67:643

Gall SA, Constantine L, Koukol D: Therapy of persistent human papillomavirus disease with two different interferon species. Am J Obstet Gynecol 1991;164:130

Krebs H: Treatment of vaginal condylomata acuminata by weekly topical application of 5-fluorouracil. Obstet Gynecol 1987;70:68

Krebs H, Helmkamp F: Chronic indications following topical therapy with 5-fluorouracil for vaginal human papillomavirus-associated lesions. Obstet Gynecol 1991;78:205

Shah K, Kashima H, Polk F, et al: Rarity of cesarean delivery in cases of juvenile-onset respiratory papillomatosis. Obstet Gynecol 1986;68:795

45
Genital mycoplasmas

By William M. McCormack, MD

Background and incidence

Mycoplasmas are microorganisms that differ from viruses in their ability to grow on cell-free media. They differ from bacteria in lacking a cell wall.

Only three species of mycoplasmas have been isolated with any frequency from human genital mucosal surfaces. One, *Mycoplasma genitalium*, is a newly recognized species of uncertain significance. The other two, *M hominis* and *Ureaplasma urealyticum*, are common isolates that have been extensively studied.

The genital mucosa of infants may be colonized during passage through the birth canal. Ureaplasmas can be recovered from vaginal cultures from about one third of infant girls. *M hominis* is isolated less often from girls. Boys are less likely than girls to be colonized by either species.

Neonatal colonization tends not to persist. Ureaplasmas can be isolated from about 10% of 1-year-old girls. Colonization continues at this low level until puberty.

Following puberty, colonization is influenced primarily by sexual experience. Sexually inexperienced adolescents have low rates of mycoplasmal and ureaplasmal colonization, similar to those seen in prepubertal children. After the onset of sexual intercourse, colonization rates increase in relation to the number of sexual partners.

Rates are higher among socially disadvantaged groups. *M hominis* has been isolated from about 50% of patients attending public clinics and from about 20% of patients visiting private obstetricians and gynecologists. Ureaplasmas have been recovered from about 80% of patients seen in public clinics and from about 50% of private patients.

Thus, both *M hominis* and *U urealyticum* are common inhabitants of the genital mucosa of normal sexually experienced adult men and women. It is against this background that their role in human disease must be viewed.

Pathophysiology

Both *M hominis* and *U urealyticum* are prominent components of the abnormal flora of bacterial vaginosis (BV). Both species have also been isolated from patients who have intra-amniotic infection, post-partum endometritis, and pelvic inflammatory disease.

In each of these conditions, mycoplasmas and ureaplasmas have rarely been isolated in pure culture, but rather have been isolated along with other organisms. Often these other organisms were also components of the abnormal flora of bacterial vaginosis. These data suggest that organisms found in bacterial vaginosis may be responsible for the aforementioned infections of the upper genital tract in women and that the isolation of *M hominis* or *U urealyticum* may be a marker for BV or a BV-related infection.

Ureaplasmas have also been associated with such disorders of reproduction as habitual spontaneous abortion, unexplained involuntary infertility, and low birthweight. More data, especially from placebo-controlled, double-blind treatment studies are needed to establish a role for *U urealyticum* in these disorders.

Diagnosis

As noted earlier, both *M hominis* and *U urealyticum* can be isolated from the vaginal mucosa of a significant proportion of normal sexually experienced women. Also noted was both the infrequency with which either species is isolated in pure culture from patients who have upper genital tract infection and the lack of conclusive evidence of a role for these organisms in disorders of reproduction.

It follows that cultures for *M hominis* or *U urealyticum* have no place in clinical practice. Examination of vaginal or other specimens for mycoplasmas or ureaplasmas is justified only in the context of a research protocol. Specimens from the vaginal mucosa are more likely to yield an isolate than are specimens from the endocervical canal or periurethral area.

Treatment

Although most isolates of *U urealyticum* are susceptible to tetracyclines and erythromycins, it is difficult to eradicate these organisms from the vagina. *M hominis* is susceptible to tetracyclines but not to erythromycins. However, because tetracycline-resistant isolates of *M hominis* are increasing in prevalence, clindamycin is more effective against this agent.

Examining cultures for genital mycoplasmas is seldom justifiable in clinical practice. However, any treatment regimen for the upper genital tract syndromes with which *M hominis* and *U urealyticum* have been associated ought to contain an antimicrobial agent that has in vitro activity against these organisms.

Prevention

Regular use of barrier contraceptives retards genital colonization by mycoplasmas, but these organisms are so widespread that it is difficult to visualize any approach that would prevent a significant portion of sexually experienced adults from eventually becoming colonized.

SUGGESTED READING

Glatt AE, McCormack WM, Taylor-Robinson D: Genital mycoplasma, in Holmes KK (ed): *Sexually Transmitted Disease*, ed 2. New York, McGraw-Hill, 1989, p 279

McCormack WM, Rosner B, Lee Y-H: Colonization with genital mycoplasmas in women. Am J Epidemiol 1973;97:240

Platt R, Lin J-S, Warren JW, et al: Infection with *Mycoplasma hominis* in post-partum fever. Lancet 1980;2:1217

Wasserheit JN, Bell TA, Kiviat NB, et al: Microbial causes of proven pelvic inflammatory disease and efficacy of clindamycin and tobramycin. Ann Intern Med 1986;104:187

46

Acute salpingitis: incidence and diagnosis

By Pål Wölner-Hanssen, MD, DMS

Background and incidence

Acute salpingitis is an infection of the fallopian tubes. Making a diagnosis on clinical grounds is unreliable because the clinical manifestations are often nonspecific. By direct observation of the tubes—for example, through a laparoscope—the diagnosis can be confirmed. For women with suspected but unconfirmed acute salpingitis, acute pelvic inflammatory disease (PID) is a more appropriate diagnosis than acute salpingitis.

Investigators have estimated the annual number of women developing acute salpingitis in the United States at the end of the 1970s to be about 857,000. It is difficult to assess the fraction who actually had acute salpingitis. Moreover, the estimate did not include what we today call silent or atypical PID. No recent survey based on verified cases of salpingitis is available. Silent PID is an undefined condition, the effects of which are felt in the numbers of infertile women with scarred tubes who have not had PID diagnosed previously. The importance of silent PID among infertile US women is unknown, however, partly because those with the highest risk of sexually transmitted diseases cannot afford infertility evaluations. Therefore, the overall incidence of salpingitis remains largely unknown.

Studies have shown that incidence seems to differ for various segments of the population, depending on the prevalence of risk factors in each group. The risk of acquiring a sexually transmitted disease, and hence acute STD-related salpingitis, is highly correlated with the number of sexual partners. Youth is a risk factor for acute salpingitis among sexually active women. In Sweden, the annual incidence of acute salpingitis among 15- to 19-year-old women (1.5% to 2%) is about three times that of 25- to 29-year-old women. Young women may have less stable sexual relationships than the somewhat older ones, and therefore may expose themselves to genital infections more often. Another possible explanation is that young women have less immunity against STD agents than older ones.

In the US, ethnic origin is a risk factor for PID. Cumulative incidence of self-reported PID among blacks is almost twice that among whites (23% versus 13%). Formerly married women have a three times higher cumulative incidence of self-reported PID than never-married women. Contraceptive practice is also a risk factor for PID. For example, many consider the use of an IUD a risk factor for acute salpingitis. In contrast, oral contraceptives and barrier methods might reduce the risk for salpingitis.

In a recent study, women with confirmed PID were more likely than controls to have douched during the previous 2 months. This association was found only in nonblack women, and was strongest among women with few sexual partners.

An association between bacterial vaginosis with both adnexal tenderness and a clinical diagnosis of PID has also recently been reported. Finally, cigarette smoking has been statistically associated with PID, although a causal relationship has not been proven.

Diagnosis
Abdominal pain is the principal symptom of acute salpingitis, but is not always present. Women with acute salpingitis may have severe pain (common in women with perihepatitis) or no pain at all (silent PID). The character of the pain (aching, burning, cramping, stabbing), and side location (unilateral versus bilateral) is unspecific. The pain is usually bilateral, but it may be unilateral and indistinguishable from that caused by appendicitis.

Patients with acute PID may report several genital and extragenital symptoms. These include symptoms from the GI tract (vomiting, diarrhea, constipation, tenesmus), the urinary tract (dysuria, frequency, urgency), or the genital tract (increased discharge, abnormal odor from the vagina, abnormal bleeding). These symptoms are all nonspecific for PID. Adnexal, uterine, and cervical motion tenderness are also nonspecific signs of acute PID.

Purulent cervical discharge is another sign that suggests acute PID in a woman with acute abdominal pain. However, lack of mucopus does not rule out acute salpingitis.

In studies in which intentionally loose criteria for enrollment but stringent criteria for the final diagnosis were used, fever was an uncommon sign of PID. Among cases with acute chlamydial salpingitis, only 20% had fever.

Few laboratory tests are useful for evaluating women with sus-

TABLE 1
Clinical criteria for diagnosis of salpingitis

Necessary for diagnosis
Abdominal direct tenderness, with or without rebound tenderness
Tenderness with motion of cervix and uterus
Adnexal tenderness

One or more necessary for diagnosis
Gram stain of endocervix positive for gram-negative intracellular diplococci

Temperature >38°C

Leukocytosis (WBC >10,000)

Purulent material (WBC present) from peritoneal cavity obtained by culdocentesis or laparoscopy

Pelvic abscess or inflammatory complex on bimanual exam or by sonography

Source: Hager WD, Eschenbach DA, Spence MR, et al: Criteria for diagnosis and grading of salpingitis. Editorial. Obstet Gynecol 1983;61:113

pected salpingitis. A sensitive pregnancy test is important for sexually active women with abdominal pain because ectopic pregnancy and acute PID often have similar manifestations.

Elevated erythrocyte sedimentation rate (ESR), white blood cell (WBC) count, or serum C-reactive protein levels suggest inflammation of some sort, but none of these tests is specific or sensitive for acute salpingitis. For example, in one study, 25% of women with acute salpingitis had normal ESR, and 53% of those without confirmed salpingitis had elevated ESR. In another study, 70% of women with acute chlamydial salpingitis had normal WBC counts.

In their classic work, Jacobson and Weström could not confirm acute salpingitis in one third of women with clinical symptoms and signs suggesting the infection. Investigators from the University of Washington encountered the same difficulty in making the diagnosis. Clinical criteria for diagnosis have since been described by Hager and co-workers and endorsed by the Infectious Diseases Society for Obstetrics and Gynecology (Tables 1 and 2). These authors also outlined a severity staging system based on laparoscopic findings.

Laparoscopic examination has become the "gold standard" for making a definitive diagnosis of acute salpingitis. Certainty of diagnosis is mandatory for prudent research, but may be less important

TABLE 2
Grading of salpingitis by clinical examination

I. Uncomplicated (limited to fallopian tubes and/or ovaries)
   Without pelvic peritonitis
   With pelvic peritonitis

II. Complicated (inflammatory mass or abscess involving fallopian tubes and/or ovaries)
   Without pelvic peritonitis
   With pelvic peritonitis

III. Spread to structures beyond pelvis (ruptured tubo-ovarian abscess)

Source: Hager WD, Eschenbach DA, Spence MR, et al: Criteria for diagnosis and grading of salpingitis. Editorial. Obstet Gynecol 1983;61:113

for routine clinical care. Nevertheless, laparoscopy is useful in distinguishing between different causes of acute lower abdominal pain. Usually, you can readily see the appendix and the genital tract through the laparoscope.

Ultrasound examination is not helpful in diagnosing acute salpingitis. The fallopian tubes are difficult to see, and there are no existing standard criteria for an ultrasound diagnosis. Ultrasonography may be useful as a check on the effect of antibiotic therapy on tubo-ovarian abscesses in patients who are difficult to examine—obese women, for example.

Endometrial biopsy is a newly developed method for confirming acute PID. A disadvantage is that its results are not available for several days. Therefore, this technique may be more useful in research than in routine care.

Microbiologic evaluation
Neisseria gonorrhoeae and *Chlamydia trachomatis* cause most cases of acute PID. Therefore, take cervical culture specimens for *C trachomatis* and *N gonorrhoeae* in women with suspected PID. Antigen-detection tests such as Microtrak (Syva Co., Palo Alto, Calif.) or Chlamydiazyme (Abbott Laboratories, Abbott Park, Ill.) are adequate alternatives to chlamydial cultures. It makes no sense to take culture specimens from the cervix for anaerobic or facultative (other than *N gonorrhoeae*) microorganisms, because these are part of the normal flora.

In women undergoing laparoscopy, there is an opportunity to culture the fallopian tubes and the cul-de-sac fluid directly without contaminating the specimens with vaginal flora. Organisms isolated from the fallopian tubes probably cause the acute inflammation. Regrettably, however, most women with obvious acute salpingitis are culture negative from the tubes.

Culdocentesis includes aspiration of cul-de-sac fluid via needle puncture of the posterior vaginal fornix. Purulent cul-de-sac fluid suggests intra-abdominal infection (PID, appendicitis, or diverticulitis). Clear fluid, however, does not rule out infection. Cultures of culdocentesis material are of little value, because vaginal microorganisms may have contaminated the fluid.

If we are going to have an impact on decreasing the sequelae of salpingitis, we must improve the efficiency of our clinical criteria for diagnosis. We must maintain a high index of suspicion in young, sexually active women with abdominal pain and make use of the laparoscope to confirm or rule out the diagnosis in cases where uncertainty exists.

SUGGESTED READING

Curran JW: Economic consequences of pelvic inflammatory disease in the United States. Am J Obstet Gynecol 1980;138:484

Eschenbach DA, Hillier S, Critchlow C, et al: Diagnosis and clinical manifestations of bacterial vaginosis. Am J Obstet Gynecol 1988;158:819

Hager WD, Eschenbach DA, Spence MR, et al: Criteria for diagnosis and grading of salpingitis. Editorial. Obstet Gynecol 1983;61:113

Jacobson L, Weström L: Objectivized diagnosis of acute pelvic inflammatory disease. Am J Obstet Gynecol 1969;105:1088

Weström L: Incidence, prevalence, and trends of acute pelvic inflammatory disease and its consequences in industrialized countries. Am J Obstet Gynecol 1980;138:880.

Wölner-Hanssen P, Eschenbach DA, Paavonen J, et al: Association between vaginal douching and acute pelvic inflammatory disease. JAMA 1990;263:1936

Wölner-Hanssen P, Svensson L, Weström L, et al: Laparoscopy in women with chlamydial infection and pelvic pain: a comparison of patients with and without salpingitis. Obstet Gynecol 1983;61:299

47

Acute salpingitis: treatment

By Richard L. Sweet, MD

Background and incidence

Pelvic inflammatory disease (PID), or acute salpingitis, continues to be a major medical, economic, and public health problem for reproductive-aged US women. Among young women, it is the most common serious complication of sexually transmitted disease. More than one million cases, including 250,000 to 300,000 hospitalizations, are estimated to occur each year. Annual treatment costs are estimated to be more than $3.5 billion.

Involuntary (predominantly tubal factor) infertility occurs in 20% of PID patients—a sevenfold increase—and ectopic pregnancy increases six- to tenfold. Chronic pelvic pain, dyspareunia, pelvic adhesions, and other inflammatory residua, which often require surgical intervention, occur in 15% to 20% of cases. In addition, tubo-ovarian abscess, the major early complication associated with acute PID, occurs in 5% to 10% of hospitalized acute PID patients.

Etiology

Until recently, *Neisseria gonorrhoeae* had been considered the primary etiologic agent for acute PID in the Western world. Thus, based on cervical culture results, PID was divided into either gonococcal or nongonococcal disease. However recent advances in technology for obtaining microbiologic specimens directly from the fallopian tubes, endometrial cavity, or peritoneal fluid, combined with advances in microbiologic isolation techniques, have resulted in recovery of nongonococcal organisms, such as *Chlamydia trachomatis* and anaerobic and facultative bacteria, from both the cervix and upper genital tract of women with acute PID.

Thus, cultures from the upper genital tract have shown PID to be polymicrobial. Studies report recovery of *N gonorrhoeae*, *C trachomatis*, or both, in 50% to 60% of women with acute PID. Nongonococcal nonchlamydial microorganisms isolated from the upper genital tract include mixed anaerobic organisms (*Bacteroides* sp and peptostreptococci) and facultative bacteria (*Gardnerella vaginalis*, streptococci, *Escherichia coli*, and *Haemophilus influenzae*). While genital tract mycoplasmas, such as *Mycoplasma hominis* and *Ureaplasma urealyticum*, have also been recovered from women with PID, their role in etiology remains uncertain.

Recent studies of distribution of etiologic agents recovered from the upper genital tract of women with acute PID show 25% to 50% to be *N gonorrhoeae*, 10% to 43% to be *C trachomatis*, and 25% to 84% to consist of nongonococcal nonchlamydial bacteria. In general, mixed anaerobic bacteria are the most common group of organisms recovered, while *N gonorrhoeae* is the most common single organism, followed by *C trachomatis*.

Treatment

The goals of management are to preserve fertility, prevent ectopic pregnancy, and reduce long-term inflammatory sequelae of acute PID. Optimal treatment requires early diagnosis and prompt institution of antimicrobial agents effective against major pathogens known to be involved in the disease process.

Initially, single-agent antimicrobial therapy focused on eradication of *N gonorrhoeae*. Most often, however, these drugs failed to eradicate *C trachomatis* and mixed aerobic–anaerobic bacteria, making such regimens largely unsatisfactory. In 1982, therefore, the Centers for Disease Control established new guidelines—subsequently updated in 1985, 1989, and 1991—for inpatient and ambulatory treatment of acute salpingitis using antibiotic combinations (Table 1).

Outpatient therapy. Unblinded noncomparative studies have reported good clinical response in outpatients treated with combination regimens. However, Thompson and co-workers, in a six-hospital collaborative study of ambulatory regimens prospectively comparing ampicillin with tetracycline outpatient treatment, reported an unacceptably high clinical failure rate of 17%.

Adequate coverage of outpatients is hard to achieve even with parenteral drugs. Also, many agents known to be effective either are not available in oral form or do not reach high enough serum concentrations when taken orally. Finally, outpatient treatment is often complicated by poor compliance.

It is unclear whether ambulatory treatment or parenteral antibiotic therapy in the hospital is more likely to prevent complications and long-term sequelae. Economic and logistic considerations cause

TABLE 1
Recommended schedules for treatment of acute PID

Ambulatory management

1. Cefoxitin, 2 g IM plus 1 g probenecid orally

   or

   Ceftriaxone, 250 mg IM

   or

   Equivalent cephalosporin

   plus

   Doxycycline, 100 mg orally bid for 10–14 days

   or

   Tetracycline, 500 mg orally qid for 10–14 days

2. For patients who cannot tolerate doxycycline:

   Erythromycin, 500 mg orally qid for 10–14 days

Inpatient treatment

1. Cefoxitin, 2 g IV every 6 hours

   or

   Cefotetan,* 2 g IV every 12 hours

   plus

   Doxycycline, 100 mg every 12 hours orally or IV

   This regimen should be followed for at least 48 hours after the patient improves clinically. After discharge, continue doxycycline, 100 mg orally bid for 10–14 days.

2. Clindamycin, 900 mg IV every 8 hours

   plus

   Gentamicin, loading dose IV or IM (2 mg/kg), followed by maintenance dose (1.5 mg/kg) every 8 hours

   This regimen should be followed for at least 48 hours after the patient improves. After discharge, continue doxycycline, 100 mg orally bid for 10–14 days total, or clindamycin, 450 mg orally five times daily for 10–14 days.

*Other cephalosporins, such as ceftizoxime, cefotaxime, and ceftriaxone, which provide adequate gonococcal, other facultative gram-negative aerobic, and anaerobic coverage, may be utilized in appropriate doses.

Source: Centers for Disease Control: MMWR 1989;38(S-8).

70% to 75% of women who have PID to be treated as outpatients. However, given the high rate of ambulatory treatment failures, the considerable morbidity caused by PID, and the prevailing impression that early and effective parenteral therapy improves outcome, criteria for hospitalizing patients with PID to administer combination parenteral therapy have been liberalized. Indeed, some authorities recommend it for all women with acute PID.

Inpatient therapy. Since 1982, a number of studies have compared results of various inpatient regimens. In general, combination regimens with either clindamycin plus an aminoglycoside or an extended-spectrum cephalosporin plus doxycycline have produced excellent initial beneficial clinical responses. On the other hand, single-agent fluoroquinolone treatment has been followed by a high rate of post-treatment persistence of anaerobic bacteria in the endometrial cavity despite apparent clinical response. Needed now are randomized, prospective studies with meticulous clinical or laparoscopic grading, microbiologic analysis, and long-term follow-up to assess these regimens' effectiveness in preventing subsequent episodes of PID, as well as adverse reproductive sequelae such as infertility, ectopic pregnancy, and chronic pelvic pain.

To minimize reinfection, we recommend that all partners of women with PID be screened for *N gonorrhoeae* and *C trachomatis.* Those found positive for these pathogens should be treated with a regimen effective against both *N gonorrhoeae* and *C trachomatis*—most commonly a combination of a single dose of 250 mg of ceftriaxone IM plus 100 mg of doxycycline orally twice daily for 7 days.

It is crucial to institute treatment as soon as possible in order to maximize future reproductive potential. Whether inpatient therapy is preferable is unclear. Likewise, whether concomitant anti-inflammatory agents will prevent long-term sequelae of infertility or ectopic pregnancy remains uncertain.

SUGGESTED READING

Centers for Disease Control: 1989 sexually transmitted diseases treatment guidelines. MMWR 1989;38(S-8):31

Eschenbach DA, Buchanan T, Pollock HM, et al: Polymicrobial etiology of acute pelvic inflammatory disease. N Engl J Med 1975;293:166

Grimes DA, Blount JH, Patrick J, et al: Antibiotic treatment of pelvic inflammatory disease: trends among private physicians in the United States, 1966-1982. JAMA 1986;256:3223

Sweet RL, Draper DL, Schachter J, et al: Microbiology and pathogenesis of acute salpingitis as determined by laparoscopy: what is the appropriate site to sample? Am J Obstet Gynecol 1980;138:985

Sweet RL: Pelvic inflammatory disease and infertility in women. Infect Dis Clin North Am 1987;1:199

Sweet RL, Schachter J, Robbie M: Failure of ß-lactam antibiotics to eradicate *Chlamydia trachomatis* from the endometrium in patients with acute salpingitis despite apparent clinical cure. JAMA 1983;250:2641

Thompson SE, Brooks CA, Eschenbach DA, et al: High failure rates in outpatient treatment of salpingitis with either tetracycline alone or penicillin/ampicillin combination. Am J Obstet Gynecol 1985;152:635

Wasserheit JN, Bell TA, Kiviat NB, et al: Microbial causes of proven pelvic inflammatory disease and efficacy of clindamycin and tobramycin. Ann Intern Med 1986;104:187

Weström L: Incidence, prevalence, and trends of acute pelvic inflammatory disease and its consequences in industrialized countries. Am J Obstet Gynecol 1980;38:880

48
Chronic sequelae of salpingitis

By Mark Gibson, MD

Background and incidence

For most victims of salpingitis, the most important consequences occur only after the pain, fever, and limitation of normal activity of acute illness subside. For these patients, chronic sequelae of adnexal inflammation, in the form of tubal inflammatory damage (TID), exact the greatest cost by causing both symptoms and reproductive dysfunction.

Infertility due to TID, which accounts for approximately 20% of instances, affects an estimated 1% to 2% of all women. Peritubal and periovarian adhesions may interfere with normal tubo-ovarian relationships and by themselves account for infertility. The most sensitive targets of salpingitis are the tube's ampulla and fimbria, where minor postinflammatory changes include phimosis of the tubal orifice and subtle degrees of fimbrial agglutination. More severe damage to the distal tube results in the classic retort-shaped sactosalpinx, most typically drawn posterolaterally beneath the ovary and bound there by webs or bands of adhesions.

In tubes that are totally occluded at the fimbriated end, abnormal mucosa and muscularis are the rule. In addition, the tube's isthmic portion may be occluded by fibrosis, plugged by amorphous inspissations, or distorted by fibrosis and diverticula in a configuration known as salpingitis isthmica nodosa. We assume these proximal tubal abnormalities result from salpingitis because they are frequently associated with typical residua of salpingitis on the adnexa.

Salpingitis clearly can cause infertility because of TID. Data from Weström's group in Sweden suggest that approximately 6% of aggressively treated cases of gonococcal salpingitis and 17% of cases of nongonococcal salpingitis lead to infertility. Association of instrumentation—from intrauterine devices or pregnancy termination—with the infection, or recurrence of infection, increases the likelihood that infertility due to TID will eventually occur.

However, even advanced salpingitis, manifesting as an inflammatory tubo-ovarian complex, is associated with successful pregnancy in 33% of women who attempt childbearing after medical treatment. This fact encourages aggressive medical treatment of advanced pelvic infection when eventual childbearing is desired.

The relationship between salpingitis, defined as an acute, symptomatic illness, and TID leading to infertility is thus not as clear as at first appears. Most women experiencing a bout of salpingitis remain fertile, and only a minority with TID-associated infertility, ranging from 25% to 50% in several series, have a history of salpingitis. Therefore, because it can be estimated that 2% of all women are infertile because of TID, one or both of the following propositions must be true:

(1) There is an important incidence of asymptomatic pelvic infection that irreversibly damages the adnexa, distinct from that which is commonly clinically termed pelvic inflammatory disease (PID).

(2) Salpingitis is frequently undiagnosed or misdiagnosed because of mild symptoms or lack of patient sensitivity to symptoms' possible significance, or both.

The resolution of this conundrum is important so that progress can be made in preventing TID. Fertility in patients who have TID is not restored by surgery in most cases, and in vitro fertilization remains an expensive and frequently unsuccessful last resort.

Diagnosis

Complementary information derived by hysterosalpingography (HSG) and laparoscopy is needed for diagnosis of TID. The HSG will reveal isthmic or interstitial obstruction, although a finding of proximal tubal obstruction in a single HSG is frequently spurious. Findings of salpingitis isthmica nodosa are highly characteristic and are reliable. Phimosis of the ampullary tubal ostium is difficult to detect on HSG, but complete obstruction with sactosalpinx is shown readily and reliably. By revealing the presence or absence of rugal folds in the ampulla, the HSG helps show the degree of mucosal preservation in cases of distal occlusion—a finding predictive of the success of subsequent attempts at repair.

Laparoscopy with chromopertubation confirms HSG findings and may invalidate findings commonly falsely positive, such as unilateral proximal tubal occlusion. Laparoscopy will also identify abnormalities that usually escape detection on the HSG, such as periadnexal adhesions and tubal phimosis.

Treatment for tubal damage

When TID is the cause of infertility, surgical correction is just one therapeutic option in an array that includes in vitro fertilization and adoption. Even with the most meticulous and expert surgical reconstruction, the outlook for pregnancy is often poor, and the anguish of failure or repeated ectopic gestations serve the couple poorly and consume valuable time in their quest for a family. Frank and expert preoperative counseling is important.

Correcting isolated occlusion of the proximal tube in an otherwise normal pelvis is often successful. Microsurgical anastomosis after resection of the occluded segment yields pregnancy rates of between 50% and 75%. Recently, hysteroscopically or fluoroscopically guided cannulation of such obstruction has been successful. The use of this cannulation technique sometimes affords good results with less surgical invasiveness, morbidity, and cost.

Likewise, prognosis is often excellent when adhesiolysis alone is all that is required to restore normal adnexal relationships. The likelihood of pregnancy depends on the extent and character of the adhesions, but pregnancy generally can be anticipated in 50% to 70% of patients in this category.

By contrast, repair of distal occlusion is associated with much poorer outcomes. Advances in microsurgical technique have not improved outcomes as convincingly in this group as in others. The best outcomes are associated with occlusions amenable to simple fimbrial dissection. Sactosalpinx dimensions are inversely correlated with success, as is the extent of mucosal destruction and of associated pelvic adhesion formation. Overall, pregnancy rates of 25% to 50% are seen after surgical correction of distal tubal obstruction.

Sequelae

Ectopic pregnancy. A frequent outcome after any surgical correction of postinflammatory adnexal damage, ectopic pregnancy accounts for one third of resulting pregnancies. Both preoperative and postoperative counseling should clearly address this possibility. Early, close biochemical and ultrasonographic monitoring of pregnancies after reconstructive surgery is mandatory for patient safety and permits earlier, more conservative intervention in the event of tubal gestation.

Ectopic pregnancy occurs more often in women with a history of salpingitis. The reported increase in the incidence of ectopic pregnancy has been attributed to salpingitis, and histologic evidence of past salpingitis is often found in fallopian tubes removed because of ectopic pregnancy. Women with a history of salpingitis should be monitored closely during early pregnancy for evidence of ectopic gestation in order to reduce the risk of hemorrhage and to facilitate less invasive and more conservative management in the event of an ectopic pregnancy.

Pelvic pain. The incidence of chronic pelvic pain is higher in women who have experienced PID. Many clinicians suspect pelvic pain arises as a result of TID, but the entity has not been systematically described or characterized by appropriate studies.

Pelvic pain in women with a history of PID may be due to reinfection or exacerbation of chronic infection or from causes unrelated to pelvic infection. However, some have portions of one or both adnexa trapped by TID and are presumably experiencing pain because of this condition. Symptoms in these patients are typically sharp or nagging unilateral discomfort, as well as abrupt periovulatory or luteal exacerbation. The latter feature may reflect effects of follicular rupture, corpus luteum formation, luteal enlargement from intraluteal hemorrhage on the adhesions with resulting traction, pressure on the adjacent peritoneum or on the ovary itself, or all these occurrences. A decrease in symptoms during a trial of gonadal quiescence induced by oral contraceptives may assist in the diagnosis.

Lysing adhesions and restoring normal relationships and mobility of the tubes and ovaries may afford the patient relief. These steps are often possible at the time of diagnostic laparoscopy. A study designed to (1) confirm the existence of a pain syndrome arising specifically from TID, (2) evaluate the reliability of its diagnosis through a trial of gonadal quiescence, and (3) show the effectiveness of adhesiolysis is very much needed.

SUGGESTED READING

Brumsted JR, Clifford PM, Nakajima ST, et al: Reproductive outcome after medical management of complicated pelvic inflammatory disease. Fertil Steril 1988;50:667

Deaton JL, Gibson M, Riddick DH, et al: Diagnosis and treatment of cornual obstruction using a flexible tip guidewire. Fertil Steril 1990;53:232

Dinsmoor M, Gibson M: Early recognition of ectopic pregnancy in an infertility population. Obstet Gynecol 1986;68:859

Jacobs LA, Thie J, Patton PE, et al: Primary microsurgery for postinflammatory tubal infertility. Fertil Steril 1988;50:855

Mäkinen JI, Erkkola RU, Laippala PJ: Causes of the increase in the incidence of ectopic pregnancy: a study on 1,017 patients from 1966 to 1985 in Turku, Finland. Am J Obstet Gynecol 1989;160:642

Pauerstein CJ, Coxatto HB, Eddy CA, et al: Anatomy and pathology of tubal pregnancy. Obstet Gynecol 1986;67:301

Rosenfeld DL, Seidman SM, Bronson RA, et al: Unsuspected chronic pelvic inflammatory disease in the infertile female. Fertil Steril 1983;39:44

Weström L: Effect of acute pelvic inflammatory disease on fertility. Am J Obstet Gynecol 1975;121:707

49
Tubo-ovarian abscess

By Gilles R.G. Monif, MD

Background and incidence

An abscess is the result of an infected host's effort to combat and localize an infectious process by walling it off. A tubo-ovarian abscess (TOA) can occur after a vaginal or abdominal delivery, after a spontaneous or elective abortion, or after gynecologic surgery. This discussion will be limited to those resulting from persistence or worsening of acute salpingitis.

A careful review of the literature on management of TOAs indicates that many of the reported cases may have been tubo-ovarian complexes (TOCs). Whereas an abscess is an accumultation of inflammatory cells and bacteria within a newly created space, a complex is the agglutination and adherence of infected structures into a space-occupying mass without walled-off purulence. There is critical difference between the two, since patients with a complex respond more favorably to antibiotic therapy than do those with an abscess.

Current estimates indicate that there are 750,000 to 1.5 million cases of salpingitis in the United States each year. Of that total, approximately 350,000 involve hospitalization. Hospital-based studies indicate that 3% to 16% of women with salpingitis develop an abscess. Therefore, it's likely that 10,500 to 56,000 salpingitis-related abscesses occur annually in the US.

Etiology

Salpingitis is a polymicrobial infection ascending through the endocervix and uterus to the fallopian tubes [see Chapter 46: Acute salpingitis: incidence and diagnosis]. Inciting pathogens may include *Neisseria gonorrhoeae* and *Chlamydia trachomatis*, as well as facultative gram-negative aerobes and anaerobic bacilli and cocci. If initial damage to one or both fallopian tubes is sufficient to cause tissue necrosis and alter oxidation–reduction potential, then secondary invaders, particularly *Bacteroides* sp, may encroach and cause an abscess. Anaerobes are isolated from abscesses in over 90% of cases.

The severity of an abscess is related to the conditions causing or initiating infections, the types of bacteria involved, and the state of the host's immune defense mechanisms. The time it takes for the infection to be detected also plays a major role in the development of an abscess. Since infection by *C trachomatis* may result in serious tubal damage before significant symptoms occur, this organism may create the ideal milieu for abscess formation.

Diagnosis

The symptoms and signs of disease are essentially those of acute salpingitis—fever, chills, abdominal and pelvic pain, and occasionally abnormal vaginal discharge—plus the presence of a tender fluctuant adnexal mass. Examination of the patient frequently reveals temperature elevation, abdominal direct or rebound tenderness, and tenderness on palpation of the cervix, uterus, and adnexa, along with presence of an adnexal mass.

The clinical diagnosis of salpingitis is frequently in error, because patients may not have the classic signs and symptoms of disease; even if present, these may be mild. Laparoscopy has become the most accurate way to verify pelvic infection. Visualization of the fallopian tubes may reveal edema, hyperemia, and purulent drainage from the fimbriated ends. If the process is advanced, the fimbria may have become agglutinated, restricting drainage from the tube and resulting in hydrosalpinx or pyosalpinx formation.

Adherence of the tube and ovary and development of adhesions results in TOC formation. If a collection of purulent material and tissue necrosis is walled off, a TOA occurs.

The diagnosis of a TOA is based on the presence of a tender, fluctuant adnexal mass in a patient who meets the clinical criteria, but pinpointing the diagnosis is not always a simple matter. In many instances, patients with acute salpingitis and peritonitis, with or without TOC or TOA, are extremely difficult to examine because of marked tenderness, guarding, and abdominal rigidity.

Confirming the clinical findings is essential in making an accurate diagnosis. Ultrasound or CT scans may be helpful. An ultrasound scan of a woman with a TOC will reveal an enlarged sonolucent and sonodense mass. If the patient has an abscess, the mass will be sonolucent because it is filled with purulent material. Scans are also valuable for determining whether the mass effect is diminishing while the patient is being treated medically.

Laboratory findings will include an elevated white blood cell (WBC) count, often with a left shift and an elevated erythrocyte sedimentation rate (ESR). Specimens for culture should include endocervical and rectal swabs for gonorrhea, an endocervical sample for *C trachomatis*, and two or three sets of aerobic/anaerobic blood cultures [see Chapter 56: Techniques for isolating pelvic pathogens]. Specimens for aerobic and anaerobic endometrial cultures may be obtained by means of a double- or triple-lumen endometrial brush or by aspiration biopsy of the endometrium. Intra-abdominal cultures may be obtained from peritoneal surfaces, the fallopian tubes, or the cul-de-sac via laparoscopy or culdocentesis. Clinical examination may be better accepted by the patient once antibiotics have been started and tenderness decreases.

Treatment

Unless the surgical emergency of a ruptured abscess exists, patients should be treated with appropriate parenteral antibiotics once the diagnosis is confirmed. Although women with acute salpingitis may be treated as outpatients with parenteral antibiotics, all those with true abscess as well as those with a tubo-ovarian complex larger than 5 cm should be hospitalized.

For hospitalized patients, cultures should be taken and ultrasound and CT scans performed. Patients should be hydrated and started on a regimen of parenteral antibiotics. Since treatment must include coverage for *N gonorrhoeae*, *C trachomatis*, facultative gram-negative aerobes, and anaerobes, multiple agents or single broad-spectrum agents must be given. Possible choices include clindamycin plus gentamicin; cefoxitin plus doxycycline; metronidazole plus ampicillin and gentamicin; ampicillin/sulbactam plus doxycycline; and imipenem/cilastatin.

An excellent follow-up tool for assessment of response to parenteral antibiotics is use of the severity score index devised by Thompson and co-workers. This scoring system weighs such factors as abdominal direct and rebound tenderness, bowel sounds, cervical motion tenderness, adnexal tenderness, and presence of adnexal masses. A woman who has salpingitis with a TOC or TOA and who responds to antibiotic therapy should show fewer symptoms, a decreased WBC count and temperature, and a reduction in adnexal mass after 72 hours of adequate antibiotic therapy. If not, surgical intervention, beginning with diagnostic laparoscopy, is indicated.

Current data indicate that 47% to 74% of patients initially respond favorably to IV antibiotics. However, Ginsburg and co-workers found that disease persisted or recurred in 86% of their patients. Of 58 patients with abscesses followed by Landers and Sweet, 31% required subsequent surgery. These data demonstrate the need for careful, prolonged follow-up of these women.

Some patients will require surgical intervention. Several investigators have now reported laparoscopic drainage of abscesses by means of large-bore suction instruments and vigorous irrigation with saline and antibiotics. For this procedure, careful patient selection and thorough surgical technique are critical.

Definitive treatment of abscesses used to be total abdominal hysterectomy with bilateral salpingo-oophorectomy. However, studies by Hager and others have shown that even for patients unresponsive to parenteral antibiotics, a more conservative approach emphasizing unilateral adnexectomy may suffice. A ruptured abscess is a surgical emergency, requiring stabilization of the patient and laparotomy. However, even in this situation, unilateral adnexectomy and peritoneal lavage may be appropriate for selected patients.

Percutaneous or transvaginal CT-directed drainage of an abscess is possible, but should be done only by those experienced with the procedure. Closed suction drains should be left in place until drainage is minimal.

Sequelae

Chronic sequelae of salpingitis include chronic pelvic pain, ectopic pregnancy, and infertility caused by tubal occlusion. TOA adds the risk of rupture and increases the risk of pelvic adhesions and surgical intervention. Women with TOA appear to be at even greater risk for chronic pelvic pain and infertility than those with acute salpingitis alone.

Long-term follow-up of women who attempted to conceive after diagnosis and treatment of an abscess revealed pregnancy rates of only 7% to 14%. Among women who had unilateral abscesses, fertility rates were better after unilateral adnexectomy than after extended antibiotic therapy.

Early, accurate diagnosis of acute salpingitis and treatment with appropriate antibiotics are essential steps in preventing abscess formation.

SUGGESTED READING

Brumsted JR, Clifford PM, Nakajima ST: Reproductive outcome after medical management of complicated pelvic inflammatory disease. Fertil Steril 1988;50:667

Ginsburg DS, Stern JL, Hamod KA, et al: Tubo-ovarian abscess: a retrospective review. Am J Obstet Gynecol 1980;138:1055

Hager WD: Followup of patients with tubo-ovarian abscess(es) in association with salpingitis. Obstet Gynecol 1983;61:680

Henry-Suchet J, Soler A, Loffredo V: Laparoscopic treatment of tubo-ovarian abscesses. J Reprod Med 1984;29:579

Landers DV, Sweet RL: Tubo-ovarian abscess: contemporary approach in management. Rev Infect Dis 1983;5:876

Reed SD, Landers DV, Sweet RL: Antibiotic treatment of tubo-ovarian abscess. Am J Obstet Gynecol 1991;164:1556

Teisala K, Heinonen PK, Punnonen R: Transvaginal ultrasound in the diagnosis and treatment of tubo-ovarian abscess. Br J Obstet Gynaecol 1990;97:178

Thompson SE, Hager WD, Wong K, et al: The microbiology and therapy of acute pelvic inflammatory disease in hospitalized patients. Am J Obstet Gynecol 1980;126:179

Tyrrel RT, Murphy FB, Bernardino ME: Tubo-ovarian abscesses: CT-guided percutaneous drainage. Radiology 1990;175:87

50
Perihepatitis

By Rhoda S. Sperling, MD

Background and incidence

The clinical syndrome of perihepatitis complicating salpingitis is often referred to as Fitz-Hugh–Curtis syndrome. Although Fitz-Hugh and Curtis were not the first to recognize this syndrome, in the 1930s these two American physicians independently described perihepatic inflammation as a complication of acute gonococcal salpingitis. It is now commonly accepted that Fitz-Hugh–Curtis (FHC) syndrome is associated with both gonococcal and nongonococcal salpingitis.

The diagnosis of FHC syndrome has been made on the basis of typical clinical symptoms in as many as 20% of patients with salpingitis and on the basis of laparoscopic findings in 5% to 15% of patients with salpingitis.

Etiology

Initially, it was believed that *Neisseria gonorrhoeae* was the only organism responsible for perihepatitis. In earlier reports, one third to one half of patients with clinical FHC had cervical cultures positive for *N gonorrhoeae*. However, there were few reports in which *N gonorrhoeae* was isolated directly from the surface of the liver.

In the 1970s, growing recognition of the importance of *Chlamydia trachomatis* in salpingitis spurred investigative interest in this organism as an etiologic agent of FHC syndrome. In 1978, Muller-Schoop and co-workers reported an association in young women of laparoscopically confirmed peritonitis and perihepatitis with serologic evidence of a recent *C trachomatis* infection. Subsequently, Wölner-Hanssen and co-workers reported three cases of acute genital chlamydial infection, confirmed by culture and serology, that had laparoscopic evidence of both salpingitis and perihepatitis. None of the patients in these cases had evidence of an acute gonococcal infection.

Additional reports have strengthened the etiologic association of *C trachomatis* with FHC syndrome. A summary by Eschenbach and Wölner-Hanssen of recently published series on FHC syndrome showed *N gonorrhoeae* isolated in only 10% and *C trachomatis* in 50% of cervical cultures of women with perihepatitis; in addition, serologic evidence of acute *C trachomatis* infection was present in 81% of cases. To date, there has been no evidence that other organisms play a significant role in the pathogenesis of this syndrome.

Pathophysiology

Only a small percentage of women with salpingitis will develop perihepatitis. Host factors and microbiologic virulence factors remain undefined.

Three mechanisms of spread from the pelvis to the liver have been proposed: (1) direct intraperitoneal; (2) lymphatic; and (3) hematogenous. In direct intraperitoneal spread, purulent exudate from the fallopian tubes travels up the paracolic gutter and collects in the subhepatic space, the most dependent portion of the abdominal cavity when a woman is supine. The result is an inflammatory reaction involving the liver capsule. The gross pathology observed during the early phase of this disease includes areas of purulent and fibrinous peritonitis on the liver capsule and hemorrhagic areas on the parietal peritoneum. Characteristic "violin string" adhesions are not seen until later in the course of the syndrome; these avascular bands between the liver capsule and the anterior abdominal wall are usually found after resolution of the acute inflammatory process.

The contribution of lymphatic and hematogenous spread of microorganisms to the pathogenesis of FHC syndrome is unclear, but the occurrence of the condition in men clearly necessitates an alternative explanation for direct intraperitoneal spread. Intraparenchymal liver damage has not been reported to be a histologic feature of this syndrome.

Diagnosis

Acute FHC syndrome is confirmed when right-upper-quadrant pain accompanies the clinical diagnosis of pelvic inflammatory disease (PID) or when both salpingitis and perihepatitis are observed by direct laparoscopic inspection. The right-upper-quadrant pain described with FHC syndrome is often sudden and intense. It occasionally radiates to the shoulder and is commonly exacerbated by breathing or coughing. In the majority of cases, it occurs simultaneously with the lower abdominal pain associated with salpingitis. In many cases, however, it will occur days to weeks after the onset of pelvic pain, and in rare cases it may precede pelvic symptoms. At times, the right-upper-quadrant pain is so severe that the signs and symptoms of salpingitis are overlooked.

Other diseases with right-upper-quadrant symptoms need to be considered in the differential diagnosis. Acute cholecystitis, viral hepatitis, and pneumonia are among the most common, but hepatic and subdiaphragmatic abscesses, pleuritis, pleurodynia, pancreatitis, perforated abdominal viscus, and even appendicitis have also been mistaken for FHC syndrome.

Liver enzyme determinations should be obtained. Slight elevations of bilirubin and serum enzymes occur in 25% to 50% of those with perihepatitis. Patients with pronounced enzyme elevations need serologic testing for hepatitis A, B, and C infection as well as for agents such as Epstein–Barr virus and cytomegalovirus that can cause viral hepatitis.

Chest x-rays and abdominal ultrasound scans are often needed to make the correct diagnosis. The chest x-ray occasionally will show a small amount of pleural fluid; a large pleural effusion or a pulmonary infiltrate is not seen as part of the FHC syndrome. Ultrasound images of the gallbladder, bile ducts, and liver parenchyma should be normal in patients with FHC syndrome.

Treatment

Parenteral regimens currently recommended for acute PID are adequate for treating FHC syndrome. These include (1) cefotetan, 2 g IV every 12 hours, plus doxycycline, 100 mg every 12 hours orally or IV; (2) clindamycin, 900 mg IV every 8 hours, plus gentamicin, loading dose (2 mg/kg) IV or IM followed by maintenance dose (1.5 mg/kg) every 8 hours; and (3) ampicillin/sulbactam, 3 g IV every 6 hours, plus doxycycline, 100 mg every 12 hours orally or IV [see Chapter 47: Acute salpingitis]. Intravenous antibiotic therapy should be given for at least 48 hours after the patient improves clinically. Continuation of doxycycline at 100 mg orally two times a day for a total of 10 to 14 days is recommended. Usually, acute upper abdominal pain resolves rapidly after IV therapy is initiated. However, chronic right-upper-quadrant pain may persist even after adequate therapy.

SUGGESTED READING

Centers for Disease Control: 1989 sexually transmitted diseases treatment guidelines. MMWR 1989;38(S-8):31

Darougar S, Forsey T, Wood JJ, et al: *Chlamydia* and the Curtis-Fitz-Hugh syndrome. Br J Vener Dis 1981;57:391

Eschenbach DA, Wölner-Hanssen PA: Fitz-Hugh-Curtis syndrome, in Holmes KK (ed): *Sexually Transmitted Diseases*, ed 2. New York, McGraw-Hill, 1990, pp 621-626

Gjonnaess H, Dalaker K, Anestad G, et al: Pelvic inflammatory disease: etiological studies with emphasis on chlamydial infection. Obstet Gynecol 1982;59:550

Muller-Schoop JW, Wang SP, Munzinger J, et al: *Chlamydia trachomatis* as possible cause of peritonitis and perihepatitis in young women. Br Med J 1978;1:1022

Owens S, Yeko TR, Bloy R, et al: Laparoscopic treatment of painful perihepatic adhesions in Fitz-Hugh-Curtis syndrome. Obstet Gynecol 1991;78:542

Paavonen J, Saikko P, Von Knorring J: Association of *Chlamydia trachomatis* infection with Fitz-Hugh-Curtis syndrome. J Infect Dis 1981;1440:176

Wang SP, Eschenbach DA, Holmes KK, et al: *Chlamydia trachomatis* infection in Fitz-Hugh-Curtis syndrome. Am J Obstet Gynecol 1980;138:1034

Wölner-Hanssen P, Weström L, Mårdh PA: Perihepatitis and chlamydial salpingitis. Lancet 1980;1:901

51
Pelvic
tuberculosis

By David Charles, MD

Background and incidence

Around 1900, genital tuberculosis was common, but during the past decade in North America it has become increasingly rare. The literature on it is likewise sparse.

Tuberculosis is still endemic in some parts of the world, and pelvic tuberculosis is frequently observed in India, the Far East, the Caribbean, and South America. With increasing immigration into the United States from these areas, physicians may more often encounter infertility caused by pelvic tuberculosis.

The decline of tuberculosis in the US ceased in 1984, and in 1986 incidence rose 2.6%. The excess of 3,900 cases was confined to communities where acquired immunodeficiency syndrome was prevalent. In Florida, tuberculosis has been found in 10% of AIDS patients, but 30% of new tuberculosis patients have AIDS. Although pulmonary tuberculosis accounts for most of these infections, as many as 25% of patients have extrapulmonary disease.

The relationship between HIV infection and tuberculosis has added to concern over the increasing prevalence of tuberculosis. In the early stages of AIDS, the decline in immunity is sufficient to allow for a dormant mycobacterial infection to be reactivated. Moreover, the extraordinary susceptibility of AIDS patients to tuberculosis is highlighted by a recent report of its development in 44% of patients with HIV infection after exposure to a source case. Because of the recent increase in the incidence of tuberculosis, physicians must be alert for pelvic tuberculosis in women with pulmonary tuberculosis.

We cannot accurately determine the actual frequency of pelvic tuberculosis in the general US population. However, it is estimated that this condition is encountered in only one of every 5,000 gynecologic hospital admissions. Thus, most gynecologists will never see a case.

Pathogenesis

Tuberculosis of the female genital tract is a local manifestation of systemic disease and is invariably secondary to a mycobacterial infection of the lung or another organ. Spread to the pelvis is usually by the bloodstream from a primary pulmonary infection. For undetermined reasons, the hematogenous infection favors the fallopian tubes rather than other female genital tract sites. The acid-fast bacillus may occasionally be spread by the lymphatics from primary intestinal tuberculosis or by direct extension from a neighboring organ, such as the urinary bladder.

After involving the tubes, the infection spreads by direct extension to the endometrium, which is involved in 90% of cases of gynecologic tuberculosis. The ovaries are far less frequently affected, while the cervix is involved in only about 1% of cases. Tuberculosis infection of the vagina and vulva is extremely rare. Primary infection of the female genital tract is rare but can occur if the patient's partner has active genitourinary tuberculosis.

Diagnosis

Most cases of genital tuberculosis are found in premenopausal women. Involuntary infertility, abdominal pain, and abnormal bleeding are the most common reasons for office visits. About 10% of cases occur in postmenopausal women who see physicians because of bleeding or pain.

Menstrual disorders occur in about 20% of women with genital tuberculosis. However, menorrhagia and metrorrhagia are no more prevalent than in other gynecologic conditions.

The history is vital. About 20% of patients with pelvic tuberculosis report tuberculosis in the immediate family, and approximately half the patients will have some form of mycobacterial infection. It is therefore important to include a chest x-ray when investigating such patients for infertility because the physical examination may be completely normal.

The clinician usually fails to suspect the diagnosis. It becomes apparent only with discovery of granulomas and giant cells in endometrial biopsy specimens or histologic studies of fallopian tubes. Less frequently, visual examination with the laparoscope may reveal gross changes of the adnexa consistent with tubercles.

Although an irrefutable diagnosis of tuberculosis can be made only by isolating *Mycobacterium tuberculosis*, most authorities now accept an unsupported histologic diagnosis. Nevertheless, one

TABLE 1
Antituberculous therapy

Ethambutol	Usual dose 15–25 mg/kg/day initially, followed after 60 days by 15 mg/kg/day as a single daily dose
Rifampin	600 mg orally once daily
Isoniazid	300 mg orally once daily
Pyrazinamide	25 mg/kg/day orally in two spaced doses
Streptomycin	1 g IM daily; ultimately, the drug should be discontinued or reduced in dosage to 1 g two to three times weekly

should always attempt to obtain bacteriologic evidence of the infection, since granulomatous salpingitis may be secondary to conditions such as actinomycosis, schistosomiasis, sarcoidosis, pinworm, Crohn's disease, or even presence of a foreign body (talc or oil-based hysterosalpingographic contrast material). Also consider tuberculous salpingitis in the differential diagnosis when a patient is not responding to conventional antibiotic therapy for acute bacterial pelvic inflammatory disease.

Availability of effective therapy makes early diagnosis of the utmost importance in achieving a satisfactory outcome. Ironically, since wide use of such therapy in developed countries has caused the disease incidence to decline, early diagnosis has become more difficult. Therefore, although pelvic tuberculosis is infrequently encountered, strong suspicion is important in making the diagnosis.

Treatment
Primary therapy is by a combination of antibiotics to which *M tuberculosis* is sensitive (Table 1). Principles and duration of antibiotic therapy are the same as those for pulmonary tuberculosis. Consequently, one should collaborate with a chest physician versed in antituberculous therapy in planning treatment.

The duration of therapy depends on the drugs used, drug susceptibility test results, and the patient's response to therapy. Although most patients with previously untreated tuberculosis can be treated with either a 6- or a 9-month regimen, the former is preferred. Both the 6- and 9-month regimens are referred to as "short-course" regimens. All regimens of 9 months or less must contain isoniazid and rifampin.

The initial phase of the 6-month regimen must consist of at least a 2-month period of daily isoniazid, rifampin, and pyrazinamide. This combination should be supplemented with either ethambutol or streptomycin when isoniazid resistance is suspected or if extensive or life-threatening disease is present. The second phase of treatment should consist of isoniazid and rifampin, given daily or twice weekly for 4 months.

The 9-month regimen consists of an initial phase of 1 or 2 months of daily isoniazid and rifampin, followed by daily or twice-weekly isoniazid and rifampin for a total duration of 9 months. Ethambutol or streptomycin should be given initially when isoniazid resistance is suspected or if extensive or life-threatening disease is present.

Drug therapy is so effective that surgery is necessary only in certain circumstances, such as when there is an adnexal mass. In women older than 40 years of age, total abdominal hysterectomy with bilateral salpingo-oophorectomy is the operation of choice. Surgical intervention should also be considered when infection or pelvic pain is persistent or recurrent. In younger patients, one must duly consider ovarian conservation if the infection has not involved the ovaries.

When the diagnosis of tuberculosis is only established postoperatively, institute drug therapy as previously described. Whether the patient has or has not required surgery, follow her up to assess therapy and help her cope with any sexual or fertility problems connected with disease.

SUGGESTED READING

Barnes PF, Bloch AB, Davidson PT, et al: Tuberculosis in patients with HIV infection. N Engl J Med 1991;324:1644

Schaefer G: Female genital tuberculosis. Clin Obstet Gynecol 1976;19:223

Sutherland AM: Gynaecological tuberculosis: analysis of a personal series of 710 cases. Aust NZ J Obstet Gynaecol 1985;25:203

52

IUD-associated infections

By Richard H. Schwarz, MD, and Philip B. Mead, MD

Background and incidence

Although an association between the use of an intrauterine contraceptive device (IUD) and increased risk of pelvic inflammatory disease (PID) has been documented for many years, recent studies suggest that this association has been overestimated. Methodologic flaws in older studies, such as comparison with inappropriate control groups, overdiagnosis of PID among IUD users, and failure to adjust for confounding variables artifactually increased the apparent risk of IUDs. The risk of PID with the Dalkon Shield was higher than with other IUDs, and failure to exclude these cases is an additional factor in the overestimation of risk with currently available devices. (A recent, controversial review by Kronmal and co-workers has even questioned the previously reported strong association between PID and the Dalkon Shield.)

Methodologically sound studies published since the mid-1980s have clarified the association between IUDs and PID and indicate a relative risk of 1.0 to 2.6 compared with that of women using no contraceptive method.

Pathophysiology

Contamination of the endometrial cavity at insertion is felt to be responsible for most cases of IUD-related PID, and this risk appears limited to the first 4 months of use. Infections occurring after 4 months are believed to be the result of acquired sexually transmitted pathogens, not the IUD itself.

Previously it was believed that IUD infections spread through lymphatics to produce a perisalpingitis similar to postabortal or postpartum infections. Now it is thought that direct spread of microorganisms from the infected or colonized uterine cavity to the fallopian tubes is the major pathogenic mechanism. It was felt at one time that unilateral tubo-ovarian abscesses were uniquely associated with IUD infections, but this view has subsequently been disproved. Although the multifilamented tail of the Dalkon Shield was thought to act as a "wick" for endometrial contamination, the monofilament tails of currently available IUDs do not appear to be of etiologic importance in PID.

Recent pathomorphologic studies of fallopian tubes excised during sterilization of asymptomatic IUD users reveal a sterile foreign-body reaction. The relationship of this sterile reaction to infectious salpingitis, if any, has not been established.

Spontaneous midtrimester septic abortions were rare until Dalkon Shields were introduced. According to Tatum, the Dalkon Shield appeared to predispose to this serious condition when the 200 to 400 separate fibers forming its sheathed multifilament tail retracted up into the endometrial cavity early in the second trimester. In addition, the microorganisms between the sheathed fibers were not exposed to the bacteriocidal and bacteriostatic endocervical mucus, as they are with the unsheathed single or double fibers of conventional modern IUD tails.

Etiology

The microorganisms associated with non-STD-related IUD PID are those of the endogenous cervicovaginal flora. These infections are always polymicrobial, and anaerobes predominate. Infections occurring more than 4 months after insertion are felt to be due to the same sexually transmitted and endogenous pathogens that cause non-IUD-related PID [see Chapter 46: Acute salpingitis: incidence and diagnosis].

A unique role for *Actinomyces* organisms in IUD PID has been suggested, but this relationship remains unclear. Although as many as 4% to 8% of IUD users may have *Actinomyces*-like organisms identified on a Pap smear, this presence has not been equated with pelvic actinomycosis, nor has the risk of subsequent pelvic infection been quantified.

IUD use may increase susceptibility to bacterial vaginosis, a condition that may of itself increase the risk of PID. However, no studies have addressed the risk of postinsertion PID in IUD users with bacterial vaginosis.

Diagnosis

The classic syndrome of IUD-related progressive endometritis, first described by Burnhill, consists of persistent foul vaginal discharge, intermenstrual spotting, premenstrual bloating, and dull backache during menstruation. Initially, the uterine corpus is tender on bimanual palpation, but adnexal tenderness and cervical motion tenderness are late findings. This syndrome has virtually disappeared with the discontinuance of older devices such as the Dalkon Shield, Birnberg Bow, and Majzlin Spring; Burnhill feels it is largely of historical interest.

Postinsertion and STD-related IUD PID can be asymptomatic or may present with the same signs and symptoms as non-IUD-related PID. The diagnosis is established in the same way as in the latter condition, and laparoscopy should be employed if the diagnosis is uncertain.

The syndrome of midtrimester septic abortion has also essentially disappeared with the abandonment of the Dalkon Shield. Patients often progressed to severe infection with minimal signs and symptoms, and septic shock and adult respiratory distress syndrome were frequent and early complications.

Treatment

Progressive endometritis. This syndrome is rarely seen at present. In the past, patients diagnosed before adnexal involvement responded to a 7- to 10-day course of an oral tetracycline, with removal of the IUD after 24 hours of antibiotics.

Postinsertion and STD-related IUD PID. Antibiotic management of these conditions is generally the same as for any acute salpingitis. We prefer parenteral therapy (clindamycin plus gentamicin, cefotetan plus doxycycline, or ampicillin/sulbactam plus doxycycline) on an inpatient basis for IUD users with salpingitis. The IUD should be removed as soon as systemic antimicrobial levels are established. Failure to respond to therapy, including treatment for tubo-ovarian abscess, is managed exactly as with other acute PID [see Chapter 47: Acute salpingitis: treatment].

Actinomyces colonization/infection. When *Actinomyces* is identified in an asymptomatic IUD user (almost always on a Pap smear), removal of the device will result in clearing of the organism. This should be followed by a repeat Pap smear after one or two menstrual cycles to confirm the result. After a negative smear is obtained, a new device may be reinserted.

Symptomatic patients should be treated with parenteral antimicrobial therapy and the IUD removed. The exact role of *Actinomyces* agents in abscess formation remains unclear, as does the mechanism of its apparent relationship to the IUD. Whether *Actinomyces* is a sole pathogen or a marker for mixed aerobic–anaerobic infection is unclear. We favor the likelihood of mixed infection and prefer to use broad-spectrum antibiotic coverage. If *Actinomyces* is demonstrated in association with a tubo-ovarian abscess, antibiotic therapy for 1 to 3 months must follow surgical extirpation of the infected tissue. Penicillin is the drug of choice; cephalosporins, clindamycin, or chloramphenicol are alternative agents. It should be remembered that metronidazole, although extremely active against most anaerobes, is not effective against *Actinomyces*.

IUDs and pregnancy. If a patient conceives with an IUD in place and wishes to continue the pregnancy, the device should be removed if the string is visible. If it cannot be removed, the patient must be advised of the potential problems and carefully monitored throughout the pregnancy. In the rare event of septic midtrimester abortion, management involves aggressive evacuation of the uterus by the most expeditious means, broad-spectrum parenteral antibiotic therapy, and intensive cardiovascular and respiratory monitoring. Failure to recognize the problem and to treat it aggressively can lead to a high mortality rate.

IUDs and bacterial vaginosis. Bacterial vaginosis should be treated in an IUD user (metronidazole, 500 mg orally twice daily for 7 days), but the IUD does not need to be removed unless signs or symptoms of PID are present [see Chapter 32: Bacterial vaginosis].

Sequelae

The greatest concern following IUD-related PID is for tubal damage. Two case–control studies of tubal infertility showed the risk highest with the Dalkon Shield and lowest with copper devices. In the study of Cramer and co-workers, the increased risk of primary tubal infertility was statistically significant for users of the Dalkon Shield (3.3), Lippes Loop or Saf-T-Coil (2.9), and copper IUDs (1.6). For secondary tubal infertility the risk associated with copper devices was not statistically significant. Of note, women with only one sexual partner had no increased risk of primary tubal infertility associated with IUD use.

In the study of Daling and co-workers, the relative risk of primary tubal infertility was 6.8 for users of the Dalkon Shield, 3.2 for users of the Lippes Loop or Saf-T-Coil, and 1.9 for users of copper devices. The risk associated with the copper devices was not statistically significant. As with PID, the risk of infertility appears to be largely related to the likelihood of exposure to sexually transmitted diseases.

Prevention

The IUD, unlike barrier methods of contraception and birth control pills, offers no protection against sexually transmitted diseases. This is a critical issue in contraceptive choice for a woman who desires fertility in the future. Careful selection of candidates for IUDs appears to offer the greatest opportunity for infection prevention. Only women at low risk for acquiring sexually transmitted infections should use an IUD. They should be in a stable, mutually monogamous relationship, have no evidence of acute cervicitis, and have no prior history of ectopic pregnancy, salpingitis, or any STD. Mishell has suggested that IUDs should not be used by any nulliparous woman who may want to conceive in the future, because of the slight possibility of postinsertion PID and its associated tubal infertility risk.

Optimally, the physician should confirm the absence of cervical infection with *Neisseria gonorrhoeae* and/or *Chlamydia trachomatis* before insertion. Frequently this is not feasible. However, if a mucopurulent discharge from the cervix is noted, insertion should be deferred until the etiology has been investigated and treated. The presence of the typical bacterial vaginosis syndrome, confirmed microscopically, should also lead to delay of insertion until treatment has been completed.

Aseptic technique must be maintained during the insertion process. The vagina and cervix are routinely cleansed with an antiseptic.

The manufacturers of currently available IUDs suggest considering antibiotic prophylaxis for IUD insertion using either doxycycline (200 mg orally 1 hour before insertion) or erythromycin (500 mg orally 1 hour before insertion and 500 mg orally 6 hours after insertion). A single study of the doxycycline regimen showed a nonsignificant decrease in PID from 1.9% to 1.3%, and a highly significant 31% reduction in IUD-related office visits.

SUGGESTED READING

Burnhill MS: Syndrome of progressive endometritis associated with intrauterine contraceptive devices. Adv Planned Parent 1973;8:144

Cramer DW, Schiff I, Schoenbaum SC, et al: Tubal infertility and the intrauterine device. N Engl J Med 1985;312:941

Daling JR, Weiss NS, Metch BJ, et al: Primary tubal infertility in relation to the use of an intrauterine device. N Engl J Med 1985;312:937

Hager WD, Douglas B, Majmudar B, et al: Pelvic colonization with *Actinomyces* in women using intrauterine contraceptive devices. Am J Obstet Gynecol 1979;135:680

Kessel E: Pelvic inflammatory disease with intrauterine device use: a reassessment. Fertil Steril 1989;51:1

Kronmal RA, Whitney CW, Mumford SD: The intrauterine device and pelvic inflammatory disease: the Women's Health Study reanalyzed. J Clin Epidemiol 1991;44:109

Lee NC, Rubin GL, Borucki R: The intrauterine device and pelvic inflammatory disease revisited: new results from the Women's Health Study. Obstet Gynecol 1988;72:1

Lee NC, Rubin GL, Ory HW, et al: Type of intrauterine device and the risk of pelvic inflammatory disease. Obstet Gynecol 1983;62:1

Sinei SKA, Schulz KF, Lamptey PR, et al: Preventing IUCD-related pelvic infection: the efficacy of prophylactic doxycycline at insertion. Br J Obstet Gynaecol 1990;97:412

53
Cystitis

By Mark G. Martens, MD

Background and incidence

Cystitis, or lower urinary tract infection (UTI), is a common malady, estimated to occur at least once in 20% of all women in their life-times. The incidence of bacteriuria varies between 4% and 6% in the reproductive-aged group, and increases 1% to 2% per decade, bring-ing the rate to approximately 10% by the early postmenopausal years.

Pathophysiology

Colonization of the vaginal introitus and periurethral region by Enterobacteriaceae from the bowel is thought to be the initial step in the pathogenesis of urinary tract infections in women. Progression to cystitis appears related to several factors, including intercourse, personal hygiene, and diaphragm use.

Etiology

The most common cause of simple cystitis is *Escherichia coli* (80% to 85%), with other gram-negative bacteria such as *Klebsiella*, *Proteus*, *Enterobacter*, and *Pseudomonas* species also contributing. The most common gram-positive bacterium recovered is *Staphylococcus sapro-phyticus* (11%). *Staphylococcus epidermidis*, the enterococci, and group B ß-hemolytic streptococci are also possible pathogens.

Diagnosis

Asymptomatic bacteriuria is identified by two consecutive urine samples of 100,000 colony-forming units (cfu) per milliliter of urine collected by the clean-catch method from a patient with no com-plaints. However, unless the patient is pregnant and undergoes pre-natal urine analysis, asymptomatic bacteriuria usually goes undetected unless she is screened for other reasons, has a voiding difficulty, or experiences suprapubic pain. Examination of the urine in an infected patient reveals evidence of pyuria and hematuria approximately 50% of the time.

Initially, UTI is diagnosed in a patient with clinical symptoms by demonstrating large numbers of bacteria and white blood cells (WBC) in the urine. The bacteria should be visible by microscopic examination of an unspun specimen, and more than 50 WBC should be seen per high-power field in a spun specimen. Samples can then be sent for Gram staining and culture, and treatment initiated.

Urine containing more than 10^5 bacteria/mL in a woman with clinical symptoms is diagnostic of cystitis. However, 30% to 50% of women with acute lower tract infections will harbor fewer than 10^5 bacteria/mL. Stamm and co-workers, using suprapubic aspiration, found $\geq 10^2$ bacteria per milliliter was the best diagnostic criterion, with a sensitivity of 95%.

Treatment

Cost analyses have demonstrated that 90% of cystitis cases are uncomplicated and respond readily to the empiric antimicrobials chosen, without the use of a culture. However, cultures are indicated and helpful in several circumstances: complicated UTI or uncertain diagnosis, recent previous UTI (less than 3 weeks), symptoms lasting more than 7 days, recent catheterization, genitourinary surgery, pregnancy, and diabetes.

Gram stain of the urine sample can help direct initial therapy. Penicillin and ampicillin, though inexpensive and effective first-line UTI agents in the past, have become less effective in some areas because of increasing resistance of several gram-negative organisms, including *E coli*. If the Gram stain demonstrates gram-positive organisms, then these agents can still be given with relative assurance. They provide continued excellent activity for gram-positive species.

For initial therapy, one of several relatively inexpensive oral agents should be utilized. These include trimethoprim/sulfamethoxazole, 1 to 2 tablets every 12 hours; nitrofurantoin macrocrystals, 50 to 100 mg every 6 to 12 hours; and sulfamethoxazole or sulfisoxazole, 2 g initially, then 500 mg to 1 g every 6 to 8 hours.

The recently released quinolone antibiotics (norfloxacin, ciprofloxacin, ofloxacin), the ß-lactamase-inhibiting combination of amoxicillin and clavulanate, and the extended-spectrum agents cefuroxime and cefixime are not first-line agents. They should be reserved for resistant or complicated UTI. [For treatment in pregnancy, see Chapter 4: Lower urinary tract infections in pregnancy.]

Approximately 20% of women treated for simple cystitis will have a recurrence. These newer agents can be given if resistance to first-line agents is documented by culture. At the same time, do a work-up to rule out upper urinary tract anomalies or obstruction.

Length of initial therapy is controversial. Several recent reports demonstrate adequate efficacy with single-dose therapy. However, the morbidity associated with recurrences and retreatment still requires further evaluation of this abbreviated regimen. Therefore, the traditional 3 to 7 days should still be followed in most instances.

Initial or recurrent infections in which an organism is not isolated by culture and symptoms persist should be evaluated for conditions such as trichomoniasis, which can produce similar symptoms. Also, nonbacterial urethritis or sterile pyuria may be present but caused by organisms not routinely cultured, such as *Neisseria gonorrhoeae* and *Chlamydia trachomatis*, and perhaps *Mycoplasma hominis* and *Ureaplasma urealyticum*.

As many as 95% of recurrences represent reinfection with a different organism. Reinfections usually occur more than 2 to 3 weeks after cessation of previous therapy. Radiographic and endoscopic examinations of the urinary tract are rarely revealing and generally are not indicated. Strategies for managing frequent reinfections include prophylaxis, intermittent self-start therapy, and postcoital prophylaxis.

Relapse or persistence with the same pathogen represents about 5% of cases. These usually occur within 1 to 2 weeks of cessation of antimicrobial therapy and are often associated with structural abnormalities of the urinary tract. Strategies for managing relapse include evaluating the urinary tract radiologically and endoscopically, and continuing courses of chemotherapy for 2 to 6 weeks or longer.

SUGGESTED READING

Harris RE, Curole DN: Urinary tract infections, in Faro S (ed): *Diagnosis and Management of Female Pelvic Infections in Primary Care Medicine*. Baltimore, Williams & Wilkins, 1985, pp 185-202

Parsons CL: New standards for UTI. Urology 1988;325:1

Stamm WE: Dysuria: establishing a diagnostic protocol. Contemp Ob/Gyn 1988;32(October):81

Stapleton A, Latham RH, Johnson C, et al: Postcoital antimicrobial prophylaxis for recurrent urinary tract infection. JAMA 1990;264:703

54
Acute urethral syndrome

By Michael G. Gravett, MD

Background

Symptoms associated with lower urinary tract infection are among the most frequent for which young women visit a physician. In the United States, more than 5 million women seek health care for such infections annually. Although frequency and dysuria are usually attributed to cystitis, these symptoms can also be associated with urethritis or vaginitis. The term "acute urethral syndrome" has been used to refer to acute dysuria or frequency without marked bacteriuria, which is defined as $\geq 10^5$ bacteria/mL urine.

Acute urethral syndrome should not be confused with the general term "urethral syndrome." This phrase is used to denote lower urinary tract symptoms that are usually of extended duration. However, they tend to appear in the absence of obvious bladder or urethral abnormalities.

The possible etiologies for urethral syndrome include not only infection but also hypoestrogenism, mechanical or functional urethral obstruction, traumatic insult, and neurologic or psychiatric disturbances.

Pathophysiology

The urethra normally plays an important role in preventing ascending urinary tract infection (UTI). In addition to a midurethral high-pressure zone that acts as a mechanical barrier preventing the ascent of genital microorganisms, mucus-secreting periurethral glands in the posterior portion of the urethra may aid in trapping bacteria and secreting immunoglobulin A. Although an average of six to eight species of microorganisms can usually be recovered from the distal urethra, the proximal 1 cm of the urethra is normally sterile.

Acute urethral syndrome may represent the earliest stages of an ascending lower UTI after periurethral colonization by coliform bacteria or other uropathogens. This hypothesis is supported by the observation of O'Grady and co-workers that over 50% of women with the syndrome followed prospectively develop significant bacteriuria. The bacteria recovered from urine cultures of these women are identical with those recovered from women with acute cystitis. The reasons why periurethral colonization progresses to acute cystitis in some women remain speculative, but may have more to do with the arbitrary clinical distinction between the two conditions than with true differences in pathophysiology.

Clinicians have adopted $\geq 10^5$ bacteria/mL of urine as the major criterion for the diagnosis of cystitis. This is based on early work by Kass. However, he used this criterion to distinguish bacteriuria in women with acute pyelonephritis from asymptomatic women or contaminated urine specimens, and he did not study women with lower urinary tract symptoms only.

More recent data suggest that among women with dysuria the demonstration of $\geq 10^2$ uropathogens/mL urine is the most sensitive and specific criterion for the diagnosis of cystitis. Thus, there is a continuum of the same disease process. It is arbitrarily designated as cystitis when associated with $\geq 10^5$/mL and as acute urethral syndrome when associated with $< 10^5$/mL.

Etiology
Studies using either suprapubic bladder aspiration or sterile urethral catheterization have demonstrated microorganisms from bladder urine of many patients with acute urethral syndrome. Stamm, Wagner, and co-workers recovered uropathogens from bladder urine of 27 (46%) of 59 women, including *Escherichia coli* in 24 (41%) and *Staphylococcus saprophyticus* in three (5%), all in concentrations of $\leq 10^4$/mL. Pyuria (defined as ≥ 8 leukocytes/mm^3 of uncentrifuged midstream urine) is strongly correlated with the recovery of uropathogens from the bladder. Pyuria was found in 26 (96%) of 27 of those patients from whom a bacterial uropathogen was recovered and in only seven (20%) of 34 of asymptomatic comparison patients.

Sexually transmitted organisms may also cause the disorder. Both *Neisseria gonorrhoeae* and *Chlamydia trachomatis* are common causes of urethritis in men, where infection is usually associated with frank urethral discharge. Similarly, both may cause acute urethral syndrome in females, although frank urethral discharge is infrequent.

Dysuria and frequency are common among women seen at sexually transmitted disease clinics who have genital infection with *N gonorrhoeae* and *C trachomatis*. Particularly intriguing is the role of

C trachomatis. Stamm and associates found evidence of chlamydial infection in 11 of 32 women with acute urethral syndrome and sterile bladder urine. Pyuria, as previously defined, was noted in 10 of these 11 patients. The correlation between *C trachomatis* infection and sterile pyuria is also important.

Among 16 patients with sterile bladder cultures and pyuria, evidence of chlamydial infection was found in 10 (62.5%) in contrast with only one (6%) of 16 patients with sterile cultures and no evidence of pyuria. Thus, infection with *C trachomatis* must be considered in a patient with acute urethral syndrome and sterile urine and pyuria.

The role of genital mycoplasmas is controversial. There is no evidence that *Mycoplasma hominis* is associated. A possible role for *Ureaplasma urealyticum* is suggested by recovery of this organism in concentrations of $\geq 10^3$/mL in first-voided urine of 60% of women with acute urethral syndrome of uncertain etiology and pyuria, and in only 31% of asymptomatic control women.

Diagnosis

Dysuria or frequency may be associated with acute urethral syndrome, cystitis, vaginitis, or primary herpetic genital infection. All patients should be carefully evaluated by appropriate physical examination, microscopic examination of the midstream urine, and appropriate urine, urethral, or genital cultures taken (Figure 1).

Approximately 10% of women with dysuria have vaginitis or genital herpes. Dysuria that is associated with vaginitis is usually described as external, and is characterized as a burning sensation when urine comes into contact with the inflamed genitalia. Vaginitis or primary genital herpes can be excluded on the basis of careful physical examination and microscopic examination of vaginal discharge. The cervix should also be inspected for mucopurulent cervicitis, as an indicator of chlamydial infection, and a Gram stain from the cervix examined for gram-negative intracellular diplococci, indicative of gonococcal infection. Urethral discharge expressed by gentle pressure on the urethra suggests infection with *N gonorrhoeae* or *C trachomatis*.

In the absence of vaginitis, carefully collected midstream urine should be cultured for usual uropathogens and also examined microscopically. Cystitis, associated with $\geq 10^5$ bacteria/mL urine, occurs in approximately 50% of women with dysuria and acute urethral syndrome occurs in another 40% of patients.

Initially, uncentrifuged urine should be microscopically examined. When examining uncentrifuged urine, the presence of one bacterium per oil immersion field correlates well with $\geq 10^5$/mL and

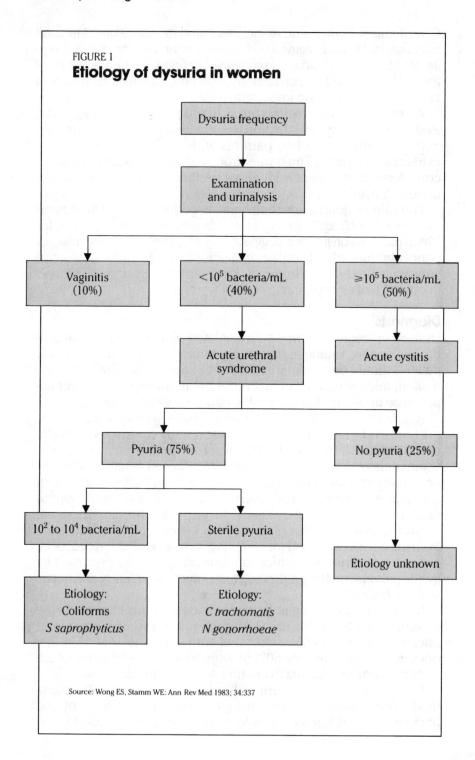

FIGURE 1
Etiology of dysuria in women

Dysuria frequency

Examination and urinalysis

| Vaginitis (10%) | <10^5 bacteria/mL (40%) | ≥10^5 bacteria/mL (50%) |

Acute urethral syndrome

Acute cystitis

Pyuria (75%)

No pyuria (25%)

10^2 to 10^4 bacteria/mL

Sterile pyuria

Etiology unknown

Etiology: Coliforms *S saprophyticus*

Etiology: *C trachomatis* *N gonorrhoeae*

Source: Wong ES, Stamm WE: Ann Rev Med 1983; 34:337

the diagnosis of acute cystitis can be made. The absence of bacteria in several oil immersion fields suggests a bacterial colony count of $\leq 10^4$/mL. Urine should also be centrifuged and the sediment examined microscopically under the high dry objective field (400×).

Pyuria, defined as ≥ 8 leukocytes/mm^3 midstream urine, corresponds approximately to 5 to 10 leukocytes per high dry microscopic field when 10 mL of urine has been centrifuged and the sediment resuspended in 1 mL of urine. Alternatively, leukocytes may be directly counted in a hemocytometer, using uncentrifuged urine. The detection of 100 bacteria per high dry objective field of unstained centrifuged urinary sediment also correlates well with the recovery of $\geq 10^5$/mL. Midstream urine should also be cultured. Patients in whom pure cultures of between 10^2 and 10^4 uropathogens/mL are recovered and who also have pyuria or dysuria should be considered to have acute urethral syndrome and treated.

If the patient has pyuria without bacteriuria and is considered to be at risk for sexually transmitted disease, or if on speculum examination has cervicitis, specimens should be taken from both the cervix and urethra and cultured for *N gonorrhoeae* as well as tested for *C trachomatis* by culture, direct immunofluorescence, or ELISA.

Several biochemical tests developed to detect bacteriuria (nitrite tests) or pyuria (leukocyte esterase tests) are helpful in diagnosing cystitis. Their role in detecting acute urethral syndrome has not been established, but these tests may be useful in screening women with dysuria.

Treatment
Uncomplicated cystitis may be effectively treated with single-dose therapy (usually trimethoprim/sulfamethoxazole, two double-strength tablets orally) or with a 3-day regimen (trimethoprim/sulfamethoxazole, one double-strength tablet twice a day; amoxicillin/clavulanic acid, 250 mg three times a day; norfloxacin, 400 mg twice a day; or ciprofloxacin, 500 mg twice a day). Sulfonamides, ampicillin, and amoxicillin can no longer be primarily recommended for the treatment of UTI because of a high frequency of *E coli* resistance to these agents.

These shorter regimens have cure rates comparable with conventional 7- to 10-day antibiotic regimens for uncomplicated cystitis. However, clinical trials comparing single-dose or 3-day regimens with longer conventional therapy for acute urethral syndrome have not been reported. It is likely that women with acute urethral syndrome associated with *E coli* or *S saprophyticus* can be treated with these shorter regimens. However, women in whom either *N gonorrhoeae* or *C trachomatis* is suspected on epidemiologic grounds or urinalysis (pyuria without bacteriuria) should be treated in accordance with current CDC guidelines for at least 7 days.

Current therapeutic recommendations for chlamydial infections include tetracycline, 500 mg orally four times a day; doxycycline, 100 mg orally twice a day; or erythromycin stearate, 500 mg orally four times a day. In addition, patients with suspected gonococcal infections should receive ceftriaxone, 250 mg IM.

Although norfloxacin and ciprofloxacin have only limited activity against *C trachomatis*, ofloxacin has excellent activity against *C trachomatis* as well as against other uropathogens. Preliminary studies of ofloxacin for the treatment of urethritis, including chlamydial urethritis, suggest clinical and microbiologic cure rates in excess of 90% in patients treated with 200 to 300 mg orally twice a day for 7 days. This fluoroquinolone antibiotic may have an important role in the treatment of acute urethral syndrome.

Patients with acute dysuria without bacteriuria or pyuria do not benefit from antibiotic therapy. These patients may be symptomatically treated with phenazopyridine HCl and reevaluated if symptoms persist. Women with persistent UTI or with chronic dysuria not associated with infection should be referred for urologic evaluation.

SUGGESTED READING

Centers for Disease Control: 1989 sexually transmitted disease treatment guidelines. MMWR 1989;38(S-8):22,28

Latham RH, Stamm WE: Urethral syndrome in women. Urol Clin North Am 1984;11:95

O'Grady FW, Richards B, McSherry MA, et al: Introital enterobacteria, urinary infection, and the urethral syndrome. Lancet 1970;2:1208

Stamm WE, Counts GW, Running KR, et al: Diagnosis of coliform infection in acutely dysuric women. N Engl J Med 1982;307:463

Stamm WE, Running KR, Hale J, et al: Etiologic role of *Mycoplasma hominis and Ureaplasma urealyticum* in women with acute urethral syndrome. Sex Transm Dis 1983;10(suppl 4):318

Stamm WE, Wagner KF, Amsel R, et al: Causes of acute urethral syndrome in women. N Engl J Med 1980;303:409

Wong ES, Stamm WE: Urethral infection in men and women. Ann Rev Med 1983;34:337

55
Evaluation of the infected postoperative patient

By Joseph G. Pastorek II, MD

Background

The typical patient cared for by an obstetrician–gynecologist is, as a rule, younger and healthier than the usual medical or general surgical patient. For this reason, mortality due to infection is rare in ob–gyn practice. However, infectious complications of such procedures as cesarean section (C/S) and hysterectomy may prolong hospital stay, increase medical expense, and extend recovery time. Therefore, the physician assessing the condition of a woman with suspected postoperative infection must be methodical and thorough to assure prompt and accurate diagnosis leading to appropriate and timely therapy.

Patient evaluation

Since most postoperative ob–gyn patients have a rather straightforward, obvious history—pregnancy, labor, C/S, fever—you must take care not to overlook important medical background. Illnesses such as postpartal lupus flare and drug fever, whose symptoms mimic postoperative infection, may mislead you.

The physical examination is paramount in evaluating the postsurgical ob–gyn patient. It is important not to concentrate exclusively on the abdomen and pelvis, nor to assume the infection is always directly related to a surgical site such as the uterus or vaginal cuff. While this is usually true, there are extrapelvic sources of postoperative symptoms. A systemic head-to-toe survey is necessary to exclude such entities as pneumonia, coincidental cold or flu, hepatitis (perhaps caused or aggravated by anesthetic agents), urinary tract infection, pyelonephritis, and puerperal mastitis.

Most sources of postoperative ob–gyn infection will be encountered in the pelvis, especially at the operative site. Therefore, the pelvic exam and the abdominal wound exam are the most fruitful areas for investigation. When you suspect infection, follow a standard method for evaluating the abdomen and pelvis. Assess, by auscultation and then palpation, the entire abdomen, including the flanks and hypochondria. Look for and define tenderness, rebound tenderness, organomegaly, and abnormal masses or fluid collections. Investigate the abdominal wound, if present, for general appearance and texture, including the classic signs of rubor, dolor, calor, and abnormal drainage. Manually express or aspirate by needle any apparent abnormal fluid collections as you search for seroma, hematoma, or abscess.

In cases of puerperal fever, examine the uterine fundus for evidence of endomyometritis. After vaginal delivery, since the uterus projects out of the pelvis nearly to the level of the umbilicus, this step is easily accomplished in most cases. Therefore, the fundus is easy to palpate through the lax and attenuated abdominal wall. However, the inexperienced examiner may have some difficulty distinguishing normal postoperative incisional pain from that due to infection. The experienced physician will palpate the fundus of the uterus from above the umbilicus, pressing in an inferior direction, all the while staying well above the most cephalad point of the usual lower abdominal incision. The adnexa of a woman who has had a bilateral tubal ligation after delivery may generate tenderness that may be mistaken for adnexitis.

After examining the abdomen, incision, and uterine fundus, turn to the pelvic examination. To perform it appropriately, arrange the patient optimally. A suitable pelvic examination table is a must. Insert the speculum, note the quantity and quality of the vaginal discharge or lochia, and check the amount of blood or pus contained therein. Inspect the vaginal barrel for evidence of inflammation, especially in proximity to vaginal lacerations or suture lines.

For patients with puerperal infection, especially those who have undergone C/S before ample cervical dilation, gently dilate the cervix (for example, with a ringed forceps) to allow any "lochial block" to drain. In patients after hysterectomy, visualize the vaginal cuff incision and pay attention to erythema, purulent discharge, or other signs of infection. Follow the speculum examination with a bimanual examination. When inserting the examining fingers, you may detect increased vaginal temperature in the patient with true pelvic infection. With this hand, palpate for abnormal fluid collections along the vagina, in the fornices, and even into the ischiorectal fossae. After hysterectomy, you may note induration and tenderness of the vaginal cuff incision, as well as fluctuance indicative of abscess or hematoma. Use the abdominal hand to delineate any unusual masses or loculations, as well as tenderness.

Laboratory evaluation

After the physical examination, perform a complete blood count and white blood cell differential, as well as general chemistry profile and urinalysis. Radiologic techniques are generally unnecessary if the pelvic examination is complete. However, in some cases of suspected pelvic infection—in particular, cases of salpingitis—ultrasonography or CT scanning may be helpful. In general, reserve the more elaborate imaging techniques for especially difficult or unusual cases, or for patients who need preoperative evaluation before surgery for suspected abscess.

In any case of suspected infection, take cultures of possible infected sites [see Chapter 56: Techniques for isolating pelvic bacterial pathogens]. Generally, in the patient with moderate infection, take blood, catheterized urine, and operative site cultures. In such patients, blood cultures are positive only 5% to 10% of the time. However, organisms found in the blood are frequently pathogens.

There is controversy about the value of culturing specimens from the endometrium or vaginal cuff. The chance of vaginal contamination is high. It is more prudent, however, to perform some type of genital culture, since you can retrospectively use the antibiotic sensitivity data generated. While these genital cultures may not directly aid in treating a particular patient, knowledge of local bacterial isolation rates and antibiotic sensitivities may guide you in future choices of antibiotic therapy.

When taking cultures from sites of possible infection, be aware that most cases will yield a polymicrobial flora. Therefore, collect and transport specimens in media or tubes appropriate for both anaerobic and aerobic microorganisms. This is true whether the specimen comes from the vaginal cuff after hysterectomy, the endometrial cavity after parturition, or an abscessed wound. It is also important that if any fastidious organisms such as *Neisseria gonorrhoeae* are suspected, appropriate transport or culture media must be available.

In any event, collect the materials for bacterial processing before beginning antibiotics. Specimens taken after several doses of medication have been given are a waste of time and money.

Summary

Infection may become manifest in the postoperative patient in a number of ways: unusual pain, leukocytosis, and loss of function (for example, paralytic ileus). The most common apparent indication of an infectious process is an elevated temperature, with oral temperature ≥38.0°C (100.4°F) on two occasions, excluding the first 24 hours, or ≥38.3°C (101.0°F) anytime. However, not all febrile morbidity is infectious morbidity. It is incumbent upon the physician to evaluate every febrile postoperative patient and determine the most likely diagnosis. Only then can appropriate therapy be instituted for the patient's ultimate cure, whether that therapy includes antibiotics or not.

SUGGESTED READING

Cox SM, Gilstrap LC: Postpartum endometritis. Obstet Gynecol Clin North Am 1989;16:363

Hemsell DL: Infections after gynecologic surgery. Obstet Gynecol Clin North Am 1989;16:381

Hemsell DL, Nobles B, Heard MC: Recognition and treatment of post-hysterectomy pelvic infection. Infect Surg 1988;7:47

Pastorek JG, Miller JM: Post-cesarean section infection. Infect Surg 1987;6:532

56

Techniques for isolating pelvic bacterial pathogens

By Gale B. Hill, PhD

Background

Knowledge of the likely etiologic agents in various female pelvic infections serves as a guide to proper collection and transport of patient specimens for microbiologic culture and for institution of appropriate empiric therapy. This information is also helpful in anticipating patterns of antibiotic resistance.

Most obstetric and gynecologic infections, with the exception of uncomplicated endocervical gonococcal or chlamydial infection, involve anaerobic and aerobic bacteria. These mixed infections include chorioamnionitis, endometritis, postabortal sepsis, bacterial vulvovaginal infections, salpingitis, pelvic peritonitis, tubo-ovarian and pelvic abscesses, postoperative wound infections, pelvic cellulitis, and pelvic thrombophlebitis. Septicemia usually involves only one species but also can be polymicrobic.

Source of infections

In general, the source of mixed infections in the female pelvis is the endogenous microflora of the lower genital tract (endocervix and vagina). The external genitalia and urethra also contain a resident aerobic/anaerobic microflora. The types may vary considerably from one individual to another, and not all organisms have the same potential to cause infection. In some women, lactobacilli are the predominant microflora; these, along with diphtheroids and coagulase-negative staphylococci, have almost no pathogenic potential in this setting. In other women, the resident flora includes potentially pathogenic microorganisms, such as *Bacteroides* sp, anaerobic gram-positive cocci, and *Escherichia coli*. Women with bacterial vaginosis characteristically have high vaginal concentrations of numerous opportunistic pathogens. The resident microflora can change markedly in species type and in their relative concentrations.

Settings for infection

Opportunistic pathogens among the endogenous flora can produce infection in tissue when local host defense mechanisms are interrupted or diminished by natural causes or medical intervention. Lowered oxygen tension and oxidation–reduction potential in tissue are critical for invasion by anaerobic organisms. Settings that predispose to infection usually involve tissue necrosis or impaired blood supply and include trauma, surgery, malignancy, foreign bodies, vascular disease, irradiation, shock, edema, and vasoconstrictive agents. Under these circumstances, aerobes and anaerobes in the vagina and endocervix may directly invade contiguous tissue structures in the normally sterile upper genital tract or be spread by hematogenous, lymphatic, or other routes.

Etiologic agents

Certain species of microorganisms are prevalent in female pelvic infections, most often present in various mixtures of aerobes and anaerobes. Others are unusual or to be expected only in particular, perhaps rare, settings.

Aerobic. Among aerobic gram-negative rods, *E coli* is most common and species of *Klebsiella, Enterobacter,* and *Proteus* are less common. Antibiotic-resistant species such as *Pseudomonas* and *Serratia* are infrequently isolated except in occasional cancer patients. Among the aerobic cocci species of *Streptococcus,* α- and nonhemolytic streptococci are particularly common. Group B ß-hemolytic streptococci colonize up to one third of women and are important pathogens in gynecologic infections as well as in maternal/neonatal disease. Group A ß-hemolytic streptococci are rarely isolated and are exogenously acquired. *Staphylococcus aureus* is infrequently isolated except in occasional abdominal wound infections, where it likely derives from an exogenous source. It is the causative agent in toxic shock syndrome, which, although rare, is a risk for the low percentage of women who carry the organism. *Gardnerella vaginalis* (previously *Haemophilus vaginalis*) is common in the genital microflora of sexually active women and can be isolated from upper genital tract infections, but its pathogenic role is not yet certain.

Anaerobic. Among the anaerobic gram-negative rods, *Bacteroides* species such as *B bivius,* the black-pigmenting *Bacteroides,* and *B disiens* are most frequently isolated. The *B fragilis* group is occasionally present. Among the anaerobic gram-positive cocci, *Pep-*

tostreptococcus anaerobius, P asaccharolyticus, P magnus, P prevotii, and *P tetradius* are most common. *Actinomyces* species or *Eubacterium nodatum* are gram-positive rods that are isolated usually only when a foreign body, particularly an IUD, is present. *Clostridium perfringens* is common in the GI tract and also is ubiquitous in the environment. The importance of its presumptive presence or isolation from a pelvic source must be carefully but speedily weighed in the context of the clinical setting. The patient's condition is important as you evaluate for the presence of cellulitis or myonecrosis.

Other organisms. Certain of the bacteria mentioned earlier are the usual agents in infections such as postoperative infectious complications and endometritis. The etiology of salpingitis, in particular, is more complex. Sexually transmissible agents such as *Neisseria gonorrhoeae* and *Chlamydia trachomatis* may be present with or without the endogenous organisms already discussed [see Chapters 7, 8, 9, 33, 34, and 35]. Genital mycoplasmas also are correlated with sexual activity, yet are so commonly present in women that they conveniently can be considered part of the mixed microflora. *Mycoplasma hominis* and *Ureaplasma urealyticum* are etiologic in perhaps 5% to 10% of cases of salpingitis and may be present in other settings such as chorioamnionitis, postpartum endometritis, and bacteremia [see Chapters 1, 3, and 67].

Collecting specimens for culture
Useful information from microbial culture initially depends upon careful site preparation and collection of an appropriate specimen, followed by protected and timely transport of the specimen to the laboratory. Whenever feasible, procure specimens for microbiologic culture before initiating antimicrobial therapy.

Avoid contaminating specimens with the anaerobic and aerobic endogenous flora of the endocervix and vagina. Certain members of the lower genital tract flora may be causing upper genital tract infection, but the *infected site* alone must be sampled to obtain the specific etiologic agents and thus avoid contamination with extraneous microorganisms. Otherwise, culture reports will be impossible to interpret and may be misleading. Thus, the vagina and endocervix would not be acceptable sites for unrestricted culture of aerobes and anaerobes. Culture should be limited to seeking specific infectious agents such as gonococci or chlamydiae from the cervix, in appropriate clinical settings. With some specific exceptions, then, appropriate specimens for culture generally are from normally sterile body sites.

Communicate with laboratory personnel before you collect specimens and culture for unusual organisms. Also, not all laboratories have the facilities or trained personnel to perform all types of culture, such as for mycoplasmas, *C trachomatis*, and occasionally anaerobes.

Specimen types

The most productive types of specimens for microbiologic culture and diagnosis are tissue samples and aspirated fluid. Samples collected on swabs are less desirable for three reasons: (1) often they do not provide sufficient material for inoculation of cultures for all likely etiologic agents; (2) they may promote loss of viability of microorganisms prior to culture because of drying and exposure of anaerobes to the toxic effects of oxygen; and (3) they are prone to contamination by extraneous bacteria if the infected site is near normally colonized sites in the vagina and endocervix or on the skin.

Many of the problems with a swab specimen can be circumvented by using a swab transport device that provides for a moist, anaerobic environment in transit to the laboratory and by making sure the swab is well saturated with infected material. Extraneous contamination generally is not a problem for swabs collected in an operating room setting, but, in this instance, the more appropriate tissue or aspirated sample usually should be available. The advancing edge of a soft-tissue infection and the wall of an abscess are examples of tissue samples. Aspirated specimens can be obtained if there is a collection of fluid or loculation present; otherwise, it may be necessary to inject a small volume of sterile, nonbacteriostatic saline to aspirate fluid back from infected tissue. Send 1 to 3 mL of aspirated fluid, if available.

The following should serve as a guide for collection of specimens from particular sources:

Body fluids. Collect by aspiration whenever possible. Amniotic fluid can be collected by transabdominal amniocentesis, by aspiration at the time of cesarean section, by needle amniotomy of intact membranes after povidone-iodine disinfection, or through a pressure catheter (discard the first 5 to 7 mL drawn) as clinically appropriate. Specimens obtained through a pressure catheter should be cultured and screened only for unusual or predominant organisms or for specific agents such as group B ß-hemolytic streptococci. Microorganisms from the lower genital tract will be introduced into the amniotic sac when the catheter is inserted.

Blood culture. Carefully prepare the venipuncture site with antiseptic to prevent skin organisms from contaminating the culture. Collect at least two blood cultures several hours apart in the setting of pelvic infection and clinical signs of possible septicemia. The yield in intra- and postpartum infections and septic abortion is higher than for salpingitis.

Decidua, membranes, or placenta. These tissues may be cultured directly at the time of C/S. After vaginal delivery, the surface of the placenta should be decontaminated, and a wedge of tissue procured. For chorioamnionic membranes, culture in between the placental amnion and chorion ≥4 cm back from torn membrane edge, avoiding the contaminated outer membrane surfaces.

Endometrial culture. Sample the decidua beyond the endocervix after first cleansing the cervical area. Protected (double- or triple-lumen) endometrial collection devices are highly desirable and should be used if available to prevent contamination by vaginal or cervical secretions. Protected devices designed for aspirating, brushing, or swabbing the endometrium can be prepared in house or can be obtained commercially. The Endometrial Pipelle suction curette (Unimar, Inc., Wilton, Conn.) provides for more specimen volume (tissue and fluid) and some protection against contamination compared with an unprotected swab. A brush sampling device sheathed within a plastic cannula is available (Uterine Sampling Device; Medi-tech, Watertown, Mass.).

Culdocentesis. For aspiration, cleanse the vaginal wall with antiseptic, leaving it in contact for 1 minute. Then wipe with a sterile gauze pad before inserting the needle. Be careful that aspiration occurs only in the cul-de-sac and not in the vagina (or bowel).

Abscesses. Where applicable, decontaminate unbroken skin or mucosal surface and aspirate pus with a syringe. In an operating room setting, aspirate abscesses or obtain abscess wall tissue.

Wound cultures. Cleanse exposed surfaces at the collection site with alcohol or dry sterile cotton pads—depending on the situation. Be sure to dry the area before collection if antiseptic is used. Preferably, collect specimen by tissue biopsy or aspiration. Swabs are prone to contamination by extraneous microorganisms and, if used, must be carefully collected from *deep* within the wound.

Vaginal cuff infection. Obtain drainage from the peritoneal cavity through an opening in the cuff, attempting to avoid vaginal secretions. This type of specimen is subject to background contamination by vaginal microflora and thus should be cultured and screened only for any unusual or predominant organism that may not respond to empiric therapy. If a loculation is present, try to aspirate directly after decontamination of the mucosal surface.

Drain effluent. Take fresh material by needle and syringe from as far up drain as possible after antiseptic cleansing of the surfaces at the site of entrance. Do not send an old accumulation of drainage material from the lower portion of drain or collector.

Specimen transport

Deliver specimens for culture to the laboratory as soon as possible to avoid degradation of the specimen and loss of viability of pathogens. Over time, important pathogens may be overgrown with other organisms. In polymicrobic infections, the presence of nutritive material and delay in transit may so alter the proportion of species that the resultant culture will not reflect the relative concentrations of organisms at the infected site. Therefore, avoid transport in nutritive (growth) media. Special transport formulations are available that preserve the viability of microorganisms and do not promote indiscriminant growth. Some are designed to select for survival or enhancement of only particular species.

In general, all specimens from infections located in sites normally sterile should be cultured at least for aerobic and anaerobic bacteria. Specimens should be transported in an anaerobic transport device to preserve the viability of anaerobic bacteria. Aerobic bacteria survive well in anaerobic devices and their numbers are somewhat more stabilized than in aerobic transport. Use transport methods and devices designed especially for sexually transmitted organisms whenever clinically appropriate.

The following are examples of special transport methods:

Anaerobic transport. Special tubes and vials containing oxygen-free gases should be used for transport to avoid exposure to oxygen and drying. These devices optimally should be transported at room temperature to arrive in the laboratory within 30 minutes. In an anaerobic environment microbial populations will remain nearly stable for 12 hours. Some examples of anaerobic transport devices:

- Port-A-Cul vials (BBL Microbiology Systems, Cockeysville, Md.): To be used for liquid specimens (body fluids or aspirated pus).
- Port-A-Cul tube (BBL Microbiology Systems): Contains reduced transport media to receive a swab specimen.
- Vacutainer Anaerobic Specimen Collector (Becton Dickinson, Rutherford, N.J.): Can be used for swab, liquid, or small pieces of tissue. A catalyst system removes oxygen.
- ANA TRANS (Carr Scarborough Microbiologicals, Inc., Stone Mountain, Ga.): Can be used for liquid specimens.
- Anaerobic Transport Medium Surgery Pack (Anaerobic Systems, San Jose, Calif.): Can be used for liquid, tissue, or swab. Caution: If the top is removed, oxygen enters system.
- Capped syringe: Can be used if no transport system is available. Expel all air from the syringe, cap the needle with a sterile stopper, and send the specimen to laboratory immediately.

Mycoplasmal transport. The genital mycoplasmas are seldom isolated in pure culture and are easily overgrown by competing microbes. Genital mycoplasmas can be cultured from specimens delivered for aerobic/anaerobic culture in an anaerobic transport device if sufficent sample is available and transport takes place within 2 to 3 hours. Special mycoplasmal transport broth contains antibiotics and therefore cannot be used for any other type of culture. Rapid delivery to the laboratory is best; if a delay occurs, however, the specimen can be maintained on wet ice for several hours. A3B Mycoplasmal Transport Broth (Remel, Lenexa, Kan.) is an example.

Laboratory request slip
On the laboratory requisition, provide (1) the specific collection site; (2) how the specimen was collected; (3) time and date of collection; (4) antimicrobial therapy given, if any; (5) clinical diagnosis; and (6) name of the physician to be consulted and to receive the report. If a specific organism is being sought (for example, *Actinomyces* in the presence of an IUD or *Listeria* in an appropriate perinatal setting), specifically note this on the slip to alert the laboratory to provide appropriate culture techniques.

SUGGESTED READING
Isenberg HD, Washington JA II, Balows A, et al: Collection, handling, and processing of specimens, in Lennette EH, Balows A, Hausler WJ, et al (eds): *Manual of Clinical Microbiology.* Washington, DC, American Society for Microbiology, 1985, pp 73-98

Knuppel RA, Screbo JC, Mitchell GW, et al: Quantitative transcervical uterine culture with a new device. Obstet Gynecol 1981;57:243

Ledger WJ: *Infection in the Female.* Philadelphia, Lea & Febiger, 1986, pp 35-56

Martens MG, Faro S, Hammill HA, et al: Transcervical uterine cultures with a new endometrial suction curette: a comparison of three sampling methods in postpartum endometritis. Obstet Gynecol 1989;74:273

Sweet RL, Gibbs RS: *Infectious Diseases of the Female Genital Tract.* Baltimore, Williams & Wilkins, 1990, pp 1-17

57
Prophylactic antibiotics

By William J. Ledger, MD

Background and pathophysiology

The pathophysiology of soft-tissue infection that occurs after obstetric and gynecologic operations is well known. These postoperative infections are caused by the diverse bacterial flora of the vagina and endocervix that overgrow and invade tissue in the postoperative environment of destruction resulting from clamps and the placing of sutures in the wound. The response in the human to these multiple bacterial invaders mimics that reported by Bartlett and co-workers in the animal model of a mixed bacterial intraperitoneal infection.

In the animal, there is an early-onset phase of infection that can be associated with bacteremia. In humans, this is paralleled in women who develop endomyometritis and associated bacteremia after an emergency cesarean section (C/S). After hysterectomy, a vaginal cuff infection or a pelvic cellulitis can be seen early in the postoperative course.

In the human, as in the animal model, there is also a late-onset phase of infection in which abscesses form and anaerobic bacteria seem to be the dominant bacterial pathogens. An example is formation of microabscesses in the uterus after C/S. The best parallel with the animal model, however, is adnexal abscess following vaginal hysterectomy. This serious problem occurs late in the clinical course. Fortunately, the frequency of these early and late events can be reduced by the use of prophylactic antibiotics.

Prevention of these postoperative-site infections by the use of antibiotics is based on well-established scientific principles. When Burke evaluated the role of systemic antibiotics in preventing local infections caused by bacteria, he found there was a measurable response after 24 hours to the injection of live and killed staphylococci at a skin site in animals. If he used IV penicillin effective against this strain of staphylococci, timing of antibiotic administration was important in determining response.

If penicillin was given before or at the time of the injection of the bacteria, it effectively decreased the extent of the host response (that is, it reduced the area of induration). If administration was delayed 3 hours or more after the injection of bacteria, it was ineffective (that is, the area of induration was the same as when no antibiotics had been given).

That timing is critical has been the underlying principle of all successful studies of antibiotic prophylaxis in obstetric and gynecologic operations. Improved postoperative results with prophylactic antibiotics have all involved administration of these agents at the time of operation.

Guidelines

There are a number of principles that can be applied to the use of prophylactic antibiotics in obstetric–gynecologic operations. If they fit a particular operation, a good case can be made for their use in that instance.

(1) *The operation should have a significant risk of postoperative-site infection.* The important aspect of this guideline is operative-site infection. For the obstetrician–gynecologist, this means postoperative infections such as vaginal cuff infection, pelvic cellulitis, adnexal abscess, abdominal wound infection following hysterectomy, or endomyometritis following C/S. If the postoperative infection problem centers on an organ system distant from the operative site (for example, lungs in a postoperative pneumonia), prophylactic antibiotics will not be the solution.

The significant risk in this guideline includes the frequency and severity of the infection at the operative site. Infections often follow hysterectomy and C/S, and they can be serious. This is an important clinical problem for obstetrician–gynecologists. In contrast, infections after pregnancy termination and reconstructive tubal surgery are much less common. Even with these, however, the outcome, can be serious for the occasional patient who becomes infected, because the tubal damage can prevent future pregnancies.

(2) *The operation should be associated with endogenous bacterial contamination.* One of the realities of any operation for an obstetrician–gynecologist is contamination of the operative field by the endogenous bacteria of the vagina and endocervix. These are also the source of bacterial contamination in vaginal hysterectomy, pregnancy termination, and C/S in the patient in labor.

Some novel ways to reduce this contamination have included hot conization of the cervix just before hysterectomy and antibiotic lavage of the uterine wound at the time of C/S. In other gynecologic operations, unexpected bacterial contamination can occur.

Recent studies by Henry-Suchet and co-workers have demonstrated the presence of *Chlamydia trachomatis* in the pelvic adhesions of women undergoing operations to restore fertility, with no gross evidence of inflammation. Clearly, endogenous bacterial soiling exists in most obstetric–gynecologic operations. Careful prehysterectomy preparation of the vagina with an antiseptic solution can reduce the number of surface organisms, but it does not eliminate the problem. Bacteria can be recovered from the surface of the vagina at the end of the operation.

(3) *The prophylactic antibiotic should have laboratory evidence of effectiveness against some of the contaminating microorganisms.* This is the most controversial of all the guidelines. The controversy relates to the general success of prophylactic antibiotics in the most widely studied operations, cesarean section and vaginal hysterectomy. Prophylactic antibiotics work and there appears to be little difference whether penicillin, tetracycline, a cephalosporin, or metronidazole is used. However, this seeming lack of difference may be related to problems with study design in the evaluations reported to date.

Serious infections, such as postoperative adnexal abscesses, occur infrequently, and the small numbers of patients in many of these studies do not permit discrimination of differences in infrequently seen complications, a statistical problem of type II error. Thus far, all reports of postoperative adnexal abscesses after vaginal hysterectomy have dealt with occurrences in patients who received prophylactic antibiotics with little activity against gram-negative anaerobic bacteria. There are similar concerns about the choice of antibiotics for prophylaxis in C/S. Antibiotics with gram-negative anaerobic activity have the best results. For pregnancy termination and reconstructive tubal surgery, the clinical concern is *C trachomatis* and the best antibiotic to prevent infection with this organism is a tetracycline. Although there is a wide range of possibilities, a preferred list of antibiotics for prophylaxis can be made for each procedure.

(4) *There should be clinical evidence of effectiveness.* This is the most important guideline. Unless prophylactic antibiotics prevent postoperative infection, there is no justification for their use. Table 1 lists the operative procedures in which prophylactic antibiotics are used. Reports give a wide variety of responses: unequivocal success in operations with high rates of postoperative infection, such as vaginal hysterectomy, C/S for the patient in labor, and radical hysterectomy for genital malignancy; general success in pregnancy termination, which has a much lower rate of infection; and mixed

TABLE 1
Results with prophylaxis

Operation	Results
Abdominal hysterectomy	Mixed
Cesarean section—patient in labor	Unequivocal success
Cesarean section—patient not in labor	Mixed
Pregnancy termination	General success
Radical hysterectomy	Unequivocal success
Vaginal hysterectomy	Unequivocal success

results for elective C/S and abdominal hysterectomy. No study has shown an increase in the infection rate when prophylactic antibiotics have been given, but some studies have shown no benefit.

(5) *The prophylactic antibiotic should be present in the wound some time during the operation.* The timing of administration of the prophylactic antibiotics is crucial for success. For most operations, the antibiotic should be administered just before the operation begins so it will be present in tissue as pedicles are clamped, cut, and ligated with a foreign body suture. If the operation lasts more than 3 hours and a prophylactic antibiotic with a short half-life has been administered, then a second dose should be given intraoperatively. Antibiotics with a short half-life include ampicillin and cefoxitin. Those with a long half-life include cefazolin, cefoperazone, tetracycline, doxycycline, and metronidazole.

There is a different clinical consideration with C/S. To avoid administering antibiotics to the baby, which could mask early signs of neonatal sepsis, they should be given after the cord is clamped.

(6) *A short course of antibiotic prophylaxis should be used.* This is one of the most important guidelines for the rational use of prophylactic antibiotics. A short course has been shown to be just as effective as prolonged administration in vaginal hysterectomy and C/S. A short course reduces the risk that the patient will have an adverse reaction and lessens the risk of colonization with resistant organisms. If the patient becomes febrile after the use of prophylactic antibiotics, a different antibiotic should be used for treatment because the

failure can be due to the presence of resistant organisms.

(7) *First-line antibiotics should be used for prophylaxis if results are superior.* This guideline has recently been revised because of clinical observations. A number of studies show that antibiotics with gram-negative anaerobic bacterial coverage provide superior results in vaginal hysterectomy and the patient in labor undergoing C/S.

In contrast, for the patient undergoing pregnancy termination or tubal reconstructive surgery, a tetracycline should be employed to cover *C trachomatis.* This serious pathogen can cause irreversible tubal damage even when there are minimal symptoms.

(8) *Benefits of antibiotic prophylaxis should outweigh risks.* Prophylactic antibiotics are clearly indicated for vaginal hysterectomy, C/S in the patient in labor, radical hysterectomy, and pregnancy termination. On occasion, they may be employed for those patients requiring abdominal hysterectomy and tubal reconstructive surgery. For the patient undergoing elective C/S, more study is needed to confirm the appropriateness of their use.

Antibiotic selection

The frequency and severity of postoperative infections have been reduced by antibiotic prophylaxis. For vaginal hysterectomy, I favor the use of cefoxitin, cefotetan, or metronidazole. In C/S, cefoxitin, cefotetan, or mezlocillin gives good results. For radical hysterectomy, cefoxitin, cefotetan, mezlocillin, and metronidazole are helpful. For pregnancy termination and reconstructive tubal surgery, doxycycline should be administered because of its effectiveness against *C trachomatis.* For the elective C/S and abdominal hysterectomy, a first-generation cephalosporin such as cefazolin will probably suffice.

SUGGESTED READING

Bartlett JG, Louie TJ, Gorbach SL, et al: Therapeutic efficacy of 29 antimicrobial regimens in experimental intra-abdominal sepsis. Rev Infect Dis 1981;3:535

Burke JF: The effective period of preventive antibiotic action in experimental incisions and dermal lesions. Surgery 1961;50:161

Ford LC, Hammill HA, Lebherz TB: Cost effective use of antibiotic prophylaxis for cesarean section. Am J Obstet Gynecol 1987;157:506

Henry-Suchet J, Catalan F, Loffredo V, et al: *Chlamydia trachomatis* associated with chronic inflammation in abdominal specimens from women selected for tuboplasty. Fertil Steril 1981;36:599

Ledger WJ, Campbell C, Taylor D, et al: Adnexal abscess as late complication of pelvic operations. Surg Gynecol Obstet 1969;129:973

Livengood CH III, Addison WA: Adnexal abscess as a delayed complication of vaginal hysterectomy. Am J Obstet Gynecol 1982;143:596

Osborne NG, Wright RC, Dubay M: Preoperative hot conizations of the cervix: a possible method to reduce postoperative febrile morbidity following vaginal hysterectomy. Am J Obstet Gynecol 1979;133:374

58
Prophylactic antibiotics for hysterectomy

By Patrick Duff, MD

Background and incidence

Because the frequency of infection after hysterectomy is relatively high, pelvic surgeons have shown great interest in the subject of antibiotic prophylaxis. The purpose of this chapter is to review the frequency and pathophysiology of postoperative infection and then evaluate results of multiple clinical trials using prophylactic antibiotics in women undergoing vaginal and abdominal hysterectomy.

Each year approximately 600,000 to 800,000 hysterectomies are performed in the United States. Two thirds of these procedures are done abdominally. Infection, incidence of which can exceed 60%, is the most common complication (Figure 1).

Etiology

The principal microorganisms responsible for posthysterectomy infections are aerobic streptococci, mainly groups B and D; anaerobic streptococci; aerobic gram-negative bacilli, most notably *Escherichia coli*; and *Bacteroides* species. Although *Neisseria gonorrhoeae* and *Chlamydia trachomatis* are important in the pathogenesis of acute salpingitis, they are not common isolates from women with immediate postoperative infections. The genital mycoplasmas also do not appear to be important in this clinical setting. Infection with particularly virulent aerobic gram-negative bacilli, such as *Pseudomonas*, *Enterobacter*, and *Serratia*, is distinctly uncommon except in immunocompromised patients.

Pathophysiology

All these organisms are normal inhabitants of the genital tract flora. During pelvic surgery, they are introduced into the upper genital tract

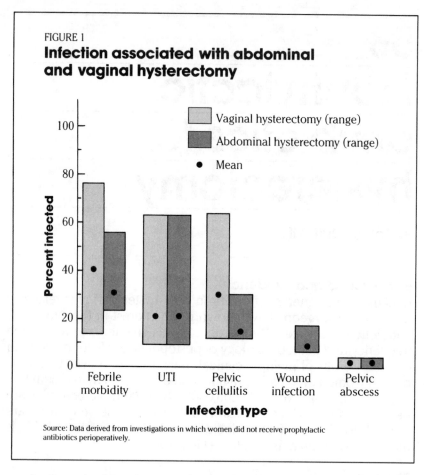

FIGURE 1

Infection associated with abdominal and vaginal hysterectomy

Legend:
- Vaginal hysterectomy (range)
- Abdominal hysterectomy (range)
- Mean

Y-axis: Percent infected

X-axis (Infection type): Febrile morbidity, UTI, Pelvic cellulitis, Wound infection, Pelvic abscess

Source: Data derived from investigations in which women did not receive prophylactic antibiotics perioperatively.

and, often, the bloodstream. Inoculation of bacteria is particularly high in women undergoing vaginal hysterectomy, since the entire procedure is performed through a contaminated surgical field. Other risk factors for infection after both vaginal and abdominal operations are low socioeconomic status, premenopausal age, extended duration of surgery, excessive intraoperative blood loss, preoperative anemia, and concurrent debilitating systemic disease.

Mechanism of action

Three conditions must be met before using prophylactic antibiotics routinely. First, the operation must be performed through a contaminated surgical field. Second, in the absence of prophylaxis, there should be a high incidence of operative-site infection. Third, it should be possible for serious sequelae, including bacteremia, septic shock, septic pelvic vein thrombophlebitis, and pelvic abscess, to

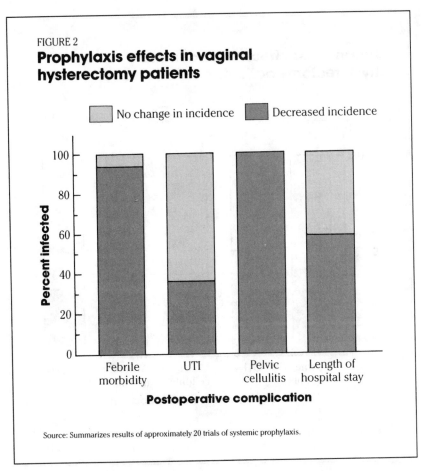

FIGURE 2
**Prophylaxis effects in vaginal
hysterectomy patients**

No change in incidence ☐ Decreased incidence ☐

Source: Summarizes results of approximately 20 trials of systemic prophylaxis.

develop from the primary infection. All three conditions are fulfilled
in patients having vaginal hysterectomy, as well as in selected groups
of abdominal hysterectomy patients.

Prophylactic antibiotics appear to exert their effect through four
basic mechanisms. Of greatest importance is their ability to reduce
the size of the bacterial inoculum introduced into the pelvic cavity. In
addition, antibiotics alter the culture medium at the surgical site so
that it does not support the growth of pathogenic bacteria. They also
penetrate the genital tract's epithelial tissue and render it less susceptible to invasion by bacteria. Finally, prophylactic antibiotics are
concentrated in macrophages and polymorphonuclear leukocytes
and thereby enhance phagocytosis.

Objectives
The use of prophylactic antibiotics has four objectives. The first goal

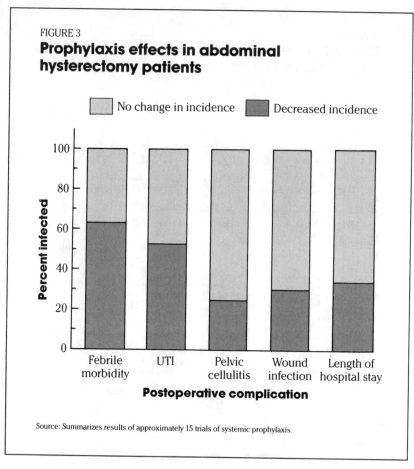

FIGURE 3

Prophylaxis effects in abdominal hysterectomy patients

No change in incidence ☐   Decreased incidence ■

Source: Summarizes results of approximately 15 trials of systemic prophylaxis.

is to reduce the frequency of pelvic cellulitis, which is the most common posthysterectomy infection and one that predisposes to more serious sequelae. In addition, patients who develop cellulitis usually have to spend 1 to 2 more days in the hospital than uninfected women.

The second objective is to prevent wound infection, which predisposes to such serious complications as dehiscence and evisceration, and is likely to prolong hospitalization. A third aim is to decrease use of more expensive therapeutic antibiotics. The final objective is to decrease overall duration and expense of hospitalization.

Results of clinical trials

The first point to be made about clinical trials of prophylactic antibiotics for vaginal hysterectomy is that women who received them had significantly less pelvic cellulitis (Figure 2). This benefit is apparent regardless of the patient's age, menopausal status, phase of menstrual cycle, or requirement for concurrent adnexal, bladder, or rectal surgery. Second, single doses of antibiotics are as effective as two- and three-dose regimens. Third, limited-spectrum agents, such as cefazolin or ampicillin, are as effective for prophylaxis as the more expensive, extended-spectrum cephalosporins or penicillins.

Of note in trials of prophylaxis for abdominal hysterectomy is that fewer than a third of investigations showed reduced frequency of pelvic cellulitis (Figure 3). In large part, this effect occurred because baseline frequency of infection is lower after abdominal hysterectomy than after vaginal procedures. Therefore, most investigations had a sample size inadequate for detecting a small difference in treatment effect. However, even the largest study, incorporating more than 400 patients, was unable to show a significant reduction in the frequency of pelvic cellulitis.

Also noteworthy is a decreased frequency of wound infection in approximately 25% of the investigations. With few exceptions, these were the same studies that showed a protective effect against pelvic cellulitis, and they included indigent patient populations that had a high baseline incidence of postoperative wound and pelvic infection.

In studies able to document a beneficial effect of prophylaxis in patients undergoing abdominal hysterectomy, there was no advantage in using the more expensive, broader-spectrum cephalosporins and penicillins. Similarly, there was no therapeutic advantage in using more than two doses of antibiotic for prophylaxis.

Complications
One of the two major types of complications that can develop when prophylactic antibiotics are administered is adverse drug reactions. Isolated case reports tell of intraoperative deaths resulting from anaphylactic reactions to cephalosporins administered for prophylaxis. Although these fatal events have not been described in obstetric or gynecologic patients, you should still exercise extreme care to elicit a history of drug allergy in any patient scheduled to receive prophylaxis.

There are well-documented case reports of women who developed drug-induced diarrhea, and even pseudomembranous enterocolitis, after receiving prophylactic antibiotics for pelvic surgery. This problem appears particularly likely to occur after use of multiple doses of extended-spectrum agents, but can occur after single-dose prophylaxis.

The second major complication is alteration in the microbial flora of the genital tract. Although specific alterations depend on which antibiotic is used, a consistent finding has been increased isolation of enterococci in women who received cephalosporins. Fortunately, there is no evidence that patients who become infected despite prophylaxis respond less readily to conventional treatment regimens.

Guidelines

■ Routine use of prophylactic antibiotics appears to be justified in all women undergoing vaginal hysterectomy and in selected, high-risk patients having abdominal hysterectomy.

■ The most cost-effective antibiotics for prophylaxis are inexpensive, limited-spectrum agents, such as cefazolin or ampicillin.

■ For most procedures, a single dose of antibiotic is enough for prophylaxis. When surgery is extended (≥2 hours), it seems appropriate to give a second dose 4 hours after the initial one.

■ A gynecologic service using prophylaxis must maintain surveillance to detect the emergence of drug-resistant microorganisms and the development of superinfections.

SUGGESTED READING

Duff P, Park RC: Antibiotic prophylaxis in vaginal hysterectomy: a review. Obstet Gynecol 1980;55(suppl):193

Duff P: Antibiotic prophylaxis in abdominal hysterectomy. Obstet Gynecol 1982;60:25

Hemsell DL, Reisch J, Nobles B, et al: Prevention of major infection after elective abdominal hysterectomy: individual determination required. Am J Obstet Gynecol 1983;147:520

Ledger WJ, Gee C, Lewis WP: Guidelines for antibiotic prophylaxis in gynecology. Am J Obstet Gynecol 1974;121:1038

Polk BF, Shapiro M, Goldstein P, et al: Randomized clinical trial of perioperative cefazolin in preventing infection after hysterectomy. Lancet 1980;1:437

59
Posthysterectomy cuff and pelvic cellulitis

By David L. Hemsell, MD

Background and incidence
Prior to the widespread use of antimicrobial prophylaxis for hysterectomy, the incidence of pelvic infection, excluding abscess, ranged from 5% to 70%. With prophylaxis, this incidence has fallen to approximately 5%. Theoretically, all women undergoing vaginal hysterectomy fall into a "high risk" category because of the anatomic location of the surgical site. Individual risk factors must be used to identify those at high risk after abdominal hysterectomy.

Pathophysiology
Hysterectomy is a clean-contaminated surgical procedure. It is the inoculation of species that make up the normal flora of the genital tract into the operative site that results in the postoperative pelvic cellulitis observed after hysterectomy. Inoculation begins with the incision at vaginal hysterectomy and continues throughout the procedure. If the anus is not carefully draped out of the field, additional contamination may occur from that site as well.

These factors may explain why infection rates without prophylaxis are higher after vaginal hysterectomy than after abdominal hysterectomy and why antimicrobial prophylaxis is more effective for that procedure. Contamination with lower genital tract flora does not occur until the last step of abdominal hysterectomy.

Etiology
Pelvic cellulitis is a polymicrobial pelvic soft-tissue infection caused by lower genital tract flora. These include predominantly gram-positive aerobes (*Enterococcus faecalis*, *Staphylococcus epidermidis*, and streptococci) and anaerobes (*Peptostreptococcus* sp and *Bacteroides*

bivius). Other *Bacteroides* sp and gram-negative aerobic agents such as *Escherichia coli* and *Enterobacter* sp are less commonly isolated.

Preoperative vaginal or endocervical and intraoperative cultures of the endocervix or cardinal ligaments have not been useful in predicting who will develop a postoperative pelvic infection. Inoculum size and such bacterial virulence factors as ß-lactamase production, bacterial attachment, presence of a capsule, and ability to disseminate in tissues through production of proteases or collagenases are key variables. Cell-mediated and humoral immunity systems are important in preventing infection. Interactions between these two ultimately determine who will develop a postoperative infection.

Diagnosis

Increasing pelvic or lower abdominal pain and tenderness when we examine the pelvis are the hallmarks of cellulitis that may develop after hysterectomy. Temperature elevation alone is a poor indicator of clinically important infection. In our hospital, up to 17% of women undergoing vaginal hysterectomy and 35% undergoing abdominal hysterectomy have recurrent temperature elevations on the second to third postoperative day, but have normal abdominal and pelvic examination results and no pain. The temperature rise disappears without therapy. Although temperature elevation cannot be ignored, it should be evaluated in conjunction with other symptoms and signs of infection. It should never be used as the only indicator for infection, nor as the automatic signal for antimicrobial administration.

Cuff cellulitis. An inflammatory response is normal during healing. Surgical margins of the vagina are erythematous, edematous, and tender for several days. These findings quickly subside when there is no clinically marked infection, as do the purulent secretions that normally appear in the vagina immediately after hysterectomy. Cuff cellulitis after hysterectomy is a physiologic response to the incision occurring in a contaminated area. Host defense mechanisms and antimicrobial prophylaxis quickly resolve this cellulitis, which can be identified in the absence of spontaneous pain and tenderness, and with or without temperature elevation. We do not know whether it contributes to the asymptomatic temperature elevation frequently observed after hysterectomy.

Perhaps 1% of patients will develop cuff cellulitis after hysterectomy that requires antimicrobial therapy. Essentially, all cases occur after discharge from the hospital, but usually not later than 10 days thereafter. Women may come to the emergency room complaining of increasing spontaneous central lower abdominal or pelvic pain, and increased vaginal discharge associated with low-grade temperature elevation. Abdominal examination is normal, or there may be slight suprapubic tenderness to deep palpation. Only the vaginal surgical margin is tender, and no masses are palpable.

Pelvic cellulitis. This is the most common infection after a hysterectomy and is almost always observed during the immediate postoperative period. Patients complain of increasing lower abdominal and pelvic pain that is usually accentuated on one side. Symptoms most commonly develop late on the second or during the third postoperative day, and the temperature is usually above 38.5°C (101.3°F). At abdominal examination, gentle depression over the parametrial area elicits tenderness not previously present. It is usually maximal where the symptoms originate.

A Pfannenstiel incision makes it somewhat more difficult to locate the origin of the distress, but it can be located. Pain and tenderness are more marked with pelvic cellulitis than they are with cuff cellulitis; in addition, the temperature is higher and the patient is obviously sicker. Inspect the vagina and perform a bimanual examination to confirm the abdominal findings of parametrial tenderness. When evaluating a woman for infection after hysterectomy, be sure to exclude infections unrelated to the operative site.

Laboratory testing. History and physical examination will confirm the diagnosis of cellulitis in the pelvis after hysterectomy. Very little in the way of laboratory testing is necessary. A complete blood count with differential is useful immediately, and may be so in the future. In the absence of symptoms and positive physical findings, it is not necessary routinely to order a chest x-ray, a urinalysis with culture and sensitivity testing, or blood cultures. The incidence of septicemia is quite low at my institution.

Bacteremia does not usually prolong therapy, or predict initial antimicrobial therapy failure. Any patient who is suspected of septicemia or who does not respond to the initial therapeutic regimen should have aerobic and anaerobic blood cultures obtained from at least two sites. A positive result mandates a repeat blood culture. Confirm absence of growth after concluding antimicrobial therapy.

There is controversy about the usefulness of a culture obtained with a sterile swab from the area cephalad to the vaginal surgical margin. Some believe culturing will help determine the species most likely to be responsible for the infection, especially when an infection does not respond to the initial antimicrobial regimen. It also does allow monitoring of resistance patterns if sensitivity testing is performed. Others believe that an initial culture is unnecessary because only a few patients will fail therapy, making the culture unnecessary for over 90% to 95% of patients. A culture performed when a regimen fails should detect the pathogens since other susceptible species will have been eradicated. Bacterial identification and sensitivity testing should be available from the laboratory for a culture to provide worthwhile information.

Treatment

Women with pelvic cellulitis respond more promptly and more completely to the available treatment regimens than do patients being treated for post–cesarean section endomyometritis. Combination antimicrobial therapy is effective, but is often unnecessary. Clinical trials have shown that single-agent therapy with a second- or third-generation cephalosporin or a semisynthetic penicillin is as effective.

Successful regimens in our patients include IV cefotaxime, 1 g every 8 hours; IV cefotetan, 2 g every 12 hours; IV piperacillin, 4 g every 6 hours; IV ampicillin/sulbactam, 3 g every 6 hours; and IV cefoxitin, 2 g every 6 hours. IV therapy is continued until the patient has been afebrile for 24 to 36 hours.

If a woman is truly allergic to ß-lactam antibiotics, then combination therapy is necessary. Our choice is IV clindamycin, 900 mg every 8 hours, combined with a 2-mg/kg loading dose of gentamicin, then 1 to 1.5 mg/kg of gentamicin every 8 hours in the same diluent. If therapy is necessary for gram-positive aerobes not covered by clindamycin, vancomycin is the agent of choice for such patients.

During therapy, the patient should be monitored at least twice daily to ensure success and to detect any adverse events resulting from therapy. Although about 15% of our patients state that they are allergic to penicillin, if their allergic manifestation is not an immediate hypersensitivity reaction, we administer a cephalosporin and have done so without observing an allergic reaction. Antimicrobials should never be administered for pelvic infection without a recent pelvic examination. It has been established that an oral outpatient antimicrobial is unnecessary after successful parenteral therapy. An adequate and thorough pelvic examination is uncomfortable for the patient, but should be performed both before therapy and prior to discharge from the hospital to ensure lack of tenderness and to detect any masses that might be present.

Women with cuff cellulitis have been treated successfully as outpatients with oral antimicrobials. Some receive an initial IM dose of one of the agents given for inpatient therapy. The oral agent providing the widest spectrum of antibacterial activity is amoxicillin with clavulanic acid. It is administered at a dose of 250 to 500 mg every 8 hours for 5 to 7 days. Patients should take their temperatures at home during treatment and should return to your care if symptoms increase or if the temperature elevation persists past 72 hours. Clinical reevaluation should be done in about 72 hours even if everything is going well for the patient.

Treatment failures. If women treated for cuff cellulitis do not respond to outpatient management, the parenteral therapy I have outlined for inpatients suffering from pelvic cellulitis is necessary. Patients treated with single agents who fail initial therapy for pelvic cellulitis require altered therapy, depending in part on their initial regimen. Many women have *Enterococcus faecalis* in infection cultures, and multiple-dose prophylaxis or therapy with a cephalosporin selects for that species. In our experience, adding ampicillin has not resulted in clinical cure of this infection. Rather, we've found it necessary to add an agent with more predictable anaerobic coverage. In many instances, that can be accomplished with oral metronidazole rather than the parenteral form. However, parenteral clindamycin, given as above, is our choice.

SUGGESTED READING

Faro S, Sanders CV, Aldridge KE: Use of single-agent antimicrobial therapy in the treatment of polymicrobial female pelvic infections. Obstet Gynecol 1982;60:232

Hager WD, Pascuzzi M, Vernon M: Efficacy of oral antibiotics following parenteral antibiotics for serious infections in obstetrics and gynecology. Obstet Gynecol 1989;73:326

Hemsell DL, Hemsell PG, Heard MC, et al: Piperacillin and a combination of clindamycin and gentamicin for the treatment of hospital and community acquired acute pelvic infections including pelvic abscess. Surg Gynecol Obstet 1987;165:223

Ledger WJ: Prevention, diagnosis, and treatment of postoperative infections. Obstet Gynecol 1980;55(suppl 5):203S

Swenson RM, Michaelson TC, Daly MJ, et al: Anaerobic bacterial infections of the female genital tract. Obstet Gynecol 1973;42:538

60
Pelvic
abscess

By Sebastian Faro, MD, PhD

Background and incidence

Pelvic abscesses can be classified by anatomic site as lower genital tract (which includes the vagina and vulva) or pelvic cavity (which includes the upper genital tract as well as structures found in the pelvis). Abscesses of the lower genital tract may involve Bartholin's gland, Skene's gland, a urethral diverticulum, Gartner's duct, and episiotomies. Abscesses may also form in the perirectal tissue or the ischiorectal fossa after a pudendal block, traumatic delivery, or complicating inflammatory bowel disease.

Pelvic cavity abscesses are most frequently preceded by salpingitis, which can lead to the formation of a pyosalpinx, tubo-ovarian abscess, cul-de-sac abscess, or, infrequently, an ovarian abscess. Other common etiologies of a pelvic abscess are ruptured appendix, rectosigmoid colon diverticulitis or perforation, and abscess of Meckel's diverticulum. Pelvic abscesses can also occur as a complication of hysterectomy or, occasionally, cesarean section.

Pathophysiology

Abscesses of the lower genital tract are usually preceded by the presence of an acute infection of a gland or diverticulum. The duct draining the gland becomes inflamed and edematous. This results in obstruction of the gland or diverticulum and blockage of a route of egress. If bacteria are present in the gland, an abscess develops. The organisms most frequently involved, initially, are *Neisseria gonorrhoeae*, *Chlamydia trachomatis*, and the facultative and obligate anaerobes.

Initially, the host's defense mechanism will attempt to eradicate the infection. However, if conditions prohibit a suitable response, an attempt will be made to localize the infection by walling off the infected site. Thus the interaction between the infecting organisms and host will lead to the formation of an abscess. Frequently, there is an extensive inflammatory response involving adjacent structures. When the bowel becomes inflamed, it becomes edematous, inhibing peristalsis and distending the abdomen. The tissues become very fragile and there is a potential for rupture of the abscess.

It is important to be aware of factors that may lead to abscess formation during a surgical procedure. Both vaginal hysterectomy and cesarean section are clean–contaminated surgical procedures. The vaginal hysterectomy is performed through a contaminated operative field. Throughout the procedure, bacteria from the vagina have ample opportunity to enter the pelvis, colonize it, and invade tissue. Necrotic tissue pedicles with suture are often left behind. Attempts are made to leave these pedicles in a retroperitoneal space and then close this space, leaving an area where blood and serum collect. The abdominal hysterectomy becomes a clean–contaminated procedure when the vagina is opened. [For a discussion of the classification of wounds, see Chapter 61.]

Cesarean section performed after a patient has labored with ruptured amniotic membranes for a prolonged period (>12 hours) should be regarded as a contaminated procedure. Bacteria are capable of ascending into the uterine cavity, colonizing the amniotic membranes as well as the decidua, and invading the myometrium. An incision is then made through the uterine musculature, either vertically (which involves the corpus and fundus) or transversely (in the lower segment). The uterine incision is closed either in a single or double layer, which can result in strangulation of the tissue because of the tendency to pull the suture tightly. This, in effect, reduces the blood flood and oxygen supply in this area. Reduced blood and oxygen, tissue necrosis, and presence of a foreign body (suture) all contribute to establishment of an infection.

Etiology

The bacteria most frequently involved in these infections are gram-positive and gram-negative facultative, as well as obligate, anaerobes. The facultative anaerobic bacteria probably play a more important role as initiators of the infectious process. However, it is synergistic activity between the facultative and obligate anaerobes that eventually results in abscess formation.

Another potential source of bacteria is the rectosigmoid. Pelvic infection causes the bowel to become inflamed and, as a consequence, leads to tissue edema. This, in turn, leads to microscopic breaks in the mucosal lining, allowing for the migration of bacteria across the bowel wall. A larger inoculum of pathogenic organisms, including agents such as *Bacteroides fragilis* and *Fusobacterium*, then becomes part of the infection process.

Diagnosis

Initially, review the patient's history to determine whether any complications were encountered during the operative procedure. Was antibiotic prophylaxis given? If so, which antibiotic was used and at what dosage? If the patient received a cephalosporin, an increased colonization by *Enterococcus faecalis* in the lower genital tract may have occurred. This bacterium, along with *B fragilis* and *B bivius*, may act synergistically to produce abscesses.

Review of the fever curve may suggest the presence of an abscess. Typically, patients with an acute abscess have high spiking temperatures with marked diurnal variation. The white blood cell (WBC) count is often in the 20,000/mm^3 range.

The physical examination may reveal the presence of peritonitis. Bowel sounds tend to be infrequent, of low intensity to absent. Pelvic examination may reveal a pelvic mass that may be solid or cystic.

Ultrasonography, CT scan, or x-ray of the pelvis may reveal characteristics of the mass that facilitate a diagnosis and treatment. Pelvic x-ray may show gas within a mass. An IV pyelogram will yield such additional information as displacement of the ureter, a partial or complete obstruction, and position of the abscess. Ultrasonography and CT scans will help determine whether or not the mass is loculated, related to an intraperitoneal structure, or drainable percutaneously.

Treatment

If the abscess is in the posterior cul-de-sac and colpotomy drainage can be attempted, ultrasonography should be used to guide the approach. Initially, insert a needle through the posterior cul-de-sac, which may require general anesthesia or, at least, local infiltration of the epithelium overlying the cul-de-sac. Purulent material aspirated from the abscess should be placed in an anaerobic transport vial. The aspirate should be Gram stained and then cultured for aerobic and anaerobic bacteria. The needle should remain in place to ensure proper placement of the incision, and the incision should be made adjacent to it.

The abscess cavity should be completely evacuated. Often, loculations will be present and will need to be disrupted if the patient is to respond satisfactorily. Ultrasonography can assist in determining whether the entire abscess has been evacuated and all loculations disrupted. The cavity should be irrigated until clear. A drain, such as a Foley catheter or Malecott drain, should be placed and connected to suction to ensure complete evacuation and prevent reaccumulation of fluid.

Abscesses not located in the cul-de-sac may be drained percutaneously, if located adjacent to the abdominal wall or determined to be accessible by CT scan. Placement of a pigtail or equivalent catheter is facilitated by ultrasound. The catheters should remain in place until the drainage ceases. The abscess cavity should be reexamined by CT scan to ensure there are no remaining collections of fluid. The cavity should be irrigated with bacteriostatic saline, and the saline should be aspirated and cultured.

If the patient is not taking antibiotics at the time the procedure is started, these should be administered immediately after obtaining the initial aspirate. Since abscesses are likely to involve gram-negative and gram-positive facultative as well as obligate anaerobes, broad-spectrum antimicrobial therapy is indicated.

If the tissue adjacent to the abscess is infected and the vessels supplying this area are thrombosed, antibiotic levels in the tissue will be absent to below an effective level. Therefore, to treat this infection successfully, you may need surgical removal of the involved tissue. This situation is encountered in patients who develop suppurative myometritis and necrosis of the uterine incision site. Similarly, patients who have tubo-ovarian abscesses, which have a thick abscess wall and are multiloculated, usually require surgical intervention. It is not uncommon to find the vessels supplying blood to the lower uterus completely thrombosed.

If the patient is not receiving antimicrobial agents at the time an abscess is diagnosed, the choice is between a single antibiotic and combination therapy. However, there are no large, prospective studies that support the use of any specific antibiotic regimen. Since pelvic abscesses are predominantly polymicrobial, the use of an antibiotic or combination of antibiotics requires that these agents be active against a variety of bacteria, including streptococci, *Enterococcus*, members of the Enterobacteriaceae family, and obligate anaerobes, including the *Bacteroides fragilis* group. Three agents fulfill this requirement: ticarcillin/clavulanic acid, ampicillin/sulbactam, and imipenem/cilastatin. The penicillins have been combined with a ß-lactamase inhibitor that broadens the spectrum of ticarcillin and ampicillin by inhibiting the activity of a variety of ß-lactamases. Imipenem, a carbapenem, is not affected by the activity of ß-lactamases.

If a patient fails to respond to therapy with one of these agents, the customary response would be to discontinue the agent and institute combination therapy. However, it would be more logical to build on the agent in use and expand the spectrum of activity. These agents have good gram-positive coverage, and anaerobic activity that is comparable to and may exceed that of clindamycin. The only weakness is the Enterobacteriaceae. Thus, the addition of an aminoglycoside, aztreonam, cefuroxime, or ceftriaxone would enhance activity against facultative gram-negative anaerobes.

If initial therapy consists of combinations of antibiotics (clindamycin or metronidazole plus an aminoglycoside) and the patient doesn't respond, drainage of the abscess should be considered. Clindamycin has activity against such gram-positive organisms as streptococci, staphylococci, and peptostreptococci, whereas metronidazole does not have activity against the aerobic cocci. Neither of these agents is effective against *Enterococcus faecalis*. Patients who are allergic to penicillin should be given vancomycin if the enterococcus is known or strongly suspected of being present. If material can be aspirated from the abscess, the fluid should be placed in an anaerobic transport vial. The fluid should be Gram stained and cultured for aerobes and anaerobes. Once specific bacteria are identified and antibiotic sensitivities are known, antibiotic therapy can be modified.

Parenteral antibiotics should be administered until the patient becomes and remains afebrile for 72 hours; WBC count should be normal, the patient should be tolerating oral liquids, and signs and symptoms should have resolved. The abscesses should be measured by ultrasonography, and measurements should be obtained serially until there is resolution of the mass. Hager and co-workers have shown that giving oral antibiotics after parenteral antibiotic treatment of serious soft-tissue infections is not beneficial in preventing immediate or delayed recurrence of infection. If one chooses to treat with oral antibiotics after parenteral therapy, however, a combination such as amoxicillin/clavulanate provides suitable broad-spectrum coverage, or metronidazole and trimethoprim/sulfamethoxasole may be used.

These types of abscesses are unlikely to respond to medical therapy and will require surgical intervention. In those cases where the abscess has been surgically removed, antibiotic therapy should be maintained until the patient has been afebrile and clinically well for 48 to 72 hours. If the abscess has ruptured and there is free purulent material in the abdominal cavity, the abdomen should be cleansed with copious amounts of saline. It is imperative that the subhepatic and subdiaphragmatic compartments be examined for the presence of purulent material. The patient should be reexamined in 2 to 3 weeks to determine whether there is a recurrence of the infection process.

SUGGESTED READING

Graham D, Sanders RC: Ultrasound-directed transvaginal aspiration biopsy of pelvic masses. J Ultrasound Med 1982;1:279

Hager WD, Pascuzzi M, Vernon M: Efficacy of oral antibiotics following parenteral antibiotics for serious infections in obstetrics and gynecology. Obstet Gynecol 1989;73:326

Johnson WC, Gerzol SG, Robbins AH, et al: Treatment of abdominal abscesses: comparative evaluation of operative drainage versus percutaneous catheter drainage guided by computed tomography and ultrasound. Ann Surg 1981;194:510

Loy RA, Gallup DG, Hill JA, et al: Pelvic abscess: examination and transvaginal drainage guided by real-time ultrasonography. South Med J 1989;82:788

Martin EC, Karlson KB, Fankuchen EJ, et al: Percutaneous drainage of postoperative intra-abdominal abscesses. Am J Roentgenol 1982;138:13

Seder MI, Wellman JL, Haaga JR, et al: Role of surgical and percutaneous drainage in the treatment of abdominal abscess. Arch Surg 1983;118:273

61
Wound infections

By David A. Eschenbach, MD

Incidence

Despite use of prophylactic antibiotics, wound infections are common. From 5% to 7% of patients undergoing primary cesarean section (C/S) develop a postoperative abdominal wound infection. In addition, wound infections after abdominal hysterectomy or adnexal surgery occur in 2% to 6% of patients. Surprisingly, few women develop infection after episiotomy. The wound infection rate depends largely on (1) type of operation, (2) local and systemic factors affecting resistance, and (3) degree of bacterial contamination, as estimated in the wound classification system (Table 1).

Wound infections are the most common cause of serious postoperative morbidity. They are also costly because they add several days to the average hospital stay and consequently an estimated $5,000 to $10,000 to hospital charges.

Wound categories

Patients having clean wounds have the lowest rate of wound infection. In clean wounds, no inflammation is present in the operative field, no break occurs in aseptic technique, and the gastrointestinal or respiratory tract is not entered.

In a clean–contaminated wound, the vagina or the gastrointestinal, respiratory, or uninfected urinary tract is entered, or minor breaks occur in sterile technique. Wound infection rates generally increase three- to fivefold when a viscus is opened.

In a contaminated wound, there is gross spillage from a hollow viscus or major breaks in sterile technique. Dirty and infected wounds are associated with pus, acute inflammation, a perforated viscus, or an old traumatic wound.

TABLE 1
Classification of operative wound infections*

Definition	Percentage infected†
Clean	**1.5%**
Nontraumatic, no inflammation	
No break in aseptic technique	
Respiratory, GI, GU tracts not entered	
Clean–contaminated	**7.7%**
Minor break in technique	
Respiratory, GI, GU tracts entered without significant spillage and in absence of infected contents	
Appendectomy	
Contaminated	**15.2%**
Major break in technique	
GU tract entered in presence of urinary infection	
Gross GI spillage	
Dirty–infected	**40.0%**
Acute bacterial inflammation with or without pus	
Transection of "clean" tissue for surgical access to drain pus	
Perforated viscus encountered	

*From Altemeier WA, Burke JF, Pruitt BA, et al (eds): Definitions and classifications of surgical infection. In *Manual on Control of Infection in Surgical Patients*. Philadelphia, Lippincott, 1976, p. 20.
†From Cruse PJE, Foord R: The epidemiology of wound infection: a 10-year prospective study of 62,939 wounds. Surg Clin North Am 1980;60:27.

Surgeons tend to underdiagnose wound infections. A wound can be considered infected when pus is identified (despite sterile cultures). Possible infection occurs without discharge or when culture-positive serous fluid is present. Uninfected wounds are those in which primary healing occurs without wound discharge.

Risk factors
Surgeons. The rate of clean wound infections varies greatly among surgeons performing the same operation. It is quite possible to achieve clean infection rates of less than 1%. Concern should arise if

an individual surgeon's clean infection rate exceeds 2%. Regular publication and discussion of wound infection rates is a powerful motive for surgeons to reduce clean infection rates.

Clean wound infection rates reflect a complex interaction of surgical technique and attention to asepsis. Rates are lowest among groups with a strong interest in applying aseptic techniques and often rise dramatically when attention to these techniques is relaxed. Other major factors contributing to wound infection by hospital personnel include failure to wash hands between caring for patients in labor and delivery and on the postpartum floor, moving freely from infected to noninfected patients, wearing soiled scrub clothes and shoes, and operating after cleaning an infected wound. Up to 25% of postcesarean wound infection is caused by *Staphylococcus aureus* acquired from the skin of the surgical team or the patient through possibly faulty surgical technique.

Between 25% and 50% of surgeons' gloves become perforated during an operation. Rates are especially high for C/S. Thus, preoperative hand scrubbing is important to reduce skin contamination from surgeons in the event of glove perforation.

Disinfectants further reduce counts of skin flora. Povidone-iodine has a large immediate effect, and hexachlorophene inhibits skin flora for at least 1 hour after application. Skin flora is adequately reduced after a 3- to 5-minute scrub for a first operation and 2 minutes for a second consecutive one. Longer scrub times do not further reduce it.

Patients. Data showing that wound infections occur in proportion to the number of days of hospitalization before surgery suggest the hospital environment increases colonization of the skin, vagina, urinary tract, and gut with virulent microorganisms. Clinical infection remote from the surgical site increases wound infection rates threefold. Wound infections are also associated with factors that reduce wound defenses, such as reoperation, increasing age after 50, obesity, malnutrition, diabetes, severe pulmonary disease, cirrhosis, uremia, and malignancy.

Shaving the skin increases wound infections compared with no shaving or with clipping. Shaving done more than 2 hours before surgery is particularly harmful because small skin nicks can be colonized with bacteria. Preoperative hexachlorophene showers reduce wound infection.

Skin scrubs ideally should be a two-step process: an initial scrub with soap or a fat solvent followed by an antiseptic scrub with 1% iodine or 0.5% chlorhexidine in 70% alcohol. Mechanical friction is advised for the skin, to remove a layer of nonviable cells, and for the vagina, to thoroughly remove discharge from between vaginal folds.

The importance of adequate vaginal preparation cannot be overemphasized. Despite popular misconception, the vagina can usually be decolonized with an adequate prep. In contrast, it is difficult to totally eliminate cervical bacterial flora.

Operating room personnel. Surgical personnel need to adhere closely to aseptic technique. Special training may be especially necessary for labor and delivery nurses called on to act as scrub nurses or nurse circulators for C/S. Personnel dedicated to practicing aseptic techniques have a major impact on reducing wound infection rates. Those with known skin infection, particularly with staphylococci, should not participate in surgery. Finding staphylococcal infections among patients in clean wound categories should prompt widespread staff cultures in an attempt to identify asymptomatic (usually nares) staphylococcal carriers.

Use drapes impervious to fluids because soaked drapes help absorb bacteria. Impervious cloth or disposable drapes are advised. Plastic adhesive drapes are associated with increased rates of clean wound infections because bacteria proliferate under the drape, and antiseptic solution on the skin needs to be removed before the drape is applied. However, these drapes are useful for reducing contaminated fluid from sinuses and fistulas.

Surgical wounds. In experimental infection, approximately 1 million bacteria per gram of tissue are required to produce infection in the normal wound. The type of bacteria inoculated is not as important as their number.

The more abnormal the local wound condition, the fewer the bacteria required to produce infection. Approximately 1,000 times fewer bacteria are required to cause a wound infection when suture or shock decreases local wound resistance.

Devitalized tissue, hematomas, shock, and a foreign-body effect from suture all act to reduce local tissue resistance to infections. Wounds torn or opened with great force have increased areas of devitalized tissue. One should keep electrocoagulation currents at a minimum and grasp blood vessels with fine tissue forceps to minimize tissue devitalization.

The tissue effect of electrocautery depends directly on the current's magnitude. Heat, and subsequently damage to tissue surrounding the blood vessel, is markedly increased at high current. Compared with scalpel wounds, those made by electrosurgical knives have a threefold increased susceptibility to infection.

One must avoid hematoma formation because blood collections allow bacteria to grow in fibrin spaces not accessible to white blood cell defenses. Shock, by reducing the local blood supply, weakens local defenses and markedly reduces the number of bacteria required to cause infection.

Sutures create a foreign-body effect by allowing bacterial attachment. Bacteria become buried on the surface of suture beneath a mucopolysaccharide covering. Sutures also act to devitalize tissue. Large-size suture increases infection rates by increasing bacterial colonization and tissue devitalization volume.

Nonabsorbable nylon sutures and then Dacron braided-plain polyester sutures have the least potential for causing infection. Of absorbable suture, polyglycolic material is the least likely to potentiate infection, perhaps because it inhibits bacterial growth in a low-pH environment. Silk, cotton, and chromic gut are most likely to potentiate infection. For skin closure, tape is least, staples next, and suture most likely to cause infection. Infection is least likely with an interrupted percutaneous technique and most likely with continuous subcutaneous skin sutures.

Drains remove potentially harmful fluid collections but also act as sources of retrograde bacterial contamination. If drains are necessary, closed drains brought out away from the wound edge assure the lowest wound infection rate. In contrast, Penrose drains exiting through the wound provide the highest infection rate because of retrograde bacterial contamination from the skin into the wound. Penrose drains also provide only limited drainage because particulate matter is trapped within accumulated fibrin deposits.

Each hour of surgery doubles the clean-wound infection rate. This phenomenon is undoubtedly related to an increase over time in such factors as bacterial contamination, wound injury, chance of wound damage from suture and coagulation, and difficulty of operations, particularly those involving blood loss.

In brief, wound infections develop from contamination of a wound with bacteria and from systemic and—more important—local factors in the wound that reduce resistance. Simply put, an increase in bacteria or a decrease in wound resistance creates potential for wound infection.

Prevention

Mechanical bowel preparation. This step reduces bulk and, more importantly, the number of bacteria present in stool. Use such preparation if the bowel may be entered.

The old method consisted of 3 days of low-residue diet, laxatives, and enemas. One of two newer, preferable techniques is more comfortable whole-gut lavage with isotonic saline and potassium administered through a nasogastric tube. Rectal effluent usually becomes clear within 3 hours. The second method employs commercially available, orally administered, balanced electrolyte solution and polyethylene glycol taken in 250-mL increments every 10 minutes until 4 L are consumed.

Oral antibiotics. Nonabsorbable oral antibiotics further reduce bowel flora. They should be given in conjunction with mechanical bowel preparation when bowel entry is likely. Administer 1 g each of neomycin and erythromycin base orally at 1 p.m., 2 p.m., and 11 p.m. the day before an operation scheduled at 8 a.m. the next day.

Prophylactic antibiotics. In patients with marked bacterial contamination, prophylactic antibiotics reduce wound infections. However, their impact is only modest, and of little or no benefit for clean wounds. For the antibiotic to be effective, it must be given within 1 to 2 hours before the surgical incision. Cephalosporins are preferred for most procedures except those involving colonic spillage.

Delayed primary closure. Dirty wounds or those made in patients with active infection, including foul-smelling amniotic fluid, have a 40% infection rate. Because of this high rate, these patients should be subjected to delayed primary wound closure, which effectively reduces the infection rate. Don't close the wound until 4 to 7 days later, when healthy granulation tissue develops. Other postoperative wound care does not significantly affect wound infection.

Wound irrigation. Saline irrigation of the abdomen and wound washes away debris and blood clots and may reduce bacterial contamination. Remove saline from the abdomen after irrigation so that leukocyte function is not inhibited.

Surveillance. Periodic reports to surgeons combined with educational programs have a definite ameliorative effect on wound infections. Although costly, wound surveillance is a necessary part of surgical care since corrective measures markedly reduce wound infection rates.

Clinical infection

Localized wound infection. Most surgical wound infections develop within 4 to 6 days of the operation. Rapid onset within 6 to 24 hours of an operation usually indicates an especially serious infection. The wound initially tends to develop a painful, red, and edematous area. The wide variety of bacteria that can be recovered can be considered to arise from either (1) the surgical team's or patient's skin (in the case of staphylococci) or (2) patient body sites naturally contaminated with large numbers of indigenous flora (anaerobic or aerobic bacteria).

However, in patients already taking antibiotics for another postoperative infection, the first manifestation is often a secondary temperature spike without prominent wound findings. Fever and abdominal/uterine tenderness may resolve with antibiotics among patients treated for postpartum endometritis, with the first sign of a late impending wound infection often only a secondary fever spike.

Exudate ranges from thick pus in the case of staphylococcal infection to a thin, watery discharge in streptococcal infection. Abscess formation occurs with both odorless staphylococcal and foul-smelling anaerobic infection. Marked manifestation of cellulitis (sharp, red, edematous borders) beyond the wound's immediate vicinity should prompt suspicion of streptococcal infection or necrotizing fasciitis, especially in patients with prominent toxicity.

Infection is usually localized to the subcutaneous tissue in the wound's immediate vicinity, which is the area that became contaminated and damaged from the surgical wound. Surrounding areas of cellulitis tend to be limited. One should open infected wounds to provide adequate wound debridement. Most patients should have a general or regional anesthetic and sharp debridement, involving removal of pus and necrotic and heavily contaminated tissue, to help control infection. After debridement, loosely pack the wound with fine gauze soaked in an isotonic saline solution. Gentle wound handling at this point promotes healing.

Use antibiotics as adjunctive therapy of adjacent cellulitis only. Well-localized infections, particularly those caused by staphylococci, do not need antibiotic therapy. Antibiotics are particularly helpful for treating cellulitis, lymphangitis, and obviously septicemia. They are not effective in necrotic or pus-filled areas. Cephalosporins, vancomycin, or penicillinase-resistant penicillin are first-line antibiotics unless anaerobes are suspected, in which case clindamycin or ampicillin/sulbactam should be included.

Necrotizing fasciitis. Although unusual, necrotizing fasciitis is a potentially lethal wound infection. An infection of the superficial fascia (subcutaneous tissue), it arises synergistically where one bacterial agent causes an initial infection and combines with a second to cause tissue necrosis. Patients with necrotizing fasciitis are typically placed on antibiotic regimens sufficient to inhibit most aerobic and anaerobic bacteria. However, in these patients, the area of wound erythema and edema nevertheless continues to increase. Wounds with marked edema are especially painful.

Patients usually appear to be suffering from toxicity and have a significant leukocytosis, often 30,000 to 60,000/mm^3. Anemia may occur from hemolysis, but hemoconcentration also occurs when intravascular fluid extravasates into the wound, and hematocrits to 60% are common. Hypocalcemia is frequent because calcium binds with degraded fat to form soap. Fat is degraded by bacterial lipases.

The diagnosis of necrotizing fasciitis is often difficult to establish because pus typical for wound infection is characteristically not found and the presence and extent of necrosis are not usually apparent. Discharge from the wound does not contain pus, but has a thin "dishwater" appearance. Necrotic fat appears edematous rather than black. Skin changes typically occur only late in infection, when blood vessels transversing subcutaneous tissue become necrosed.

Because these clinical features are atypical of wound infection and because necrotizing fasciitis is rare, misdiagnosis is common. Additionally, there is often a failure to appreciate the seriousness of infection. Necrotizing fasciitis has occurred in C/S, episiotomy, and laparotomy and laparoscopy wounds, as well as superficial abrasions of the vulva and from Bartholin's gland infection.

Patients must undergo an exploration of the wound under anesthesia if necrotizing fasciitis is suspected. Inadequate exploration often results in missed diagnosis because the wound is usually too tender to explore adequately without anesthesia. Necrosis of the superficial fascia (subcutaneous fat) can be diagnosed when cut subcutaneous tissue does not bleed and can be easily removed by blunt dissection. The mortality rate is about 50% in surgically treated cases where debridement was adequate, but it approaches 100% in patients with necrosis who are treated medically without surgery. These patients usually die in septic shock. Thus, septic shock in patients with cellulitis should be considered due to necrotizing fasciitis unless proved otherwise.

Toxic shock. A toxigenic strain of staphylococci can give rise to toxic shock, which has occurred from wounds after surgery, breast infection, clean abdominal wounds, and laparoscopy. Typical signs, such as high fever, hypotension, multisystem failure, and eventually skin peeling, may occur even before the wound develops obvious signs of infection. One should consider patients with a recent wound and manifestations of toxic shock to have toxic shock from a wound infection. Debridement, IV fluid, and support of multisystem failure are usually sufficient treatment. When shock does occur, it is important to differentiate toxic shock from necrotizing fasciitis.

SUGGESTED READING

Altemeier WA, Burke JF, Pruitt BA Jr, et al (eds): *Manual on Control of Infection in Surgical Patients*. Philadelphia, Lippincott, 1984

Cruse PJE: Incidence of wound infection on the surgical services. Surg Clin North Am 1975;55:1269

Cruse PJE, Foord R: A five-year prospective study of 29,649 surgical wounds. Arch Surg 1973;107:206

Iffy L, Kaminetzky HA, Mainman JE, et al: Control of perinatal infection by traditional preventive measures. Obstet Gynecol 1979;54:403

Nichols RL, Condon RE, Gorbach SL, et al: Efficacy of preoperative antimicrobial preparations of the bowel. Ann Surg 1972;176:227

62
Adult respiratory distress syndrome due to infection

By F. Gary Cunningham, MD, and Thomas William Lowe, MD

Background and incidence

The first clinical description of what is now termed adult respiratory distress syndrome (ARDS) was reported in 1967. The syndrome results from diffuse injury to alveolar epithelium, capillary endothelium, or both. The resulting disruption of the alveolar–capillary membrane leads to increased permeability and accumulation of extravascular lung water despite normal or low capillary hydrostatic pressure.

Respiratory failure in these cases is caused by or is associated with a growing number of illnesses or injuries. In obstetrics and gynecology, common predisposing factors include viral or bacterial pneumonias; severe acute hemorrhage and massive transfusion associated with ectopic pregnancy, placenta previa, placental abruption, or postpartum hemorrhage; aspiration of acidic gastric contents; and septicemia resulting from septic abortion, acute pyelonephritis, chorioamnionitis, or postpartum metritis.

Pulmonary injury and ARDS develop in association with the sepsis syndrome 25% to 65% of the time whether or not bacteremia is documented. Conversely, bacteremia without systemic manifestations of infection is not a common antecedent of adult respiratory distress syndrome.

The pathogenesis of pulmonary injury is not clearly defined but may involve either the complement or coagulation cascade with activation of neutrophils and their subsequent aggregation in the lungs. Neutrophil aggregates then produce vascular damage by releasing toxic oxygen radicals into pulmonary capillaries. Additional toxic factors may include proteases and arachidonic acid metabolites.

It seems unlikely that pregnancy increases the risk for respiratory failure. However, there are some special considerations to bear in mind. For example, osmotic pressure is decreased substantially during pregnancy because albumin concentration falls. This is even more marked in women with severe preeclampsia.

Functional residual capacity also decreases progressively throughout pregnancy. Importantly, it is now appreciated that many cases of preterm labor are stimulated by occult amnionic fluid infection that, in combination with attempted tocolysis, may cause pulmonary edema.

Pathophysiology

The changes in the alveolar–capillary membrane lead not only to accumulation of extravascular lung water but also to that of plasma proteins and even red blood cells in the pulmonary interstitium and alveoli. As a consequence of these alterations, there is a decrease in both the compliance and functional residual capacity of the lung.

The presence of fluid-filled or collapsed airways leads to intrapulmonary shunting, arterial hypoxemia, and an increase in the alveolar–arterial oxygen gradient. Pulmonary vascular resistance increases and the surfactant normally present in the alveoli is destroyed.

Diagnosis

Following the inciting event, there is usually a lag phase of 12 to 72 hours before respiratory insufficiency becomes apparent. Then the woman becomes dyspneic and arterial blood gas analysis discloses progressive hypoxemia.

Tachypnea, almost invariably the first finding, should never be ignored. Typically, tachycardia also is present. At first, the chest usually is clear to auscultation, although inspiratory rales may be heard, but subsequently diffuse abnormalities are present. The chest x-ray often shows only minimal changes, and at this early stage hypoxemia can usually be corrected by oxygen.

With ultimate progression, these findings worsen and the chest x-ray demonstrates extensive alveolar infiltrates and pleural effusions that may become confluent and show up as "whited-out" lungs. As the disease continues to worsen, and shunting through collapsed or fluid-filled alveoli increases, simple oxygen administration may not correct arterial hypoxemia and mechanical ventilation becomes necessary.

Treatment

Treatment is aimed at eradicating the initiating cause and supporting respiratory function. Early and aggressive treatment of sepsis is important in improving survival. Broad-spectrum antimicrobial coverage is indicated.

Use of high-dose corticosteroid therapy is not recommended because it has not been shown to affect the outcome of ARDS due to sepsis. Operative therapy, such as prompt curettage of infected uterine contents with septic abortion or surgical debridement with necrotizing fasciitis, may be lifesaving.

Persistent sepsis complicating antepartum pyelonephritis may be due to obstruction from a calculus or an anatomic urinary malformation. In these cases, drainage, effected by stents placed via cystoscopy, or percutaneous nephrostomy may be necessary to treat urosepsis adequately. If peritonitis is apparent, an exploratory laparotomy may be performed for definitive treatment of a leaking or ruptured tubo-ovarian abscess.

Ventilation and respiratory function are supported by the simplest method and lowest inspired fraction of oxygen (FI_{O_2}) needed to maintain a P_{O_2} of around 60 mm Hg with 90% saturation. To avoid oxygen toxicity, it is desirable to maintain the FI_{O_2} below 60% and preferably below 40%. In many cases, tracheal intubation with mechanical ventilation with increased oxygen concentration is needed to reverse dangerous hypoxemia or hypercapnia.

Examples of initial ventilator settings include an FI_{O_2} of 100%, rate of 12 breaths per minute, tidal volume of 10 to 15 mL/kg of body weight, and a positive end-expiratory pressure (PEEP) of 5 cm H_2O. After stabilization, the FI_{O_2} is decreased incrementally. If arterial oxygen cannot be maintained using an FI_{O_2} of 60% or less, then end-expiratory pressure is increased. Although it is unclear whether PEEP alters the ultimate outcome of ARDS, its use allows a lower FI_{O_2} by increasing lung volume and decreasing intrapulmonary shunting. Serious side effects of PEEP include pulmonary barotrauma as well as decreased cardiac output due to diminished venous return and interventricular septum deviation.

In women with cardiopulmonary instability, or especially those in whom multiple factors are identified (for example, hemorrhage and infection), pulmonary artery catheter placement for central hemodynamic monitoring may be helpful. Its use permits measurement of the right- and left-heart filling pressures, cardiac output, and mixed venous oxygen saturation. Because of the leaky alveolar–capillary membrane, it is best to maintain the lowest pulmonary capillary wedge pressure consistent with adequate tissue perfusion as reflected by factors such as blood pressure, urine output, adequate arterial blood oxygenation, mixed venous oxygen saturation, and mentation.

Sequelae

Pulmonary failure from alveolar–capillary leaking has a reported mortality rate of 50% to 70%. However, the prognosis in otherwise healthy young women should be better if treatment for infection and respiratory insufficiency is initiated promptly and if ventilatory support can be maintained until the underlying disease is treated appropriately. Although deaths from respiratory failure occur, most often mortality is caused by the initial injury or illness or other organ system failure.

SUGGESTED READING

Bernard GR, Luce JM, Sprung CL, et al: High-dose corticosteroids in patients with adult respiratory distress syndrome. N Engl J Med 1987;317:1565

Bone RC, Fisher CJ, Clemmer TP, et al: Sepsis syndrome: a valid clinical entity. Crit Care Med 1989;17:389

Bresler MJ, Sternbach GL: The adult respiratory distress syndrome. Emerg Med Clin North Am 1989;7:419

63
Osteomyelitis pubis

By Udo B. Hoyme, MD

Background and incidence

Osteomyelitis of the pubis is a rare but serious infection that can result from bacteremia or may be secondary to a contiguous focus of infection. Parenteral drug abuse has been described as a predisposing condition for bacteremia-related pubis infection. Most cases, however, have occurred after surgical procedures such as bladder resection, urethral suspension, pelvic exenteration, or radical vulvectomy. Rarely, they have originated after obstetric procedures, such as forceps or complicated delivery.

Pathophysiology

Most cases of postoperative infection arise in an area of surgical trauma that becomes contaminated with bacteria. In vesicourethral suspension, the exposed retropubic space can be traumatized by electrocoagulation or during placement of suture into the periosteal space behind the symphysis. Also, pelvic exenteration or radical vulvectomy can cause injury to the os pubis from pressure of retractors, direct trauma of sharp dissection, or use of electrocautery for hemostasis. In addition, long operation time, large blood loss, and frequent contamination of the wound and retropubic space by urine may affect the local environment of the symphysis.

Besides trauma and impaired blood circulation, irradiation may deprive the bone or synchondrosis of vascular supply. This effect is most prominent after high-dose, poorly fractionated, or repeated courses of low-energy radiation.

Most patients enrolled in recent studies of osteomyelitis pubis received perioperative antibiotics active against the facultative and some of the anaerobic bacterial flora. Nevertheless, all patients who developed osteomyelitis of the pubis initially had a postoperative wound infection. Regardless of whether infection of the bone or necrosis occurs first, postoperative osteomyelitis of the pubis results in an infected necrotic area of the pubic bone at the interpubic disk.

Several teams of investigators have suggested that a noninfectious inflammatory process, osteitis pubis, may have pathogenic, clinical and radiologic characteristics identical to those of osteomyelitis of the pubis. Osteitis pubis has been described as a self-limited disease of unknown etiology that occurs after pelvic surgery or trauma, vigorous physical exercise, or childbirth. However, some have attributed it to unrecognized anaerobic infection.

Etiology
Documentation of an infectious process in a woman suspected of having osteitis pubis by blood culture, or culture of a bone biopsy specimen or aspirate, allows specific treatment. In most cases, bacteria recovered from the bone infection were previously isolated from wound and soft-tissue infections. In about one half of patients, infection is caused by multiple bacterial species.

Staphylococcus aureus is present in 60% of infections. Gram-negative bacteria account for about 40% of the cases, half of them in mixed infections with *Pseudomonas aeruginosa* predominating. Anaerobes are rarely isolated in these infections, but must be considered potential pathogens, especially in chronic bone infections secondary to contiguous septic foci. Use of suboptimal anaerobic transport and culture techniques in published reports may explain the rarity of anaerobic isolates.

Diagnosis
Symptoms related to osteomyelitis pubis do not usually appear until at least 8 weeks after the initial procedure, and it can take several months for the correct diagnosis to be established. The manifestations of the disease are frequently very subtle, and are commonly first attributed to wound infection. Extensive destruction of the bones may occur without obvious external signs of bone infection.

Pelvic bone tenderness and pain, avoidance of ambulation, pain of the adductor muscles, and severe pain on abduction are typical of osteomyelitis of the pubis. Drainage from the wound or from a fistula can often be seen. In addition, low-grade fever, moderate leukocytosis, an increased erythrocyte sedimentation rate, and elevated alkaline phosphatase may also be present.

The x-ray or computed tomographic scan of the pubic bone often shows rarefaction, erosion, osteolytic lesions, or irregularities of the bone margins with separation of the symphysis. These abnormalities can be misdiagnosed as metastasis from malignancy.

Later in the course of the disease, there is evidence of bone repair, with new bone formation from the periosteum or sclerosis of the symphysis. Further evidence of these changes is afforded by increased activity in the gallium scan.

Treatment

Various methods of therapy for noninfectious osteitis pubis have been recommended, including bed rest, immobilization in a spica body cast, irradiation, vitamin B, antibiotics, diathermy, surgical debridement, and injection of local anesthetic, adrenocorticotrophic hormone, or cortisone. However, classic noninfectious osteitis pubis should be self-limited, and the effectiveness of these measures is uncertain.

Start treatment of the lesion early in the course of infectious osteomyelitis with an antibiotic that has been selected according to antibiotic susceptibility data and ability to concentrate in bone. Obtain an adequate culture before beginning therapy. If a causative organism cannot be identified in a patient with suspicious clinical findings, empiric antibiotic treatment should be started to cover *S aureus*. The minimum course of therapy is 2 to 4 weeks of IV antibiotics followed by oral antibiotics for 2 to 3 additional weeks.

If blood flow to the bone is compromised, the antibiotic will not achieve a therapeutic level in the infected area. In these patients, effective treatment includes surgical decompression and evacuation of pus and infected tissue.

SUGGESTED READING

Grace JN, Sim FH, Shives TC, et al: Wedge resection of the symphysis pubis for the treatment of osteitis pubis. J Bone Joint Surg [Am] 1980;71:358

Hoyme UB, Tamimi HK, Eschenbach DA, et al: Osteomyelitis pubis after radical gynecologic operations. Obstet Gynecol 1984;63:47S

Jenkins FH, Raff MJ, Florman LD, et al: Pubic osteomyelitis due to anaerobic bacteria. Arch Intern Med 1984;144:842

64
Septic pelvic thrombophlebitis

By Alan B. Berkeley, MD

Background and incidence

Septic pelvic thrombophlebitis (SPT) is an infrequent but still serious complication of pelvic infections. It includes the entity referred to as ovarian vein syndrome and occurs in two distinct clinical forms. Although it most often follows operative obstetric surgery, it can also occur after vaginal delivery, abortion, gynecologic surgery, and pelvic inflammatory disease. The reported incidence of this disease is 1% to 2% after postpartum infection and 0.1% to 0.5% after gynecologic procedures. It is said to occur once in every 2,000 deliveries.

Although postoperative infection is still the most common complication of obstetric and gynecologic procedures, the widespread acceptance of the prophylactic use of antibiotics for cesarean section, vaginal hysterectomy, and high-risk abdominal hysterectomy has significantly reduced its incidence. Whether this reduction will also be associated with a decrease in the incidence of the most serious complications of infection, such as pelvic abscess and SPT, remains to be determined.

Etiology

Although no specific cause has been identified, the development of SPT is enhanced by conditions that promote venous stasis, vascular injury, and bacterial contamination. Among factors that may explain the predilection of SPT for the obstetric population are increased levels of circulating clotting factor and platelets in pregnant women, and of tissue thromboplastin in the placenta and amniotic fluid. In addition, the ovarian veins dilate markedly during pregnancy to accommodate increased uterine blood flow, possibly leading to venous valvular incompetence, pooling, and thrombus formation.

The dextro-rotated, gravid uterus also compresses the right ovarian vein, as well as the ureter, as it crosses the pelvic brim.

No specific microbiologic agent has been isolated as a cause of SPT. The organisms recovered from ovarian vein surgical specimens reflect the mix of both aerobic and anaerobic species usually isolated from infected pelvic sites. Thus, it is more likely that in SPT venous stasis or surgical insult allows genital tract bacteria access to already damaged endothelial and intimal cells of pelvic veins, leading to a pathologic sequence of clot formation, suppuration, fragmentation, and embolization.

Pathophysiology

The clinical presentation of SPT can be classic or enigmatic, as described by Duff and Gibbs. The classic form of the disease suggests acute thrombus formation, marked by steadily worsening lower abdominal pain, particularly on the affected side in most cases of unilateral disease. The symptoms begin 2 to 4 days after surgery and are accompanied by moderate fever, marked tachycardia, gastrointestinal distress (possibly with ileus), and cardiorespiratory compromise if embolization has occurred. A tender cord is eventually palpable abdominally in 50% to 67% of cases, arising just lateral to the uterine cornua and extending into the upper abdomen.

The enigmatic form of the disease also begins with an operative infection, but in these cases the patient continues to have spiking temperatures despite clinical improvement after the start of antibiotic therapy. Tachycardia in these cases is often present only during temperature spikes, unlike the persistent tachycardia of classic disease. Usually, no abdominal cords are palpable; rather, small thrombi are diffusely scattered in smaller pelvic veins. In some 30% of cases, a tender, thrombosed vein will be palpable in the vaginal fornix or parametrial region despite the paucity of abdominal symptoms. Duff suggests that this form of the disease usually follows vaginal delivery or pelvic surgery, whereas the classic form usually follows abdominal delivery.

In the absence of a thrombosed vessel palpable abdominally or vaginally, the diagnosis is often one of exclusion based on the clinical history and physical examination. The typical history is that of a patient who has been appropriately treated with antibiotics for a pelvic infection but continues to have temperature spikes. If symptoms persist, the differential diagnosis commonly includes appendicitis, urolithiasis, pyelonephritis, adnexal torsion, and pelvic hematoma or abscess. If the symptoms abate, drug fever or viral illness is often suspected and a trial of antibiotic discontinuation undertaken. It is not uncommon for several days to pass before these other diagnoses are discarded and appropriate treatment begins.

Diagnosis

The diagnostic dilemma often caused by SPT highlights the need for a complete evaluation of the initial pelvic infection. In addition to the usual hematologic and blood chemistries, adequate microbiologic cultures must be obtained from potentially infected sites. Since these patients often spike fevers, blood cultures are mandatory for temperatures above 38.9°C (102°F). If there is any respiratory compromise, a chest x-ray should be obtained not only to rule out pneumonia but also to check for the diffuse lower lobe densities sometimes found with SPT; the wedge-shaped defects associated with classic pulmonary emboli are rarely found. In the presence of embolization, typical ECG changes of right axis strain and deviation, coupled with ST-T segment change, may be seen.

Abdominal or vaginal sonography may identify pelvic abscess. A recent report suggests that CT scanning or magnetic resonance imaging may also play a significant role in identifying inflamed or thrombosed pelvic vessels. Lung scans and, in rare cases, pulmonary angiograms may be needed to rule out embolization. Intravenous pyelograms may be more useful in ruling out urolithiasis and pyelonephritis than in ruling in SPT, since ureteral dilatation is common in the normal pregnant and postpartum woman while gynecologic patients may have normal IVPs in the presence of SPT. Venography may identify the presence of a thrombus, especially if the inferior vena cava is involved.

Finally, one cannot emphasize enough the importance of a thorough abdominal and pelvic exam to identify masses and cords.

Treatment

For the past 25 years, anticoagulation has been the method of choice for treating persistent temperature elevations despite appropriate antibiotic therapy. The length of antibiotic therapy considered adequate before beginning anticoagulation depends on several factors: (1) whether or not resistant organisms have been isolated; (2) whether diagnostic tests to identify other disease entities have been completed; and (3) the relative potency and breadth of microbiologic coverage afforded by the antibiotics chosen. Since each antibiotic regimen usually requires at least 48 hours to evaluate, most patients are not started on anticoagulants until 4 to 7 days after their infection was initially diagnosed, unless a palpable cord is discovered.

Once the diagnosis of SPT has been made, heparin by continuous infusion pump is the treatment of choice. Antibiotic therapy should be continued concomitantly. Most investigators treat for 7 to 10 days, although exactly how long or short a course of heparin therapy is required is unknown. Some suggest maintaining anticoagulation until the patient has been afebrile for 48 to 72 hours. Data supporting a need for long-term anticoagulation with warfarin do not exist. Many physicians, however, routinely convert from IV to oral anticoagulation after a week of heparin therapy, and then maintain the patient on warfarin for 1 to 3 months if occurrence of pulmonary emboli has been documented. Bleeding complications from anticoagulant therapy are rare in these patients, especially when infusion pumps are used and carefully monitored.

Approximately 90% of patients will respond successfully to heparin therapy. Surgery should be reserved for those who fail to respond to medical therapy or experience pulmonary emboli while on therapeutic doses of anticoagulants. Operative technique should include ligation of one or both ovarian veins; ligation of the vena cava inferior to the insertion of the renal veins should be done only if that vessel is involved or emboli have occurred while the patient was fully anticoagulated. Excision of the affected ovarian vein is not necessary because isolation of the suppurative thrombus by ligation, coupled with anticoagulant and antibiotic therapy, will allow natural defense mechanisms to resolve the problem. Hysterectomy or salpingo-oophorectomy is not necessary unless those organs are involved in an inflammatory process or abscess.

Collins reported an operative mortality of 11% among patients treated with surgery alone. Operative morbidity and mortality have decreased with the advent of modern antibiotics and blood banking, and only about 10% of patients will need surgery. However, SPT can still be a fatal illness.

Sequelae

Recovery from SPT is usually rapid and complete once appropriate anticoagulant therapy has been instituted. Temporary dependent edema can occur after caval ligation but almost always resolves within 6 weeks as extensive collateralization develops. Chronic pelvic pain may develop, depending on the severity of the initial infection or operative scarring, or both.

Only one report addresses the subsequent reproductive outcome of these patients; since it deals only with patients who underwent vessel ligation, it may not fairly represent outcomes of medically managed patients. However, it does suggest decreased fertility coupled with increased fetal wastage and premature delivery in the operative group.

SUGGESTED READING

Brown TK, Munsick RA: Puerperal ovarian vein thrombophlebitis: a syndrome. Am J Obstet Gynecol 1971;109:263

Cohen MB, Pernoll ML, Gevirtz CM, et al: Septic pelvic thrombophlebitis: an update. Obstet Gynecol 1983;62:83

Collins CG: Suppurative pelvic thrombophlebitis. Am J Obstet Gynecol 1970;108:681

Duff P, Gibbs RS: Pelvic vein thrombophlebitis: diagnostic dilemma and therapeutic challenge. Obstet Gynecol Surv 1983;38:365

Josey WE, Staggers SR: Heparin therapy in septic pelvic thrombophlebitis: a study of 46 cases. Am J Obstet Gynecol 1974;120:228

65

Infections in the oncology patient

By James W. Orr, MD, and W. David Hager, MD

Background and incidence

Each year, gynecologic malignancies are diagnosed in more than 70,000 women in the United States. The majority of these women require surgery for staging or treatment of their cancer.

Postoperative febrile morbidity is common following most gynecologic procedures. In this situation, however, temperature does not correlate well with infection. In fact, an infectious etiology is documented in fewer than 30% of gynecologic patients with postoperative fever. Since the febrile morbidity rate is approximately 50% after radical surgery in gynecology, infectious morbidity would be approximately 15%. Infection following radical vulvar procedures is significantly higher.

The etiology and techniques for diagnosis of postoperative infections are discussed elsewhere [Chapters 55 and 56]. Prevention is the key to minimizing infection-related morbidity in both normal and immunocompromised women undergoing treatment of gynecologic malignancy. Many variables related to the disease process, coexisting disease, and treatment exist. The surgeon must attempt to alter or modify these associated variables, regardless of the degree of immunocompromise, in a manner that reduces infectious risk.

Yearly, more than 4 million women, including the majority of those with gynecologic cancer, undergo a surgical procedure. Regardless of their preoperative immunologic status, the operative procedure adversely affects the host defenses of these patients. The trauma of incision itself interrupts multiple epithelial or mucosal barriers. Most gynecologic operations that require vaginal entry are associated with significant bacterial contamination. In fact, the unprepared vagina has as many as 10^9 organisms per gram of vaginal fluid. Anaerobic organisms outnumber aerobes by 10 to 1. Each sutured pedicle leaves necrotic tissue distal to the suture and forms a potential nidus for infection. This occurs postoperatively, at a time when phagocytic activity is suppressed.

Risk factors and preventive measures

Many factors influence the risk of infection in a given patient. Cruse and Foord have described several risk factors for infection in surgery. They have detailed ways to alter these factors in an attempt to decrease postoperative morbidity. Other textbooks also describe these factors in detail. In this chapter, we will list the factors and preventive measures.

A significant number of hospitalized women have evidence of an existing nutritional deficit. At least 10% of women with early-stage endometrial or cervical cancer have abnormal nutritional parameters. The need for adequate preoperative nutrition must be emphasized.

Older women, obese women, and women with coexisting medical illness such as diabetes are at increased risk of developing postoperative infection. Women with gynecologic cancer are typically older. Obesity, a common finding among women with endometrial cancer, is associated with longer operative times, increased surgical blood loss, poor healing, and an increased risk of surgical wound infection. Adequate control of ancillary medical illnesses is essential in operative patients. In addition, prolonged preoperative hospitalization increases the risk of postoperative infection.

The risk of surgical site infection, even in short operations such as appendectomy, increases linearly with surgical experience. The experienced surgeon strives to decrease manipulation of tissue and operative time.

Preoperative patient preparation is important in minimizing intraoperative and postoperative morbidity. Mechanical bowel preparation with liquids and cathartics is usually well tolerated and can be completed at home by compliant patients. In contrast with bowel preparation, preoperative douching has not been shown to have a significant benefit in reducing postoperative infection. Removal of hair from the operative site is preferred by most surgeons. As compared with shaving, clipping of hair or use of a depilatory is associated with lower wound infection rates.

Electrocautery used in the cutting mode to maintain intraoperative hemostasis is associated with significant thermal damage and a potential increase in wound culture media. It also has an adverse effect on wound healing strength.

Suture material should be of the smallest caliber possible for the procedure being done. Since reactivity of suture materials varies, the least reactive material should be used [see Chapter 61: Wound infections]. To avoid tissue necrosis, sutures should not be tightly cinched down.

Intraoperative irrigation of the abdomen or incision theoretically decreases the amount of necrotic tissue, fibrin, and other materials that serve as potential culture media. Any irrigation fluid placed into the abdomen or pelvis should be removed in its entirety, since excess intra-abdominal fluid may interfere with normal macrophage function. If the surgeon deems that a drain would be beneficial in decreasing the amount of residual fluid in or near the operative site, closed suction drains should always be employed.

Antibiotic prophylaxis to prevent postoperative infectious morbidity is discussed elsewhere [see Chapters 57 and 58]. The antibiotic used should be an agent that would not be used to treat serious infections. It should be of low toxicity and low in cost, and should be given in a single dose. If operative time is extended beyond 2 hours, the dose should be repeated.

Etiology

Like most pelvic infections, those occurring in oncology patients are polymicrobial. Many cancer patients are immunocompromised because of their disease or the effects of chemotherapy on neutrophils. Approximately 80% of organisms responsible for neutropenic infection are a part of the endogenous human flora, and almost 50% of cancer-related infections are caused by hospital-acquired organisms. The latter tend to have been selected out by antibiotic pressure for their virulence and resistance. Within several days of hospitalization, the normal skin and mucosal flora may shift from penicillin-sensitive coagulase-negative staphylococci and *Corynebacteria* to methicillin-resistant *Staphylococcus epidermidis*, as well as other resistant organisms. These changes in flora increase the risk and severity of infections and suggest a benefit in decreasing the frequency and duration of hospitalization of preoperative patients and patients receiving chemotherapy.

Treatment

The successful treatment of any infection can be correlated to index of suspicion, rapidity of diagnosis, appropriate antibiotic treatment, and timely use of surgical or percutaneous drainage. Depending on the extent or location of the infection, other system support, such as mechanical ventilation, vasopressor administration, hyperalimentation, or transfusion, may be critical. The clinician must evaluate each process and the given clinical situation, and then institute appropriate treatment. In instances such as postoperative abdominal wound infection, simple drainage may be the only treatment necessary. In other instances of soft-tissue infections in neutropenic patients, extensive debridement, antibiotic treatment, and other support may be life sparing.

The availability of a variety of antibiotics sometimes makes treatment decisions difficult or almost impossible, as each new drug or drug combination has potential or reported benefits. Antibiotic therapy for intra-abdominal infection in the postoperative patient should be directed towards the mixed pattern of pathogens usually present. Anaerobic bacteria alone or in combination with aerobes will be isolated in approximately 88% of infections. There is rarely an initial need for drugs directed towards enterococci or *Pseudomonas* sp, although these organisms may be recovered more frequently in neutropenic patients. One should not reinstitute therapy with a drug given for prior, recent prophylaxis. Fortunately, fungal, viral, and protozoan infections are rare in this patient population.

The gold standard regimen of antibiotic coverage for postoperative intra-abdominal infection combines an aminoglycoside (gentamicin, 1.5 mg/kg IV every 8 hours) with clindamycin (900 mg IV every 8 hours) or metronidazole (500 mg IV every 6 hours). Although extremely successful, this regimen requires multiple drug administrations and has significant potential toxicity. During the past decade, a number of reports comparing these regimens with monotherapy suggest a single drug with broad-spectrum coverage is equally effective. Monotherapy proponents cite the advantages of decreased toxicity, lower cost, and less need for drug toxicity monitoring. Unfortunately, the majority of these studies lack significant patient numbers and fail to report their diagnostic criteria for patient inclusion or even drug failure. Often, they intermix patients with multiple diagnoses and coexisting illness.

These problems make meaningful interpretation difficult; most reports, however, suggest that treatment of a postoperative intra-abdominal infection with a single broad-spectrum antibiotic or a combination is successful approximately 90% of the time. Additional drugs and surgical or percutaneous drainage are rarely necessary. At this time, there appears to be no single antibiotic or drug combination that is ultimately superior as long as broad-spectrum (aerobic and anaerobic) coverage is initiated. The choice of drug or drug regimen must be guided by local antibiotic sensitivities, local and reported experience, and potential toxicities. Obviously, antibiotic treatment of specific infections (pulmonary, urinary) should be guided by culture results.

Antibiotic selection and treatment principles change dramatically in the febrile neutropenic patient both because the infecting pathogens differ and because unusual problems, such as perineal soft-tissue infections, are more common. The treatment of infection in neutropenic patients leaves little room for error. Immediate attention to all potential infectious sites and organisms is important. In contrast to the usual postoperative fever, as many as 80% of fevers in neutropenic patients are caused by occult bacterial processes.

Combinations of a cephalosporin with an aminoglycoside and/or an antipseudomonal drug have been the most commonly used antibiotics in neutropenic patients. In general, drug regimens should be bactericidal, synergistic, and of low toxicity. The latter property is particularly important, as these patients may require prolonged therapy.

The current trend in antibiotic treatment of neutropenic patients is to single-drug therapy. So-called "third-generation" cephalosporins have been studied intensively for this use and appear effective almost regardless of the regimen. These agents may be combined with an aminoglycoside to ensure adequate coverage of *Pseudomonas* species. As compared with results for postoperative infection, clinical cure rates for neutropenic patients are lower (60% to 80%) with primary therapy regardless of the drug or drugs used. Depending on culture results, duration of neutropenia, and infection site, modifications of the regimen will be required in 20% to 50% of patients. These patients will need to be monitored closely, as multiple infectious problems can occur that require antifungal, antiviral, or antianaerobic therapy.

Evaluation and treatment of fever in neutropenic cancer patients frequently requires empiric antibiotic therapy, after appropriate cultures have been obtained. While gram-negative bacteria have prevailed as the major infectious pathogens, gram-positive organisms have recently assumed a more prominent role in primary or secondary neutropenic infections. There is no apparent benefit in adding vancomycin to the initial "empiric" antibiotic regimen unless there is a high local incidence of methicillin-resistant staphylococcal infection. The institution of vancomycin with either known (culture proven) primary or secondary infection is uniformly successful and allows nontreatment of 80% of patients.

More focused therapies, based on culture results, are required in patients with prolonged neutropenia because of the high rate (47%) of secondary infections. Once initiated, antibiotics should be continued until the neutropenia resolves. Discontinuing antibiotics earlier, even if temperature is normal, results in a recrudescence of fever (40%) and hypotension (12%) in a significant number of patients.

Evaluation and treatment of fungal infections continue to be problematic in granulocytopenic patients. While occasionally they occur as primary infections, they commonly are seen in persistently febrile granulocytopenic patients. While a number of antifungal medications exist, amphotericin B remains the drug of choice. While its toxicity prohibits empiric use, early therapy is essential in patients who are persistently febrile and granulocytopenic despite 4 to 7 days of antibiotic treatment or who have a positive blood culture for fungi.

SUGGESTED READING

Cruse PJE, Foord R: A 5-year prospective study of 23,649 surgical wounds. Arch Surg 1973;107:206

Cunningham FB, Gilstrap LC, Kappus SS: Cefamandole for treatment of obstetric and gynecologic infections. Scand J Infect Dis 1980;suppl 25:75

Deitch EA: Infection in the compromised host. Surg Clin North Am 1988;68:181

Orr JW: Sutures and incisions: an update. Ala J Med Sci 1986;23:36

Orr JW, Shingleton HM: Importance of nutritional support in the surgical patient. J Reprod Med 1984;29:635

Orr JW, Taylor PT: Reducing postoperative infection in the patient with gynecologic cancer. Infec Surg 1987;12:666

Shapiro M, Munoz A, Tager IB, et al: Risk factors for infection at the operative site after abdominal or vaginal hysterectomy. N Engl J Med 1982;307:1661

66
Toxic shock syndrome

By Roger Bawdon, PhD

Background and incidence

Since 1984, fewer than 300 cases of toxic shock syndrome (TSS) have occurred each year. During the peak of the TSS outbreak in 1980, the case rate was three for every 100,000 menstruating women, and in California, 9.1 for every 100,000. Women using high-absorbency tampons who had had an episode of TSS had a recurrence rate of up to 30%. Even after removing certain brands of tampons from the market, some states reported that they observed no change in the TSS case rate.

More recently, 20% to 40% of TSS cases have been unrelated to menstruation. In addition, because other diseases mimic TSS, as many as 53% of reported cases did not meet all the criteria for TSS, suggesting marked overdiagnosis. Clinicians probably fail to uncover cases of TSS because they try to relate TSS to menstruation and tampon use. Menstruation-related TSS, however, is only one aspect of what remains a clinically challenging disease entity.

Although the incidence of menstrual-related TSS has dropped since 1980, nonmenstrual cases are still reported. These cases may be associated with vaginal infections, vaginal delivery, cesarean section, spontaneous abortion, diaphragm use, postpartum endometritis, CO_2 laser treatment of condyloma acuminatum, and complications of salpingitis. Consequently, clinicians should continue to focus attention on this entity.

Etiology

TSS is caused by a microbial infection or colonization with bacteriophage-specific strains of *Staphylococcus aureus* in a body cavity or on a foreign object in a body orifice, associated with the production of an epidermal toxin, toxic shock syndrome toxin-1 (TSST-1). This toxin and staphylococcal enterotoxin B (SEB), and perhaps other staphylococcal toxins, cause the clinical symptoms. TSST is generally associated with the group I bacteriophage, which is found in approximately 10% of all *S aureus* strains.

Pathophysiology

The pathogenesis of TSS and host defense comprises a number of complex variables. The following factors have been implicated:

■ Most TSS patients have little or no preexisting antibody to TSST-1.

■ *S aureus* strains that do not produce TSST-1 are isolated from 40% of patients with non-menstrual-associated TSS, suggesting that other toxins produce TSS.

■ The antibody titer to TSST-1 is variable, and may not be elevated even in convalescent patients who have had TSS.

■ Some patients may be antibody(IgG)-deficient for TSS, and TSST-1 may suppress B cell response in vitro.

■ It is possible to have patients with a high TSST-1 antibody titer who have never had the disease and are carriers of the toxin-producing strain of *S aureus*.

■ Patients with a generally low hormonal state who are menstruating or postpartum and are young are at risk for TSS.

The toxic response mechanism activates macrophages and produces interleukin; then, in the acute phase, white blood cell (WBC) counts drop, plasma fibronectin levels rise, and C-reactive protein appears. Many other general clinical responses to small quantities of TSST-1 and SEB are also evident.

Diagnosis

In 1980, the Centers for Disease Control compiled the most commonly used diagnostic criteria for TSS. They include the following clinical signs:

■ temperature above 38.9°C (102°F);

■ erythematous rash during acute illness;

■ desquamation of the palms and soles 1 to 2 weeks after onset of the illness;

■ hypotension;

■ three or more of the following: (1) vomiting or diarrhea during acute illness; (2) severe myalgia or elevated creatine phosphokinase; (3) vaginal, oropharyngeal, or conjunctival mucous membrane hyperemia; (4) elevated blood-urea nitrogen, elevated creatinine, or more than five WBCs in a high-power field in the absence of a urinary tract infection; (5) a platelet count of less than 100,000/mm^3; (6) elevated serum glutamic pyruvic transaminase; and (7) disorientation or alteration in consciousness without focal neurologic signs;

- negative blood, throat, and cerebrospinal fluid cultures; and
- negative serologic tests for Rocky Mountain spotted fever, leptospirosis, and measles.

These findings, complicated by shock and multisystem failure, may result in death. The pathology of TSS includes changes in the vagina, cervix, kidneys, liver, and lungs. The cervical mucosa may show desquamation and ulceration. Pulmonary changes consist of congestion, alveolar hemorrhage, and possibly hyaline membrane formation. Kidney pathology is consistent with tubular necrosis. Liver findings include variable periportal inflammation and microvesicular fatty changes.

Additional laboratory findings may show that *S aureus* has not been isolated from culture sites. Since several other diseases may mimic TSS, one must evaluate the history, physical examination, and laboratory findings to assure accurate differentiation.

Treatment

Hospital management of TSS cases associated with tampon use involves vaginal examination, including close observation for erythema and—less frequently—ulcerations. Tampons should be discontinued. It is also necessary to search for foci of *S aureus* infection elsewhere in the body. Culture specimens for *S aureus* should be taken from the vagina, cervix, blood, and any lesions, whether inflamed or not. In nonmenstrual TSS, wound and blood cultures should be done.

The most important treatment is fluid replacement with crystalloid solutions. The pulmonary, cardiovascular, and renal systems should be carefully monitored. Although antibiotics don't help shorten the duration of acute disease, they may reduce the incidence of recurrence. Antibiotics should include penicillinase-resistant penicillins, such as oxacillin or nafcillin, and should be given early in case the diagnosis of TSS is incorrect. Recurrence rates in patients with a previous episode of menstrual-related TSS are about 30%. They may drop to 5% if the patient is treated with ß-lactamase-resistant antibiotics.

Prevention

Steps for preventing recurrences include parenteral antibiotic treatment of first episodes as described, education of the patient, and avoidance of tampons. Prevention of first episodes probably requires minimal use of high-absorbency tampons.

SUGGESTED READING

Centers for Disease Control: Summary—cases of specified notifiable diseases, United States. MMWR 1989;38:392

Centers for Disease Control: Toxic shock syndrome, United States, 1970-1982. MMWR 1982;31:201

Davis JP, Chesney PJ, Wand PJ, et al: Toxic shock syndrome: epidemiologic features, recurrence, risk factors and prevention. N Engl J Med 1980;303:1429

Petitti D, D'Agostino RB, Oldman MJ: Non-menstrual toxic shock syndrome: Methodologic problems in estimating incidence and delineating risk factors. J Reprod Med 1987;32:10

Todd JK: Toxic shock syndrome. Clin Microbiol Rev 1989;1:432

Todd JK, Ressman M, Caston SA, et al: Corticosteroid therapy for the patients with toxic shock syndrome. JAMA 1984;252:3399

67
Bacteremia and septic shock

By Bernard Gonik, MD

Background and incidence

The incidence of bacteremia in obstetric and gynecologic infections is 8% to 10%, and that of septic shock in bacteremic ob–gyn patients 0% to 12%, quite low overall. Conditions identified as predisposing to septic shock include chorioamnionitis, postpartum endometritis, upper urinary tract infection, septic abortion, cuff cellulitis, pelvic inflammatory disease, pelvic abscess, and toxic shock syndrome.

Fortunately, risk of death from septic shock, in contrast to other medical and surgical fields, is low in the otherwise healthy ob–gyn patient. Incidence of death from sepsis is estimated at 0% to 3%.

Pathophysiology

Septic shock comprises vascular collapse, cellular hypoxia, and end organ dysfunction caused by infection, which can result from a wide variety of microorganisms. Most attention has been given to gram-negative sepsis. Endotoxin, a complex lipopolysaccharide present in the cell wall of gram-negative bacteria, appears critical in producing the pathophysiologic derangements associated with septic shock. Shock, apparently closely related to release of a variety of exotoxins, can also develop in patients with gram-positive sepsis.

The series of events initiated by bacteremia or endotoxemia is complex. Macrophage activation leading to release of the cytokine cachectin is central.

Triggering of the complement cascade by endotoxin also initiates critical immune responses. Leukocyte exposure to the invading pathogen results in release of vasoactive histamine, serotonin, and bradykinin. These substances increase capillary permeability, induce endothelial damage, and promote vasodilation. Phagocytosis of gram-negative bacteria by host leukocytes also increases release of intracellular toxins such as superoxide free radicals, lysosomes, and hydrogen peroxide into the systemic circulation.

Diagnosis

In early septic shock, the patient experiences a shaking chill, sudden rise in temperature, tachycardia, and warm extremities ("warm" shock). Although she appears "infected," the diagnosis of septic shock may elude the clinician who neglects a careful evaluation for hypotension.

Laboratory findings vary substantially during this early phase. The white blood cell count may show marked leukocytosis or be somewhat depressed. One sometimes sees transient hyperglycemia, caused by catecholamine release and tissue underuse of glucose as a substrate. Early evidence of disseminated intravascular coagulation (DIC) may take the form of a decreased platelet count and fibrinogen and elevated fibrin split products and thrombin time. Initial arterial blood gas determinations tend to reflect a mild respiratory alkalosis.

As shock progresses, intact neuronal reflex responses (transmitted by sympathetic activation) produce profound vasoconstriction in all organ systems. This vasoconstriction further reduces tissue and organ perfusion. Clinical manifestations of this later stage include cold extremities, oliguria, and peripheral cyanosis ("cold" shock). The resultant cellular hypoxia and acidosis disrupts the ability of individual cells to use oxygen. This effect leads to capillary bed dysfunction with marked reductions in peripheral vascular resistance due to extensive capillary pooling of blood.

The classic complex of hypotension, cardiovascular collapse, and hypoxia is usually referred to as secondary, or "irreversible," shock. A central feature of this stage is profound myocardial depression related to systemic release of a myocardial depressant factor. Subsequent widespread end-organ failure is invariably followed by coma and death.

In most cases, the approach to diagnosis should include microbiologic evaluation of specimens from blood, urine, sputum, and wound. Even though mixed flora is usually identified in transvaginal cultures, careful sampling of the endometrial cavity should be carried out if this area is the suspected source of infection. In patients thought to have chorioamnionitis, transabdominal amniocentesis or cultures taken from a free-flowing internal pressure transducer catheter may be useful.

Appearance in pregnancy. Physiologic adaptations to pregnancy occur in practically every organ system. These changes can theoretically influence the presentation and course of septic shock.

In experiments by Beller and co-workers involving endotoxin-induced septic shock, pregnant animals had a much more pronounced metabolic acidosis and earlier cardiovascular collapse than did controls.

Interestingly, the fetus and newborn are much more resistant to the direct deleterious effects of endotoxin than the mother. Fetal and newborn lambs proved capable of tolerating endotoxin doses ten times larger than those proving to be lethal in adult pregnant sheep. However, Morishima and co-workers, after giving endotoxin to pregnant baboons, reported profound asphyxia and rapid deterioration in the fetus. These effects were thought to result primarily from maternal factors, such as hypotension and increased myometrial activity, contributing to reduced placental perfusion.

Treatment

Initial intervention for septic shock strives to accomplish the following:

- improve functional circulating intravascular volume;
- establish and maintain an adequate airway to make management of respiratory failure easier;
- determine the septic focus through diagnostic evaluation; and
- institute empiric antimicrobial therapy to eradicate the most likely pathogens.

When dealing with a pregnant patient, strive foremost for maternal well-being, since fetal compromise results primarily from maternal cardiovascular decompensation. Improvements in maternal status will have positive effects on fetal condition. Furthermore, attempts at delivering the fetus of a hemodynamically compromised mother may increase the risk of fetal distress and the need for more aggressive surgical intervention.

However, an exception is the fetal compartment that is the source of sepsis (as when there is chorioamnionitis). In such circumstances, therapy includes stabilizing the mother while starting antibiotic therapy and beginning attempts at delivery.

Fluid management. The mainstay of acute management of septic shock involves volume expansion to correct absolute or relative hypovolemia. At times, considerable fluid is needed because of profound vasodilation, increased capillary permeability, and extravasation of fluid into extravascular spaces. The best monitoring method is to use a flow-directed pulmonary artery catheter, which also allows for the determination of cardiac output and oxygen-related variables.

One method of monitoring fluid given the patient is to administer up to 200 mL IV over 10 minutes. If pulmonary capillary wedge pressure increases by more than 7 mm Hg, withhold additional fluid. Otherwise, administer a repeat dose. Isotonic crystalloid solutions, such as normal saline, are most often used. However, some have recommended the use of colloid solutions, such as 5% normal human albumin, to maintain a normal colloid osmotic–pulmonary artery wedge pressure gradient (more than 4 mm Hg), thus reducing the risk of pulmonary edema.

Vasopressor therapy. If fluid resuscitation alone proves inadequate for restoring optimal cardiovascular function, vasoactive agents are indicated. The most useful is dopamine hydrochloride, which has dose-dependent α- and ß-adrenergic effects. Administer dopamine as a continuous infusion started at 2 to 5 µg/kg per minute and titrated according to clinical and hemodynamic responses.

Most of the various other pressor agents available produce cardiac output increase at the expense of undesirable vasoconstriction. Therefore, indications in septic shock for these agents are limited to patients in whom blood pressure cannot be supported by dopamine alone.

Assessment of tissue oxygenation. Oxygenation at the lungs can be assessed easily by arterial blood gas determinations. However, oxygen consumption or use is harder to gauge. In the patient with septic shock, peripheral tissue use of oxygen is frequently reduced.

An indirect measurement of poor tissue oxygen extraction is the finding of a high mixed-venous oxygen saturation or determination of a reduction in arteriovenous oxygen content difference. Actual peripheral oxygen consumption can be calculated using the Fick equation: the normal indexed nonpregnant range is 120 to 140 mL O_2/min/m^2. Clinical improvement in the patient's condition should be reflected in an increase or normalization of peripheral oxygen consumption.

Antibiotic therapy. Because the course of septic shock can be short and fulminant, a diagnostic workup must be done without delay and empiric antimicrobial therapy started immediately.

Empiric therapy in the obstetric patient should include coverage for numerous aerobic and anaerobic bacteria, including both gram-negative and gram-positive organisms. Parenteral therapy combining aqueous penicillin (3,000,000 U every 4 hours) or ampicillin (1 g every 4 hours), an aminoglycoside (loading dose of 2 mg/kg, followed by maintenance doses of 1.5 mg/kg every 8 hours for patients with normal renal function), and clindamycin (900 mg every 8 hours) is recommended. If *Staphylococcus aureus* infection is suspected, a semisynthetic penicillin may be substituted for the aqueous penicillin agent.

Because nephrotoxicity is a well-established complication of aminoglycoside usage, monitor peak (6 to 10 µg/mL) and trough (less than 2 µg/mL) aminoglycoside levels. When available, use culture results and organism sensitivities to guide subsequent therapy more selectively. Other alternative antimicrobial regimens may be substituted for those listed above, depending on the individual clinician's experience.

Surgical therapy. In patients with septic abortion, attempt to evacuate the uterus promptly after initiating antibiotics and stabilizing the patient. Septic shock in association with chorioamnionitis in a gestationally viable fetus also is treated best by expeditious evacuation of the uterus. Evacuation can be accomplished vaginally if maternal hemodynamic parameters are stable and labor is progressing adequately.

In the postpartum patient, hysterectomy may be needed if microabscess formation is identified within the myometrial tissue or if there is clinical evidence of deterioration despite appropriate antibiotic therapy. Similarly, when overwhelming sepsis is associated with PID, suspect abscess formation. Under these circumstances, an operative approach to drain the abscess is frequently needed to effect stabilization.

Additional supportive measures. Other needed measures include management of electrolyte imbalances, correction of metabolic acidosis, stabilization of coagulation defects, and monitoring of renal function. Monitor lactic acidosis stemming from anaerobic metabolism by serial arterial blood gas and serum lactate level determinations. Administer normal saline infusions with one to two ampules of sodium bicarbonate periodically to help correct severe acidosis.

Laboratory coagulation abnormalities tend to reflect generalized DIC. Unless there is clinical evidence of bleeding or need for surgical intervention, don't aggressively attempt to correct DIC. Spontaneous amelioration will occur once the overall clinical status improves.

Renal function is best monitored with an indwelling Foley catheter and serial creatinine and blood urea nitrogen determinations. With acute renal failure, tests of tubular function show increased fractional excretion of sodium (urinary sodium greater than 40 mEq/L) and impaired concentrating ability (urine osmolality less than 400 mOsm/kg H_2O). Provided irreversible acute tubular necrosis has not occurred, correction of underlying hemodynamic and perfusion deficits should restore renal function.

Sequelae

A common complication encountered in the septic shock patient is adult respiratory distress syndrome [see Chapter 62]. The diagnosis is made on the basis of progressive hypoxemia, a normal pulmonary capillary wedge pressure, diffuse infiltrates on chest x-ray, and decreased pulmonary compliance.

Treatment involves intubation and ventilatory support to maintain an adequate gas exchange at nontoxic levels of inspired oxygen. Positive end-expiratory pressure (PEEP) is often necessary to accomplish this goal. Serial monitoring of arterial blood gases is essential.

SUGGESTED READING

Beller FK, Schmidt EH, Holzgreve W, et al: Septicemia during pregnancy: a study in different species of experimental animals. Am J Obstet Gynecol 1985;151:967

Blanco JD, Gibbs RS, Castaneda YS: Bacteremia in obstetrics: clinical course. Obstet Gynecol 1981;58:621

Bryan CS, Reynolds KL, Moore EE: Bacteremia in obstetrics and gynecology. Obstet Gynecol 1984;64:155

Gonik B: Intensive care monitoring of the critically ill pregnant patient, in Creasy RK, Resnik R (eds): *Maternal-Fetal Medicine: Principles and Practice*, ed 2. Philadelphia, WB Saunders, 1989, pp 845-874

Lee W, Clark SL, Cotton DB, et al: Septic shock during pregnancy. Obstet Gynecol 1988;159;410

Morishima HO, Niemann WH, James LS: Effects of endotoxin on the pregnant baboon and fetus. Am J Obstet Gynecol 1978;131:899

Rackow EC, Astiz ME: Pathophysiology and treatment of septic shock. JAMA 1991;266(4):548

Index